Death Education

Related Titles from

●HEMISPHERE PUBLISHING CORPORATION

Davidson   The Hospice: Development and
Administration

Wass   Death Education: Pedagogy •
Counseling • Care—An International
Quarterly

Wass   Dying: Facing the Facts

Death Education

An Annotated Resource Guide

Hannelore Wass University of Florida, Gainesville

Charles A. Corr Southern Illinois University, Edwardsville

Richard A. Pacholski Millikin University, Decatur, Illinois

Catherine M. Sanders University of South Florida, Tampa

● Hemisphere Publishing Corporation

Washington   New York   London

DEATH EDUCATION: An Annotated Resource Guide

1 2 3 4 5 6 7 8 9 0   B C B C   8 9 8 7 6 5 4 3 2 1 0

This book was set in Century by Hemisphere Publishing
Corporation. The editors were Jeanne Ferris and Christine
Flint; the designer was Sharon Martin DePass; the production
supervisor was Rebekah McKinney; and the typesetter was
Linda Holder.
BookCrafters, Inc. was printer and binder.

Library of Congress Cataloging in Publication Data

Main entry under title:

Death education.

    Includes indexes.
    1. Death—Study and teaching—Audiovisual aids
—Catalogs. 2. Death—Study and teaching—
Bibliography. 3. Death—Information services.
I. Wass, Hannelore.
HQ1073.D42   016.1559'37   79-27707
ISBN 0-89116-170-8

To Harry, Donna, Phyllis, and Herschel

Contents

Preface / ix

Part I
Printed Resources

Articles and Books / 3
    General / 5
    Death Education for Children and Adolescents / 7
    Death Education for College Students / 21
    Death Education for Health Professionals / 25
    Death Education for Adults / 40
    Death Education for Counselors and Therapists; Self-Help Groups / 46

Selected Text and Reference Books / 51

Bibliographies / 95

Periodicals / 123

Research and Assessment of Death Attitudes / 133

Part II
Audiovisual Resources

Introduction / 149
  Sources of Media / 150
  Costs / 150
  Selecting Educational Audiovisuals for the Classroom / 151
  Using Feature Films in Death and Dying Courses / 151
  Keeping Up / 154

Listings / 159

Distributors / 237

Part III
Organizational Resources

Introduction / 249

Listings / 251

Part IV
Community Resources

Text / 271

Appendix: Additional Entries / 277
  Printed Resources / 277
  Audiovisual Resources / 279
  Audiocassettes / 285
  Distributors / 286
  Organizational Resources / 286

Topical Index: Audiovisual Resources / 289

Topical Index: Organizational Resources / 295

Index / 299

Preface

The impetus for this volume arose from our realization that the resources available to those who are involved in death education are not adequate. This need results in part from the growing interest in this field among many educators and private individuals. As death education continues to expand and increase in sophistication, new instructors are moving into this area while those already involved are striving continually to improve the quality of their work. Both groups seek information and guidance for achieving their goals. This desire is particularly acute since there are few, if any, formal programs to prepare people for death education, and until now there has been no single, comprehensive resource guide to which they could turn.

In addition, death education embraces an unusually wide range of instructional programs and settings. It can be initiated by parents at home, by teachers from preschool through high school and college, by those who teach in professional schools, and by those who conduct continuing education programs for various groups. Programs in death education require information about resource materials and guidance in determining teaching tactics. Such information and guidance should be available in a manageable form. It should also intersect all educational levels since death educators at one level can benefit from knowing what is useful and achievable at other levels.

The most direct reason for preparing this guide is the tremendous increase that has occurred over the past few years in both volume and variety of resources for death education. Books, articles, and audiovisual materials have appeared on the market at a staggering rate. New journals have begun publication, numerous bibliographies have been compiled, and many organizations have come into being or expanded their services to meet new needs. A wealth of new information and ideas has dramatically altered our appreciation of what can be attempted in education about death, dying, and bereavement, and how that instruction might be conducted effectively. However, this information is widely scattered and in many instances not well organized. Even under the best of circumstances, few individuals have the time or the energy to examine all of these separate resources. Yet educators wish to draw upon those materials that are best suited to their goals and student population.

Our intention in this resource guide is to assist death educators at all levels, beginners and seasoned instructors alike, in identifying and assessing materials that may help them in their educational efforts. Much of these materials may also be useful for counselors, caregivers, and those pursuing research, individual study projects, or their own private interests. We have sought to provide assistance in two primary ways: first, by gathering together in one convenient place relevant information that is, at best, available from a wide variety of independent sources; and, second, by providing descriptive and evaluative comments on this information. These comments appear in our introductory remarks to each section, in the annotations to all individual reference items, and in various narrative passages throughout our text. We wish to emphasize that our comments are intended only to provide guidance in evaluating and using the reference items; they reflect our own assessments and are not meant to preempt the judgment of individual readers. Cross-references are provided where appropriate, and in a few cases we offer multiple listings for a particular item when they seem necessary.

Our work is based on the conviction that death education is a multidisciplinary field and that death educators draw upon a variety of resources in order to know and teach the subject adequately. For this reason we have crossed without hesitation topical, thematic, disciplinary, and professional boundaries to construct a comprehensive guide to the many diverse resources that are currently available. The result is a series of annotated lists of 384 journal articles and books on death education, 28 detailed descriptions and evaluations of selected textbooks and reference works, 147 bibliographies, 28 journals and newsletters, 67 references concerned with research and measurement of death attitudes, 588 audiovisual entries, and 99 organizations, together with a summary of suggested community resources.

This volume is the result of a team effort. We have collaborated in various ways by pointing out and exchanging materials, by editing and commenting on each other's work, and by giving each other encouragement. Each of us assumed major responsibility for certain parts of the book. Hannelore Wass is responsible for the overall organization of the volume, for the annotations in the section "Articles and Books," and for Part IV, "Community Resources"; Charles A. Corr is responsible for the sections "Selected Text and Reference Books," "Bibliographies," and "Periodicals"; Richard A. Pacholski, for Parts II and III, "Audiovisual Resources" and "Organizational Resources"; and Catherine M. Sanders, for the section "Research and Assessment of Death Attitudes." The Appendix contains additional entries received too late for inclusion in the annotated text.

Although we have made every effort to be as thorough and as complete as possible in compiling these lists, we realize that some items will have eluded our search. Further, new materials are continually being generated and some may have appeared by the time this book has been published. We intend to continue our work of identifying resources and will be grateful to readers who bring items to our attention. Meanwhile, we hope that our readers will find this guide useful in locating information and resources for their endeavors in death education.

Hannelore Wass
Charles A. Corr
Richard A. Pacholski
Catherine M. Sanders

Death Education

PART I

Printed Resources

Articles
and Books

Anyone who endeavors to produce an annotated bibliography of articles and books on death education confronts several immediate problems. One has to do with the relative recency of death education as a distinct, identifiable field within the broader range of human concerns with death, dying, and bereavement. The field of death education is still fluid and lacking in the clarity and crystallization that characterize a well-established professional discipline. This problem cannot be solved here. It will take further concerted effort on the part of many workers to give this field the kind of stability that it needs. In a sense, this section—and indeed this entire resource guide—is intended as a partial contribution to that major task.

A second and closely related problem concerns the proper definition of death education. "What is death education?" appears to be a simple enough question. However, there is, to date, no single, agreed-upon answer. Death education can be defined as the science of formal teaching or instruction of a group or groups about topics related to the subject of "death." This includes goals and objectives, curriculum content, materials and organization, teaching methods and techniques, and evaluation of teaching outcomes or effectiveness. A broader definition of death education (or any kind of education) would include consideration of the group to be taught, that is, it would consider certain special conditions, characteristics, and needs of the members of the group that may be relevant to the goals and purposes, the subject matter, and the methodology used. Moreover, a broader definition of death education goes beyond formal instruction to include informal, incidental, spontaneous, periodic, occasional, and indirect teaching. This wider definition of death education might include, for example, aspects of socialization or the kind of "teaching" done by parents and other significant others, or done simply by the way in which a system, say, the hospital, is organized and the manner in which it operates. In addition, death education can under certain circumstances be understood to include counseling of individuals and/or groups that is both therapeutic and informational. We subscribe to the broadest definition of death education and have used it throughout this resource guide. It has also served as the basis for criteria for the inclusion of bibliographical materials in the present section.

An additional problem that needs to be considered here concerns the "target" group, or the persons at whom death education is directed. For example, in a death education program at the high school level the target group is obviously high school students. By contrast, a course on death education for nursing students is not merely directed at those students but is also intended to benefit dying patients and their families. Similarly, death education for parents, teachers, and counselors is intended to have a beneficial effect on their children and clients. One might conceptualize primary, secondary, and other subordinate target groups for death education, but for simplicity's sake we are assuming that a target group is any group that potentially benefits from death education.

This brings us to the internal organization of the bibliographical materials that we have assembled in the present section. Here we have been guided by two factors. First, there are two major thrusts in death education materials, one dealing with death education for young people in general, the other dealing with death education for the health professional and other caregivers. The former is concerned with a variety of goals and purposes. The latter is concerned with improved care for patients as well as support for family. A third less obvious thrust concerns death education for parents, teachers, counselors, clergy, elderly persons—in fact, all adults. We have followed these trends in grouping our materials by target audiences.

Second, since death education is a relatively new field, much of the literature is concerned with describing a need or formulating a rationale for it at the various levels and for various target groups. Most frequently, statements of the need for death education are based on descriptions of conditions and/or characteristics of the target group. For example, a number of articles and books point to the need for death education for nursing students based on findings that show nurses have difficulty coping with death and, given a cure-oriented institutional ethos and organization, are not effective in caring for dying patients. Since nurses are the single group most likely to be present at the institutionalized dying common in our society today, preparatory education in this field is critical. Other articles simply describe existing conditions and/or characteristics without discussing their implications for death education. We have included both kinds of pieces—those dealing with conditions and characteristics of the target group and those going beyond to argue the need for death education—under the major categories in our bibliography. Obviously, we have included materials that address questions of curriculum, teaching method and particular techniques, and evaluation of teaching effectiveness under the major categories. In addition, we have listed and annotated articles that discuss children's literature on death. Children's books about death have received much attention, and their educational and therapeutic potential for children is stated explicitly in a number of articles and is implied in others. We have included these articles under the appropriate major category. We have grouped together books and articles that deal broadly with death education under a "general" category. Articles discussing self-help groups and counseling concerns are under a separate heading.

It would be foolish to claim comprehensive coverage for the bibliography that follows. Not even the most sophisticated computer search program could yield such results in a new and rapidly changing field. In addition, in a few cases when we could not ourselves confirm their existence or locate copies for our review, we have had to omit titles that had been reported to us. However, in view of the breadth and volume of the materials that we have assembled, we do not believe that such omissions will ultimately be of great significance. We shall continue to search for additional materials; some items may be available in print by the time this resource guide is published. Finally, it should be noted that we have attempted in this section to avoid judgmental statements in our annotations, leaving such evaluations to the reader.

GENERAL

Agatstein, F. Attitude change and death education: A consideration of goals. *Death Education*, 1980, *3*(4), 323-332. This paper critically examines the goals of death anxiety reduction and the development of positive attitudes toward death in death education courses. Well argued.

Bugen, L. A. Appendixes: Structured exercises for death education. In L. A. Bugen (Ed.), *Death and dying: Theory/research/practice.* Dubuque, IA: Brown, 1979, 425-474. A number of exercises for death education classes are described, including goals, recommended group size, physical setting, time required, as well as variations. It lists the contributors of each exercise and often references and is useful for those who seek directions for experiential class activities.

Bugen, L. A. Death education: perspectives for schools and communities. In L. A. Bugen (Ed.), *Death and dying: Theory/research/practice.* Dubuque, IA: Brown, 1979, 237-249. Reviews both writings of death educators and studies on the effects of death education at the college level. Recommends death education for the general public.

Callas, M. A. *The effect of an experience of death education on death attitudes and concepts and on self-perception.* Unpublished, doctoral dissertation. The Catholic University, 1976. This dissertation includes a section that reviews rationales and goals for death education (pages 35-41). For a description of the research see (page 135).

Crase, D. The need to assess the impact of death education. *Death Education,* 1978, *1*(4), 423-431. This article discusses the need for evaluation of death education, cites studies done thus far, and stresses the need to attend to basic questions concerning curricular matters.

Crase, D., & Crase, D. R. Emerging dimensions of death education. *Health Education,* 1979, *10*(1), 26-29. A brief overview of current concerns in death education at all levels including some projections for the future.

Green, B. R., & Irish, D. P. (Eds.). *Death education: Preparation for living.* Cambridge, MA: Schenkman, 1971. This is the proceedings of the symposium of the same title sponsored by Hamline University, St. Paul, Minnesota, February 1970. It consists of addresses by Herman Feifel, John Brantner, Dan Leviton, and Donald Irish, and excerpts from workshop discussions prepared by Betty Green. A selected bibliography appears on pages 126-143.

Kastenbaum, R. We covered death today. *Death Education,* 1977, *1*(1), 85-92. The author argues that death education may be manipulated to serve as yet another, though more sophisticated, form of denial rather than an open and disciplined inquiry into our relationship with death, and recommends that the death educator be aware of social pressures to make death education merely comforting.

Knott, J E. Death education for all. In H. Wass (Ed.), *Dying: Facing the facts.* Washington, DC: Hemisphere, 1979, 385-403. The author discusses the why, where, when, how, and by whom of death education. He stresses the need for careful deliberation, well-defined objectives, and appropriate methods.

Kurlychek, R. T. Death education: Some considerations of purpose and rationale. *Educational Gerontology,* 1977, *2*, 43-50. The author discusses the major issues and concerns of death educators, including ethical concerns and the problem of evaluating the effectiveness of death education programs.

Leviton, D. The scope of death education. *Death Education,* 1977, *1*(1), 41–55. Stating that death education should promote the quality of life, the author outlines impersonal and emotional topics for discussion in a college course and lists goals for such a course including those that can be therapeutic-interventive.

Pine, V. R. A socio-historical portrait of death education. *Death Education,* 1977, *1*(1), 57–84. In this paper the author attempts a historical analysis of the evolution of death education over the past 50 years. He lists some problems of the current status of the field and makes recommendations for improvement.

Schulz, R. Death education. In. R. Schulz, *The psychology of death, dying, and bereavement.* Reading, MA: Addison-Wesley, 1978, 162-169. This is a very brief discussion of death education programs for various groups, including medical students.

Simpson, M. A. Death education—Where is thy sting? *Death Education,* 1979, *3,* 165-173. The author considers basic questions for planning death education at any level, cognitive and affective objectives, and some principles regarding teaching method and evaluation. He warns that death is exploitable and ability to recognize this phenomenon should be a major objective.

Ulin, R. O. *Death and dying education.* Washington, DC: National Education Association, 1977. This booklet touches briefly on most of the significant issues in death education, e.g., why there should be death education, whether the schools are the proper place for it, what should be taught, and teacher qualification.

DEATH EDUCATION FOR CHILDREN AND ADOLESCENTS

Agree, R. H., & Ackerman, N. J. Why children must mourn. *Teacher,* 1972, *90*(10), 15-16. This is a loose discussion touching upon a variety of topics related to death and the child.

Alexander, I. E., & Adlerstein, A. M. Affective responses to the concept of death in a population of children and early adolescents. *Journal of Genetic Psychology,* 1958, *93,* 167-177. The authors found a significant response was elicited by "death words" in a word association test. Affective responses were measured by galvanic skin responses.

Ames, L. Death: Ways to help children get perspective. *Instructor,* 1969, *78,* 59; 118. Ames offers some ideas and methods teachers can use to help children understand and cope with death.

Anthony, S. *The child's discovery of death.* New York: Harcourt, 1940. The author concludes that to the child death is primarily related to fear of retaliation for aggressive behavior and that changing concepts of death parallel other developing concepts in Piaget's theory of cognitive development.

Anthony, S. *The discovery of death in childhood and after.* New York: Basic Books, 1972. This is a complex discussion using Freudian and Piagetian concepts, and incorporating the author's earlier research as well as that of others.

Arnstein, F. J. I met death one clumsy day. *English Journal*, 1972, *61*(6), 853–858. This paper stresses problems that arise when students are discouraged from expressing their ideas and fears about death. It includes poems written by students in the author's English classes.

Atkinson, T. L. Teacher intervention with elementary school children in death-related situations. *Death Education* (in press). Atkinson addresses the questions of death education for elementary children in the context of death-related situations and the influence the teacher's death attitudes may have upon such education.

Ayalon, O. Is death a proper subject for the classroom? Comments on death education. In A. deVries and A. Carmi (Eds.), *The dying human*, Ramat Gan, Israel: Turtledove, 1979, 97–105. The article argues for death education in the classroom in cognitive, anthropological, emotional, and social areas and recommends approaches through literature, creative writing, and psychodrama and role-playing.

Bailis, L. A. Death in children's literature: A conceptual analysis. *Omega*, 1977-1978, *8*(4), 295–303. A sample of 40 children's books was used to examine the concepts of death presented in literature. Death was viewed most frequently as temporary and inevitable. No book considered death as the termination of all existence. The author speculates about the absence of this death concept.

Bailis, L. A., & Kennedy, W. R. Effects of a death education program upon secondary school students. *Journal of Educational Research*, *71*(2), 1977, 63–66. Two groups of high school students who participated in death education modules were compared with a control group using The Collett-Lester Fear of Death Scale. No significant differences between groups were found. The authors asserted that death education was of doubtful value to high school students.

Balkin, E., Epstein, C., & Bush, D. Attitudes toward classroom discussions of death and dying among urban and suburban children. *Omega*, 1976, *7*, 183–189. The researchers found that white suburban upper-middle-class children were more often in favor of classroom discussions of death than black inner-city children. Black children expressed greater fear of discussing death.

Bensley, L. B., Jr. (Ed.). *Death education as a learning experience.* Washington, DC: ERIC Clearinghouse on Teacher Education, Novmber 1975. This pamphlet outlines death education with an aim of seeing it integrated into a health education curriculum.

Berg, D. W., & Daugherty, G. G. *Perspectives on death: Student activity book.* DeKalb, IL: Perspectives on Death, 1972. This is part of an instructional package outlining a course on death and dying for high school students.

Berg, D. W., & Daugherty, G. G. Teaching about death. *Today's Education*, 1973, 46–47. This article discusses the development of an instructional unit on death and dying for high school students.

Berman, D. B. The facilitation of mourning: A preventive mental health approach. Unpublished doctoral dissertation, University of Massachusetts, 1978. This study indicated that a curriculum model can aid preschool children in the development of cognitive and affective capacities to deal with death and to mourn effectively, which is viewed as a preventive mental health concern.

Bernstein, J. E. *Loss: And how to cope with it.* New York: Seabury Press, 1977, 1-117. Written for young readers who have experienced a death, especially of someone close; deals with accompanying feelings and how to handle them. Simple, practical. (See also page 104.)

Bertman, S. L. Death education in the face of a taboo. In E. A. Grollman (Ed.), *Concerning death: A practical guide for the living.* Boston: Beacon, 1974, 333-361. The author discusses young children's interest in and concern about death, and how parents and teachers can help.

Blue, R. Mentioning the unmentionable. *Teacher*, 1975, *92*, 54-57; 105-106. The author argues for the need to discuss sensitive subjects, including divorce and death, in the classroom with young children. Discussions should be honest in a trusting, nondepressed atmosphere.

Brent, S. B. Puns, metaphors, and misunderstandings in a two-year-old's conception of death. *Omega*, 1977-1978, *8*(4), 285-293. This article reports, analyzes, and interprets a 2-year-old's conception of death through puns and misunderstandings about language.

Butler, A. F. Scratchy is dead. *Teacher*, 1978, *95*, 67-68. This is a day-care teacher's accounts of how the death of a pet gerbil provided the "teachable moment" for death education in the classroom for the young child.

Childers, P., & Wimmer, M. The concept of death in early childhood. *Child Development*, 1971, *42*(4), 1299-1301. The authors report on a study of the awareness of the universality and irrevocability of death in children aged 4-10. Older children tended to understand that death is universal, but not that it is irreversible. Younger children understood neither concept.

Clay, V. S. Children deal with death. *The School Counselor*, 1976, *23*, 175-184. In this article the author stresses that children think about death and need to be able to explore and be assisted in their understanding by their teachers.

Colarusso, C. "Johnny, did your mother die?" *Teacher*, 1975, *92*, 57. By describing a 6-year-old's loss of his mother, the author, a psychiatrist, offers the teacher practical suggestions about how to help the child in the classroom.

Crain, H. Basic concepts of death in children's literature. *Elementary English.* 1972, *49*, 111-115. This article excerpts basic ideas about death conveyed in various children's books.

Crase, D. R., & Crase, D. Live issues surrounding death education. *The Journal of School Health*, 1974, *44*(2), 70-73. The authors argue for formal death education beginning at the middle school level. They make a case for an interdisciplinary course, coordinated by the health educator and determined by the needs and interests of the students.

Crase, D. R., & Crase, D. Helping children understand death. *Young Children*, 1976, *32*, 21–25. This article suggests that teachers are significant adults in the child's life, and therefore have a responsibility in responding appropriately to the child's concerns about death. This requires self-development of the teacher, effective communication, positive use of experiences, and parent involvement.

Crase, D. R., & Crase, D. Attitudes toward death education for young children. *Death Education*, 1979, *3*(1), 31–40. The authors found that teachers of young children see the need for self-development, try to respond to children's death concerns, and are willing to help parents of bereaved children and to consider systematic death education in the early childhood curriculum.

Dahlgren, T., & Prager-Decker, I. A unit on death for primary grades. *Health Education*, 1979, *10*(1), 36–39. The article describes a unit on death for young children organized around five basic concepts. It includes objectives, materials, and procedures, and is very useful for teachers at that level who seek guidance and direction.

Deslisle, R. G., & Woods, A. S. Death and dying in children's literature: An analysis of three selected works. *Language Arts*, 1976, *53*(6), 683–687. The books are: *Charlotte's Web, The Magic Moth*, and *A Taste of Blackberries.*

Dobbelaere, C. J. A teaching strategy on tragedy. *Health Education*, 1977, *8*(6), 11–12. A teaching strategy for a death course at the high school level is proposed using Shneidman' death questionnaire and a series of open-ended statements.

Dunton, H. D. The child's concept of death. In B. Schoenberg, A. C. Carr, D. Peretz, & A. H. Kutscher (Eds.), *Loss and grief: Psychosocial management in medical practice.* New York: Columbia University Press, 1970, 355–361. This paper reviews studies of the child's concept of death, discusses family influence, and concludes that educating the child about death is a complex problem.

Fontenot, C. The subject nobody teaches. *English Journal*, 1974, *63*, 62–63. The author describes a teaching unit on death carried out with an 11th grade English class. Suitable material from the classical literature is suggested.

Formanek, R. When children ask about death. *Elementary School Journal*, 1974, *75*, 92–97. The author argues that teachers should answer small children's questions about death to prevent anxieties and to assist them in their development of a realistic concept of death.

Fredlund, D. J. Children and death from the school setting viewpoint. *Journal of School Health*, 1977, *47*, 533–537. In this paper the author advises teachers what to do and what not to do when a student, parent, other relative, or pet dies.

Freeman, J. Death and dying in three days? *Kappan*, 1978, *60*(2), 118. This brief paper presents sensitive and sensible arguments against a fifth grade teacher's approach to death education in a 3-day unit reported in the same issue. (See J. M. Mueller, p. 15.)

Furman, E. Helping children cope with death. *Young Children*, 1978, *33*(4), 25–32. This article describes how death, bereavement, and grief are dealt with in a therapeutic nursery school.

Galen, H. A matter of life and death. *Young Children*, 1972, *27*(6), 351–356. Provides preschool teachers with rationale and guidelines for handling the subject of death with young children.

Garner, A. E., & Acklen, L. Does death education belong in the middle school? *National Association of Secondary School Principals Bulletin*, 1978, *62*, 134–137. The authors argue that from a developmental point of view the middle school curriculum should include death education. They briefly describe an interdisciplinary minicourse on death at that level.

Gartley, W., & Bernasconi, M. The concept of death in children. *Journal of Genetic Psychology*, 1967, *110*, 71–85. The researchers report results of interviews with 60 children about their thoughts of death. The article includes a great deal of verbatim question-and-answer material.

Gideon (Everett), M. Criteria for evaluating curriculum materials in death education from grades K–12. *Death Education*, 1977, *1*(2), 235–239. The author outlines criteria by which death education curriculum materials can be assessed in terms of usefulness for classroom teaching at the various levels.

Gordon, A., & Klass, D. Goals for death education. *The School Counselor*, 1977, *24*(5), 339–347. The authors point at the lack of training for death education and systematic analysis of purposes. They stress the danger of death education by unqualified teachers and give an appalling illustration, suggest four goals for death education, and discuss each in some detail.

Gordon, A., & Klass, D. *They need to know: How to teach children about death.* Englewood Cliffs, NJ: Prentice-Hall, 1979. This book discusses the child's experience of death, and speaks directly to teaching about death. A set of 9 appendixes reproduces useful documents that might support this education. In general, the book seems to mark a new stage in the development of curriculum guides and handbooks for parents and teachers.

Hair, J. M. What shall we teach about death in science classes? *Elementary School*, 1965, *65*, 414–418. The author lists four reasons why death is an important topic in the school curriculum. Evidence is cited from a personal study of scientists' and physicians' beliefs about dying and death.

Harnett, A. L. How we do it. *Journal of School Health*, 1973, *43*(8), 526–527. This article describes an independent study unit compiled for advanced high school or college students based on Dan Leviton's suggested course outlines.

Harris, W. H. Some reflections concerning approaches to death education. *Journal of School Health*, 1978, *48*, 162–165. Five approaches to death education at the high school level are discussed: philosophical, sociological, psychological, medicolegal, and health educational. The author suggests that the health educator combine several approaches.

Hart, E. J. Death education and mental health. *Journal of School Health*, 1976, *46*(7), 407-412. Hart suggests that dealing with death should be one of the mental health concerns of all school health programs.

Hause, K. Outdoor education and death. *Independent School*, 1976, *36*(3), 43-44. Basing the article on a fatal accident during a hike in the mountains with his class, the teacher-author provides a set of practical questions and answers about dying and death useful for classroom teachers.

Hawkinson, J. R. Teaching about death. *Today's Education*, 1976, *65*, 41-42. A 9-week course on death at the high school level is described, and reactions to it from students and others are reported.

Holmes, J. Teaching about death: A review of selected materials. *Social Studies Journal*, 1975, *4*(1), 48-50. Books and audiovisual aids on death are evaluated. A brief description of death courses is provided.

Hymowitz, L. Creative teaching strategies in death education—thanatology. *American Secondary Education*, 1978, *8*(1), 7-18. Suggestions for use in a death education unit at the high school level include visiting a cemetery, studying funeral prices, and language arts activities.

Hymowitz, L. Death as a discipline: The ultimate curriculum. *NASSP Bulletin*, 1979, *63*, 102-106. The importance of death education as an integral part of a student's life curriculum is argued. Stresses the need for home-school cooperation in this endeavor.

Kastenbaum, R. The child's understanding of death: How does it develop? In E. A. Grollman (Ed.), *Explaining death to children*. Boston: Beacon, 1967, 89-108. The author discusses the development of ideas about death as part of intellectual growth and the total pattern of personality development that ideally continues as reevaluation and reorientation through life.

Kastenbaum, R. Childhood: The kingdom where creatures die. *Journal of Clinical Child Psychology*, 1974, *3*(2), 11-13. In this paper the author suggests that most children have death-related thoughts and experiences, although most adults pretend children are oblivious to death. Parents who have not come to terms with their own death anxieties may not be able to help their children.

Kastenbaum, R. Death and development through the lifespan. In H. Feifel (Ed.), *New meanings of death*. New York: McGraw-Hill, 1977, 18-45. This article discusses understanding of death from its discovery in childhood, through interpretations given in adolescence and adulthood in the context of cultural and subcultural patterns and special sensitivity about death in midlife, to death sensitivity in old age.

Keith, C. R., & Ellis, D. Reactions of pupils and teachers to death in the classroom. *The School Counselor*, 1978, *25*, 228-234. The authors describe six cases of the impact of death in the classroom. They conclude that in a "healthy" classroom questions about a classmate's death are discussed and children are allowed to express their feelings. Five practical recommendations for teachers, counselors, or principals are included.

Klass, D., & Gordon, A. *Goals in teaching about death.* Washington, DC: National Institute of Education, 1976. A set of guidelines and goals for death education in the schools are proposed for teachers who plan to develop curriculum materials in this area.

Koby, I. M. "And the leaves that are green turn to . . . ?" *English Journal*, 1975, *64*, 59-61. An English teacher at an intermediate school reports her success with approaching the subject of death through poetry and music.

Koocher, G. P. *Childhood, death, and cognitive development.* Unpublished doctoral dissertation, University of Missouri, 1972. Research findings indicate that death concepts develop in accordance with Piagetian developmental levels and that developmental level is a better indicator of a child's understanding of death than is chronological age.

Koocher, G. P. Why isn't the gerbil moving anymore? Discussing death in the home and in the classroom. *Children Today*, 1974, *4*, 18-36. In this paper the author discusses the development of the concept of death in children. Parents and other adults should listen to children's hidden questions about death. The author also offers suggestions for talking about death in the classroom and for introducing classroom projects on death.

Koocher, G. P. Talking with children about death. *American Journal of Orthopsychiatry*, 1974, *44*(3), 404-411. The author found that children have no severe anxiety in responding to questions about death and that responses vary with different age levels. Koocher speculates about the reason for different responses of U.S. children and the Hungarian children used in Nagy's study.

Krahn, J. H. Pervasive death: An avoided concept. *Educational Leadership*, 1973, *31*(1), 18-20. Adults' problems of talking about death with children are discussed. A good rationale for death education in the elementary school is provided.

Lasker, A. A. Telling children the facts of death. *Your Child*, Winter 1972, 1-6. This paper was not available for review.

Lowenberg, J. S. Coping behavior of fatally ill adolescents and their parents. *Nursing Forum*, 1970, *9*, 269-287. The author presents two lists of coping behaviors for adolescents developed from the author's clinical observations.

Marshall, J. G., & Marshall, V. W. The treatment of death in children's books. *Omega*, 1971, *2*, 36-41. Citing evidence that young children have a realistic concept of death, the authors argue the need for children's death literature that is consonant with conceptual development. (See also page 112.)

McConville, B. J., Boag, L. C., & Purohit, A. P. Mourning processes in children of varying ages. *Canadian Psychiatric Association Journal,* 1970, *15*, 252–255. This article reports that children's mourning patterns are determined by chronological age, developmental stage, and previous life experiences.

McDonald, M. Helping children to understand death: An experience with death in a nursery school. *The Journal of Nursing Education,* 1963, *19*(1), 19–25. The author describes children's reactions to the death of a 4-year-old's mother and the approach taken to help the children deal with this event. The author stresses the need for honesty and for helping them with their fears and anxieties.

McIntire, M., Angle, C., & Struempler, L. The concept of death in midwestern children and youth. *American Journal of Diseases of Children,* 1972, *123*, 527–532. This research report suggests that middle-class children report disease and old age as the cause of death whereas children from low socioeconomic backgrounds list violence, war, and accidents.

McLear, J. D. Children's concepts of death. *Journal of Genetic Psychology,* 1973, *123*(2), 359–360. A replication of Nagy's study with U.S. children is reported. The author concludes that death concepts develop in four stages rather than three, and assigns different age levels to the stages.

McLendon, G. H. One teacher's experience with death education for adolescents. *Death Education,* 1979, *3*(1), 57–65. The author describes the development of a teaching unit in her humanities classes at the eighth and ninth grade level. She reports great interest and the need for an emotionally nonthreatening approach.

McLure, J. W. Death education. *Kappan,* 1974, *15*(7), 483–485. The author of this article provides a good rationale for death education in the public school curriculum, but includes cautionary remarks concerning implementation.

McMahon, J. Death education: An independent study unit. *Journal of School Health,* 1973, *43*, 526–527. This paper contains a list of topics called "subunits" on death for high school students, adapted from course outlines by Dan Leviton.

Middleton, K. H. Strategies for teaching about death and loss. *Health Education,* 1979, *10*(1), 36. This is a miniarticle describing methodological considerations in teaching children the concept of loss.

Mills, G., Reisler, R., Robinson, A. E., & Vermilyer, G. *Discussing death: A guide to death education.* Homewood, IL: ETC Publications, 1976. This book essentially prescribes learning objectives and activities for students separated into four age levels: ages 5–6, 7–9, 10–12, and 13–18. It includes an adaptation of Shneidman's death questionnaire. Teachers who lack knowledge, resourcefulness, and goal-setting skills will find this book a useful guide. (See also page 113.)

Mitchell, M. E. *The child's attitude to death.* New York: Schocken, 1967. The author discusses religious, scientific, and sociological influences on British children's concepts and fears about death, immortality, and killing.

Moller, H. Death: Handling the subject and affected students in the school. In E. A. Grollman (Ed.), *Explaining death to children.* Boston: Beacon Press, 1967, 145–167. Four cases of children with death experiences are related.

Morris, B. Young children and books on death. *Elementary English,* 1974, *51,* 395–398. The author discusses several children's books on death.

Moss, J. P. Death in children's literature. *Elementary English,* 1972, *49,* 530–532. Seven books on death considered valuable for children are analyzed.

Mueller, J. M., Jr. I taught about death and dying. *Kappan,* 1978, *60*(2), 117–118. A fifth grade teacher reports on a three-day concentrated death unit he taught and how he integrated death with social studies, spelling, mathematics, language arts, and music. This is a good example of what not to do. (See J. Freeman, p. 11.)

Mueller, M. L. Fear of death and death education. *Notre Dame Journal of Education,* 1975, *6*(1), 84–91. The author reports on a study of the effect of death education on death fear among early adolescents in parochial schools. It was found that death education increased fear of death. Possible explanations are explored.

Myers, J. "Werewolves" in literature for children. *Language Arts,* 1976, *53,* 552–556. This article reports how a "werewolf" story written by a 10-year-old stimulated the class to write a death drama, suggesting that such literary experiences fit the child's developmental level in the conceptualization of death.

Nelson, R. C., Peterson, W. D., & Sartore, L. Issues and dialogue: Helping children to cope with death. *Elementary School Guidance and Counseling,* 1975, *9*(3), 226–232. The authors argue that children's exposure to death through TV, movies, radio, traffic accidents, fairy tales, and war games is rarely emotional and is apt to create distorted concepts. They urge adults to help children express their feelings and to respond to children's questions.

Noland, M., Richardson, G. E., & Bray, R. M. The systematic development and efficacy of a death education unit for ninth grade girls. *Death Education* (in press). The authors report findings of the effectiveness of a death education unit through two controlled experiments. An outline of the death education unit is included. Excellent design and assessment.

Ordal, C. C. Death as seen in books for young children. *Death Education* (in press). The author categorizes and evaluates 22 children's books on death with respect to their potential usefulness in helping 3–9-year-olds understand and cope with death. Useful for parents, teachers, and librarians.

Parness, E. Effects of experiences with loss and death among preschool children. *Children Today,* 1975, *4,* 2–7. After studying anecdotal material the author concludes that, contrary to the belief of other researchers, the preschool child may grieve with the same intensity as adults. It is suggested that working effectively with children requires adults to explore their own anxieties about death and loss.

Perkes, A. C. Classroom animal death—Its learning potential for death education. *School Science and Mathematics*, 1977, 77, 93–96. The author argues that the death of an animal can provide stimulus to death education, both cognitive and affective. Some suggestions for classroom teachers are listed.

Perkes, A. C. Teachers' attitudes toward death-related issues. *School Science and Mathematics*, 1978, 2, 135–141. This article explores teachers' attitudes particularly with respect to the sacrifice of certain kinds of organisms for teaching purposes. It was found that few teachers advocated the killing of animals for learning experiences, but use of natural and accidental death of classroom pets for death education was rarely mentioned.

Perkes, A. C., & Schildt, R. Death-related attitudes of adolescent males and females. *Death Education*, 1979, 2(4), 359–368. Significant sex differences are reported on 11 of the 22 items investigated.

Plank, E. N. Young children and death. *Young Children*, 1968, 23, 331–336. Some of the literature on children's thoughts about death is listed. The author believes that religious faith and ritual offer little reassurance for today's children.

Pope, A. J. Children's attitudes toward death. *Health Education*. 1979, May/June, 27–29. Repeats what has been said and written previously by many others.

Prouty, D. Read about death? Not me! *Language Arts*, 1976, 53(6), 679–683. A class of fourth graders initially refused to sign up for a group designed to read death-related books. After encouragement 16 students did. The teacher tells about the sessions and the books. (See also page 116.)

Reed, E. L. *Helping children with the mystery of death.* Nashville: Abingdon, 1970. This book was not available for review.

Reisler, R., Jr. The issue of death education. *The School Counselor*, 1977, 24(5), 331–337. The author discusses eight reasons why death education is a relevant subject in school.

Reynolds, J. D. A teaching program for death education. In O. J. Z. Sahler (Ed.), *The child and death.* St. Louis: Mosby, 1978, 248–278. In this chapter the author describes the development of a death education program at the high school level including behavioral objectives, content development and evaluation.

Rochlin, G. How younger children view death and themselves. In E. A. Grollman (Ed.), *Explaining death to children.* Boston: Beacon, 1967, 51–85. Clinical evidence is provided indicating that very young children can discover death. Rochlin explains how they cope with this knowledge, using Freud's theory of defense mechanisms.

Romero, C. E. Children, death and literature. *Language Arts*, 1976, 53(6), 674–678. Books for primary, intermediate, and adult reading are suggested.

Romero, C. E. *The treatment of death in contemporary children's literature.* (ERIC Document Reproduction Service ED 101 664) No. Computer Microfilm International, P.O. Box 190, Arlington, VA 22210, 1974. This is a bibliographical essay including a review of children's books on death from colonial times to the present.

Rowe, K. B., & Loesch, L. C. An affective education experience for helping children reduce their anxieties about death. *Humanist Educator,* 1978, *16*(3), 103-110. An affective experience for children consisting of seven sessions is described. The authors believe that it can be readily replicated or adapted by teachers or counselors.

Rucker, M. E., Thompson, L. M., & Dickerson, B. E. The home economics curriculum: Death education. *Journal of Home Economics,* 1977, *69*(2), 14-21. The authors offer suggestions for approaches, discussion questions, class activities, and reading assignments for the study of death in a home economics classroom.

Ruffo, V. C. Visit a mortuary. *Instructor,* 1969, *79,* 112-113. A mother recounts a field trip to a funeral home by her son's sixth grade class.

Russell, R. D. Educating about death. *Health Education,* 1977, *8*(6), 8-10. A health education professor recounts his experiences in learning and teaching about death.

Ryerson, M. S. Death education and counseling for children. *Elementary School Guidance and Counseling,* 1977, *11*(3), 165-174. The article suggests some activities for teachers and counselors to educate children about death and help them overcome fears and anxieties.

Sadker, D., Sadker, M., & Crockett, C. Death—a fact of life in children's literature. *Instructor,* 1976, *85*(7), 73-84. Ten recent books on death for children are discussed.

Safier, G. A study of relationships between life-death concepts in children's. *Journal of Genetic Psychology,* 1964, *105,* 283-294. This is a report of a study based on the three-stages formulations by Nagy and Piagetian theory of cognitive development. The author found that animism decreases with age and that there is a positive relationship between the concept formations of life and death.

Schrank, J. Death: Guide to books and audiovisual aids. *Media and Methods,* 1971, *7*(6), 32-35, 64. The author offers a rationale for death education in the high school with suggestions of topics. This article contains a useful annotated bibliography of books and films, as well as rock-folk music suitable for this level.

Schur, T. J. What man has told children about death. *Omega,* 1971, *2,* 84-90. A historical analysis of children's literature on death is presented. The author concludes that such a survey challenges the reader to examine personal and present-day ideas about the meaning of death.

Sharapan, H. "Mister Rogers' Neighborhood": Dealing with death on a children's television series. *Death Education,* 1977, *1*(1), 131-136. In this article the author discusses Mr. Rogers' approach to death for his large young television audience, using dialogue, song, and a puppet drama in a low-key, low anxiety manner.

Somerville, R. M. Death education as part of family life education: Using imaginative literature for insights into family crises. *The Family Coordinator*, 1971, *20*, 209-224. Based on surveys of textbooks and curriculum guides, the author concludes that death and bereavement have been largely ignored in family life education at the high school level as well as in teacher preparation. Somerville suggests that fiction may fill this gap and includes a list of recommended books.

Stanford, G. Miniguide: A mini-course on death. *Scholastic Teacher*, 1973, 40-44. Materials and books for use in minicourses at the high school level are suggested.

Stanford, G., & Perry, D. *Death out of the closet: A curriculum guide to living with dying.* New York: Bantam, 1976. This is a handbook for death education at the high school level. The authors suggest how to choose topics and design course outlines. They recommend materials and teaching strategies, and provide overview, synopsis and discussion questions for 19 popular paperbacks often used in this sort of teaching.

Stanford, G. Methods and materials for death education. *The School Counselor*, 1977, *24*(5), 350-360. Stanford discusses a variety of approaches, topics, activities, and resources useful for death education at the elementary and secondary school level. (See also Bibliographies, p. 33.)

Steinmetz, Ross E. Children's books relating to death. In E. A. Grollman (Ed.), *Explaining death to children.* Boston: Beacon, 1967, 249-271. It is asserted that young children have no need for material that relates to death. The author recommends death-related books for children over 10.

Stern, M. E. Death. *English Journal*, 1975, *64*, 61-62. This is a brief description of a course on death for seniors who are average, or above, in English.

Stillion, J., & Wass, H. Children and death. In H. Wass (Ed.), *Dying: Facing the facts.* Washington, DC: Hemisphere, 1979, 208-235. This chapter deals with adults' denial of death with children, and offers a historical perspective of this attitude. Studies on children's views on death are examined. The authors plead for open, honest discussion of death with the child to assist in developing a realistic understanding. (See also page 90-91.)

Sugar, M. Normal adolescent mourning. *American Journal of Psychotherapy*, 1969, *22*, 258-269. The author proposes a theory that normal adolescent mourning of separation from parents is often manifested in symptoms of depression. Eight case studies are included.

Swain, H. L. Childhood views of death. *Death Education*, 1979, *2*(4), 341-358. Based on individual interviews with 120 children aged 2-16, age was found to be the only variable that significantly differentiated between various views held by children.

Swenson, E. J. The treatment of death in children's literature. *Elementary English*, 1972, *49*, 401-404. This article reviews the history of children's literature on death and discusses four contemporary children's books on death that deal with the topic honestly.

Tallmer, M., Formanek, R., & Tallmer, J. Factors influencing children's concepts of death. *Journal of Clinical Child Psychology*, 1974, *3*(2), 17-19. This is a report of a study that assessed parental influence on children's death concepts. It was found that neither parental explanations nor the child's experiences with death as reported by parents showed any significant relationship with the child's death concept. Lower-class children were more aware of the concept of death than were middle-class children.

Thompson, M. L. Symbolic immortality: A new approach to the study of death. *Media and Methods*, 1977, *13*, 60-64. The author offers a new approach to death at the high school level: image gathering and image making based on Robert Lifton's and Eric Olson's book *Living and Dying*, in which the authors contend that the development of concepts, images, and symbols gives meaning to experience and "symbolic immortality."

Ulin, R. O. *Death and dying education.* Washington, DC: National Education Association, 1977, 44-72. Contains a syllabus for an 18-week death and dying course for high school students including topics, objectives, activities, and various resources.

Wahl, C. W. The fear of death. In H. Feifel (Ed.), *The Meaning of Death.* New York: McGraw-Hill, 1959, 16-29. It is suggested that the child's concept of death is a composite of mutually contradictory paradoxes: Death is not conceived of as a possibility for oneself, but, at the same time, if strong adults die how can the weaker child survive?

Warren, W. E. Physical education and death. *Physical Education*, 1971, *28*, 127-128. The author cites the work of existential philosophers and attempts to relate their ideas on existence to certain aspects of physical education.

Wass, H., & Scott, M. Middle school children's death concepts and concerns. *Middle School Journal*, 1978, *9*(1), 10-12. This is a report of a study of 85 students aged 11-13 in which death concepts and concerns are compared with demographic factors, sex, and self-concept. It includes a discussion of educational implications and specific recommendations.

Wass, H., & Shaak, J. Helping children understand death through literature. *Childhood Education*, 1976, *53*(2), 80-85. The authors mention the need for open discussion of death at home and suggest that children's books are a valuable source of information and comfort. The article includes a selective annotated bibliography (29 items), arranged by age groups.

Wass, H., Guenther, Z. C., & Towry, B. J. United States and Brazilian children's concepts of death. *Death Education*, 1979, *3*(1), 39-53. This article reports on a cross-cultural study involving 215

U.S. and 188 Brazilian urban, middle-class children aged 10 and 11, in which death concepts among the two groups were compared.

Watt, A. S. Helping children to mourn, part I. *Medical Insight*, 1971, *3*, 29-32. It is suggested that children proceed more slowly and for a longer period of time in their "grief work" than do adults. The article describes different mourning patterns of children and stresses the need of facilitative adults during the child's mourning period.

Watt, A. S. Helping children to mourn, part II. *Medical Insight*, 1971, *3*, 57-62. The author describes adult behaviors that impair the child's ability to mourn a death, such as restraining their own show of grief, removing the child from the event, ceasing to speak of the departed, and giving unrealistic religious explanations. In addition, the author describes signs that should alert adults that the child may need professional help.

Watts, P. R. Evaluation of death attitude change resulting from a death education instructional unit. *Death Education*, 1977, *1*(2), 187-193. The author reports preliminary results of a study involving health education students. The indication is that more favorable death attitudes were found in students who were exposed to an instructional unit on death than in those who were not.

Watts, R. G. *Straight talk about death with young people.* Philadelphia: Westminister, 1975. The need for honest talk about death is stressed. Watts suggests discussion groups and discussion topics with seventh and eighth grade students and includes photographs.

Webb, A. I. Death: The last taboo. *English Journal*, 1977, *66*, 55-56. This is a brief description of a 6-week elective course on death for high school students.

Weininger, O. How to have a funeral. *Orbit*, 1971, *2*(1), 16. The author encourages teachers of young children to allow open talk about death, or dramatic acting out such as performing a funeral rite in a psychologically safe environment.

Whitley, E. Grandma: She died. *Childhood Education*, 1976, *53*, 77-79. This article describes an "adopted grandparents" program for first and second graders and its benefit for learning about the life cycle, including death.

Yarber, W. L. Death education: A living issue. *Science Teacher*, 1976, *43*, 21-23. In this paper the author suggests study topics, learning experiences, and guest speakers for a death and dying unit in health or sciences courses at the high school level.

Yudkin, S. Children and death. *Lancet*, 1967, *7*, 37-41. The literature on children and death in the nineteenth and twentieth century is reviewed. Yudkin indicates problems of alleviating children's anxieties and the need for medical personnel to help the dying child and parents by giving empathy and understanding.

Zazzaro, J. Death be not distorted. *Nation's Schools*, 1973, *91*(5), pp. 39-42; 102. The author argues the need for death education in the schools, K-12.

DEATH EDUCATION
FOR COLLEGE STUDENTS

Barrett, C. J. The advantages of credit–noncredit gerontology courses: Widowhood as an illustration. *Death Education,* 1980, *3*(4), 333-345. Here an interdisciplinary course on widowhood sponsored by a College of Liberal Arts and Sciences and the Division of Continuing Education is described and evaluated. It was found that the course was highly successful and suggested that heterogeneity in student backgrounds and ages may be an asset and that such courses facilitate the integration of content and life experience.

Bell, B. D. The experimental manipulation of death attitudes: A preliminary investigation. *Omega,* 1975, *6*(3), 199-205. College students who had taken a death course are compared with a control group. The experimental group thought more about death and showed greater interest in death-related discussions than did the control group. There were no significant differences between the groups concerning fear of death.

Bloom, S. On teaching an undergraduate course on death and dying. *Omega,* 1975, *6*(3), 223-226. This is a brief description of an undergraduate course on death with 11 students enrolled.

Bluestein, V. W. Death-related experiences, attitudes, and feelings reported by thanatology students and a national sample. *Omega,* 1975, *6*(3), 207-218. The author compared attitudes of students enrolled in a death course with responses by *Psychology Today* readers using Shneidman's death questionnaire. She concludes that thanatology students think a lot about death, have experienced more death, and tend to be more sensitive to interpersonal relationships than *Psychology Today* respondents.

Cherico, D. J., Kutscher, M. L., Colvin, L., & Kutscher, A. H. (Eds.). *Thanatology course outlines (Vol. 1).* New York: MSS Information Corporation, 1978. This is an apparently unorganized, unedited collection of 27 outlines, syllabi, and/or selected reading lists used for courses on death at the college level. (See also O. S. Margolis, et al., p. 24.)

Chiappetta, W., Floyd, H. H., & McSeveney, D. R. Sex differences in coping with death anxiety. *Psychological Reports,* 1976, *39*, 945-946. Female college students had higher manifest death anxiety than their male counterparts.

Corr, C. A. A model syllabus for death and dying courses. *Death Education,* 1978, *1*(4), 433-457. This article outlines in detail a 13-unit model syllabus for a broad-scale, introductory course on death and dying at the college level.

Corr, C. A. What is philosophical in the death and dying course? *Death Education,* 1977, *1*(1), 93-111. It is argued that the standard college-taught death course includes a strong component of philosophical issues. For this reason, a course on death should be team-taught and a philosopher must be a key member of the team.

Cummins, V. A. *On death education in colleges and universities in the United States, 1977.* Paper read at the conference of the Forum for Death Education & Counseling, Washington, D.C., September 1978. Results of an extensive mail survey of 4-year colleges and universities with a 63.6 percent response were reported. More than 1000 death courses were reported, which enrolled nearly 30,000 students and were offered in various disciplines and professional schools.

Donohue, W. R. Student death: What do we do? *National Association of Student Personnel Administrators (NASPA) Journal,* 1977, *14*, 29-32. This author gives practical advice to student affairs deans at a university about the steps to be taken when a student dies on campus.

Embry, C. R. Love, death, and liberal education. *Liberal Education,* 1976, *62*, 444-456. A case is made for the psychological, educational, and philosophical significance of love and death and the potential of liberal education to capitalize upon the interest these topics generate in students.

Fang, B., & Howell, K. A. Death anxiety among graduate students. *Journal of American College Health,* 1976, *25*, 310-313. The authors found no sex differences and no differences with respect to religion and death anxiety. They did find that medical students showed less death anxiety than graduate students in other fields.

Golburgh, S. J., Rotman, C. B., Snibbe, J. R., & Ondrack, J. W. Attitudes of college students toward personal death. *Adolescence,* 1967, *2*, 212-229. The authors report on findings of a study of 137 college students concerning various views, feelings, and opinions about death.

Gurfield, M. On teaching death and dying. *Media and Methods,* 1977, *13*, 56-59. The author tells with candor how his need to retain a faculty position motivated him to offer a course on death at a community college, and reflects upon the success of his course. Happily, it attracted the numbers of students that assured his tenure. Hopefully no other courses are initiated by this kind of external motivation.

Hart, D. V. A measurement of the improvement of attitudes toward death. *The Journal of School Health,* 1976, *46*, 5, 269-270. Hart found that the majority of 68 students who took a death course (61 percent) showed a statistically significant improvement in death attitudes, whereas 23 percent showed a decline and 16 percent showed no change.

Hoelter, J. W., & Epley, R. J. Death education and death-related attitudes. *Death Education,* 1979, *3*(1), 67-75. This study revealed significant differences between college students enrolling in a death course and those not enrolling. No significant before and after test differences were found, indicating. that the death course did not affect death-related attitudes in a significant way.

Jeffrey, D. W. *Death education: Teaching a course on death and dying.* Paper read at the annual meeting of the American Psychological Association, San Francisco, August 1977. A course on death and dying for college students is described, with detailed class assignments and activities. The author proposes three major goals for death education.

Knott, J. E., Prull, R. W. Death education: Accountable to whom? For what? *Omega*, 1976, *7*(2), 177-181. This article reports on a study of the effects on students' death attitudes of a college course on death education and lethal behavior.

Leviton, D. The need for education on death and suicide. *The Journal of School Health*, 1969, *39*, 270-274. The author reviews studies on death thoughts and the fear of death in children and adolescents, then describes the format of the course on death he teaches at the college level.

Leviton, D. Education for death, or death becomes less a stranger. *Omega*, 1975, *6*(3), 183-191. Here the author describes a death education course designed for a large number (over 300) of college students. A report of student responses to the course is included.

Leviton, D. The stimulus of death. *Health Education*, 1976, *7*(2), 17-20. In this paper Leviton reviews the status of death education, describes a death course at the college level, and reports on a pilot study concerning the motivations of students enrolling in a death course. He suggests that the study of death can profoundly affect life.

Leviton, D. Death education. In H. Feifel (Ed.), *New meanings of death.* New York: McGraw-Hill, 1977, 254-272. The author discusses the development of death education, tentative goals, characteristics of students taking death education courses, and variations in content and methodology.

Leviton, D., & Fretz, B. Effects of death education on fear of death and attitudes towards death and life. *Omega*, 1978-1979, *9*(3), 267-277. Students taking death education courses were compared with students taking sex education and introductory psychology on a number of dimensions including beliefs, attitudes, and background. On the basis of pre-post scores it was found that students who had taken a death course viewed death as more approachable and personal rather than technological.

Lonetto, R., Fleming, S., Gorman, M., & Best, S. The psychology of death: A course description and some student perceptions. *Ontario Psychologist*, 1975, *7*(2), 9-14. A course on death at the college level is described and student opinions on various aspects of death are presented.

Magni, K. Reactions to death stimuli among theology students. *Journal for the Scientific Study of Religion*, 1970, *9*, 247-248. Theology students at Uppsala University were asked to respond to picture stimuli depicting death. Students planning to become parish priests responded more positively to the stimuli than did students planning to become researchers or teachers in theology.

Margolis, O. S., Cherico, D. J., O'Connor, B. P., & Kutscher, A. H. (Eds.). *Thanatology course outlines (Vol. 2)*. New York: MSS Information Corporation, 1978. This is a collection of 23 outlines, syllabi, and/or selected readings lists used for courses on death at the college level, plus one-item guidelines for elementary school death education, without apparent organization or editing. (See also D. J. Cherico, et al., p. 21.)

Middleton, W. C. Some reactions toward death among college students. *Journal of Abnormal and Social Psychology*, 1936, *31*, 165–173. Reported are the responses of 825 college students to a series of questions concerning personal views about death.

Sadwith, J. An interdisciplinary approach to death education. *The Journal of School Health*, 1974, *44*, 455–458. The development of a death course for undergraduate students is described.

Salter, C. A., & Salter, C. D. Attitudes toward aging and behaviors toward the elderly among young people as a function of death anxiety. *The Gerontologist*, 1976, *16*(3), 232–235. This study found that the more fearful college students were those who believed that the elderly were less likely to be able to live in their homes. Those most afraid of death were also most afraid of their own aging. Additional factors must influence attitudes and behaviors toward the elderly.

Shapiro, S. I. *Instructional resources for teaching the psychology of death and dying*. Honolulu: University of Hawaii, 1973. This 64-page pamphlet is a helpful resource for the beginning instructor of a course on the psychology of death. It lists seven pages of possible topics, a number of class exercises, films, popular musical pieces, paintings, famous sayings, poems, and quotes, and weekly reading assignments (poor students at the U. of H.!).

Shneidman, E. S. Can a young person write his own obituary? *Life-Threatening Behavior*, 1972, *2*(4), 262–267. The author presents sample obituaries written by college students at Harvard University in 1969. He concludes that young people have difficulty objectifying themselves or seeing themselves as dead.

Shneidman, E. S. *Death and the college student*. New York: Behavioral Publications, 1972. This is a collection of papers on death and related subjects written by college undergraduates enrolled in a course on the psychology of death taught by the author at Harvard University in 1969.

Shneidman, E. S. The college student and death. In H. Feifel (Ed.), *New meanings of death*. New York: McGraw-Hill, 1977, 68–86. This paper discusses conceptualizations and attitudes of college students toward death and bereavement. It includes recorded sessions between the author and terminal and bereaved students.

Stillion, J. M. Rediscovering the taxonomies: A structural framework for death education courses. *Death Education* 1979, *3*(2), 157–

164. The author suggests application of the taxonomies of the cognitive and affective domains as educational principles underlying death courses.

Thorson, J. A. Variations in death anxiety related to college students' sex, major field of study, and certain personality traits. *Psychological Reports*, 1977, *40*, 857–858. Females had higher death anxiety than males, and students majoring in social work tended to have higher death anxiety, those in business lower, than students in other fields.

Thorson, J. A. Lifeboat: social values and decision making. *Death Education*, 1978, *1*(4), 459–464. Described is a role-playing or simulation technique useful in stimulating discussion among students in a death class or seminar.

White, D. K. An undergraduate course in death. *Omega*, 1970, *1*(1), 167–174. The author describes an undergraduate course on death piloted at the University of Michigan. Included are a syllabus, and samples of students' reactions.

DEATH EDUCATION
FOR HEALTH PROFESSIONALS

Achte, K. A., & Vauhkonen, M. L. Cancer and the psyche. *Omega*, 1971, *2*, 45–56. It is concluded that the majority of patients wish to be told of their terminal condition and suffer no permanent negative consequences as a result of being informed.

Astrachan, M. Management of a staff death in a children's institution. *Child Welfare*, 1977, *56*, 380–385. Special problems of a staff member's death in a children's institution are discussed. The author suggests a program of preparation that anticipates such an event.

Baer, R. The sick child knows. In S. Standard & H. Nathan (Eds.), *Should the patient know the truth*. New York: Springer, 1955, 100–106. The author, a pediatric nurse, relates a number of instances and behaviors of young terminal children (ages 2–8) that convinced her that they knew they were dying although they were not told. She believes they quietly accepted their fate. Children whose prognosis is good should be told, but those for whom there is no hope should be denied it.

Barton, D. The need for including instruction on death and dying in the medical curriculum. *Journal of Medical Education*, 1972, *47*(3), 169–175. The author points at the paucity of formal instruction about death in the medical school curriculum. Using excerpts from small group discussions, he illustrates the concern of students regarding personal experiences and professional management of the seriously ill, and thus a need for death education to ensure optimal patient care.

Barton, D., Flexner, J. M., van Eys, J., & Scott, C. E. Death and dying: A course for medical students. *Journal of Medical Education*,

1972, *47*(12), 945–951. The authors present format, content, and goals of a course designed to teach medical students about the psychosocial aspects of life-threatening illness. The course was first offered in the 1971/72 academic year at Vanderbilt University's School of Medicine.

Barton, D. Teaching psychiatry in the context of dying and death. *American Journal of Psychiatry*, 1973, *130*(11), 1290–1291. This article suggests that death and dying education can be of benefit in the psychiatry curriculum, and offers reasons why.

Barton, D., & Crowder, M. K. The use of role playing techniques as an instructional aid in teaching about dying, death, and bereavement. *Omega*, 1975, *6*(3), 243–250. The method of role-playing is described and examples of role-playing vignettes dealing with death-related issues are presented. The authors suggest that role-playing is an effective method of teaching about death.

Beachy, W. N. Assisting the family in time of grief. *JAMA*, 1967, *202*(6), 223–224. A list of 15 do's and don'ts is presented for helping the grieving family and others who suffer.

Benoliel, J. Q. Talking to patients about death. *Nursing Forum*, 1970, *9*(3), 255–263. The author discusses the need for nurses to learn to discuss death with patients and family. This involves confronting one's own feelings and acting upon one's values by working in the best interest of the patient rather than the system.

Benoliel, J. Q. Comment: Some thoughts about the complexities of education for humanistic care in the face of death. *Omega*, 1971, *2*, 215–216. Here the author argues that faculties in health care fields need to come to grips with the issues underlying contemporary professional practice, and to be willing to find ways to help students learn to approach death with sensitivity and human concern rather than to avoid it.

Benoliel, J. Q. Nursing care for the terminal patient: A psychosocial approach. In B. Schoenberg, A. C. Carr, D. Peretz, & A. H. Kutscher (Eds.), *Psychosocial aspects of terminal care.* New York: Columbia University Press, 1972, 145–159. Hospital work is recovery-oriented and terminal care is low status work. Research evidence is cited showing that nurses feel inadequately prepared for the psychosocial matters of nursing care, particularly in dealing with the dying. The author recommends revision in educational preparation and continuing education efforts to shift emphasis from technical-oriented care to person-centered care.

Benoliel, J. Q. Dying in an institution. In H. Wass (Ed.), *Dying: Facing the facts.* Washington, DC: Hemisphere, 1979, pp. 137-157. The organization and structure of the hospital are analyzed in terms of its effectiveness in providing terminal care. The author concludes that contemporary hospitals function on an ethic of saving lives and neglect the caregiving aspects with respect to the dying.

Bergman, A. B. Sudden infant death. *Nursing Outlook*, 1972, *20*, 775-777. This article briefly describes the history and the syndrome, and discusses the effect of sudden infant death on parents.

Bloch, S. A clinical course on death and dying for medical students. *Journal of Medical Education,* 1975, *50,* 630-632. This is a brief description of course format, evaluations, and problems. In addition, the author makes a case for courses on death and dying for medical students.

Bloch, S. Teaching medical students how to care for the dying. *The Medical Journal of Australia,* 1975, *21,* 902-903. Bloch describes an experimental course for medical students that focuses on a personal and intimate relationship between student and terminal patient.

Bloch, S. Instruction on death and dying for the medical student. *Medical Education,* 1976, *10,* 269-273. Here the author outlines nine objectives for death education in medical schools, which have been reported in the literature or seem pertinent. Questions about who should teach, when, and what format could be used are discussed.

Bonine, B. N. Student's reactions to children's death. *American Journal of Nursing,* 1967, *67,* 1439-1440. The author briefly mentions the effect of children's death on nursing students. Several suggestions are made on how to help nursing students cope with their feelings and thereby become more effective.

Browning, M. H., & Lewis, E. P. (Comps.). *The dying patient: A nursing perspective.* New York: The American Journal of Nursing Company, 1972. This useful source book for nurses consists of 37 reprinted articles dealing with the issues of death and dying as they relate to nursing care. Contents are: philosophical and ethical issues; the dying process; care of the dying patient and his family; the grieving process; dynamics and personal experiences; nurses' reactions to death and dying; educating nurses to care for dying patients and their families; death during childhood and adolescence, and alternative styles of dying.

Bunch, B., & Zahra, D. Dealing with death: The unlearned role. *American Journal of Nursing,* 1976, *27*(12), 851-852. In this article the authors argue for the need of new effective role behaviors for nurses in dealing with death. They recommend that death education concern itself with the formation of such behaviors.

Burton, L. (Ed.). *Care of the child facing death.* London: Routledge, Kegan, Paul, 1974. This useful source and reference volume consists of a series of articles that deal with problems facing parents and children when terminal illness is discovered in the children. It offers ideas about how education can help, and discusses the role of grief and the rebuilding of the family after bereavement.

Butler, R. N. The need for quality hospice care, *Death Education,* 1979, *3,* 215-225. This is the author's address to the National Hospice Organization's first meeting, held in Washington, D.C., October 1978. The author reviews the crucial components of hospice care and points at the need on the part of the medical personnel to view each patient as a unique person. He discusses a number of concerns such as the dangers of commercialization and specialization.

Cairns, N. U., & Lansky, S. MMPI indicators of stress and marital discord among parents of children with chronic illness. *Death Education* (in press). In this study it was found that parents of children with life-threatening illness suffered more stress than those with healthy children but less than marriage counselees.

Caldwell, D., & Mishara, B. L. Research on attitudes of medical doctors toward dying patients: A methodological problem. *Omega*, 1972, *3*, 341–346. From a sample of 73 medical doctors, including residents and interns who were available to be interviewed during a one-week period, only 13 consented to an interview. The others refused when told they would be asked about dying patients. The authors concluded that the topic may be more of a problem to physicians than has been recognized.

Carr, A. C. Principles of thanatology. *Archives of the Foundation of Thanatology*, 1978, *7*(2), 96. (Abstract) The author states 12 principles of thanatology and a summary principle which asserts that thanatology is an art and a science. As an art it stresses humanistic approaches to dying and bereavement, and as a science it stresses the need for death education, and systematic investigation and inquiry.

Cassidy, H. Helping the social work student deal with death and dying. In E. R. Prichard, J. Collard, B. A. Orcutt, A. H. Kutscher, I. Seeland, & N. Lefkowitz (Eds.), *Social work with the dying patient and the family*. New York: Columbia University Press, 1977, 313–322. The author describes an interaction with second-year graduate social work students working on the cancer wards and pediatric intensive care unit of a general hospital. Her efforts were intended to assist the students to deal with death and dying through retrospective articulation and integration.

Crase, D. R., & Crase, D. Death and the young child. *Clinical Pediatrics*, 1975, *14*(8), 747–750. This paper offers practical suggestions for pediatricians in helping parents deal with children's questions about death.

Davis, B. . . . Until death ensues. *Nursing Clinics of North America*, 1972, 7, 303–309. This article reports on interviews with nursing home residents, and finds they indicated a need to talk about death and dying. Some suggestions on how to help prepare patients for dying are offered.

Dickinson, G. E. Death education in U.S. medical schools. *Journal of Medical Education*, 1976, *51*(2), 134–136. The author reports results of a survey of 113 medical schools conducted in 1975. A total of 107 questionnaires were returned. Only 7 had a full-term course on death; 44 had a "minicourse," and 42 a lecture or two. Only 71 percent of the schools require that at least half of their students be exposed to any death education.

Drummond, E., & Blumberg, J. Death and the curriculum. *Journal of Nursing Education*, 1962, 21–28. The need for death education in programs for nurses is argued, and some topics for lectures and discussions are suggested.

Dubrey, R. J., & Terrill, L. A. Loneliness of the dying person. *Omega*, 1974, *6*(4), 357-371. This report is based on an interview with terminal hospitalized patients. The conclusion was that patients feel lonely and will talk about their concerns if someone will stay long enough to listen.

Durlak, J. A. Comparison between experimental and didactic methods of death education. *Omega*, 1978-1979, *9*(1), 57-66. The effect of a death workshop on attitudes toward life and death of a heterogeneous group of hospital staff were studied comparing a lecture-small group discussion and experiential (death awareness exercises) methods. Pre-post data were collected and compared with a control group. The experientially taught group showed a significant fear reduction as a result of the workshop whereas the lectured group and the control group changed negatively. The author suggests that a personal, emotional approach is an important component of effective death education.

Durlack, J. A., & Burchard, J. A. Preliminary evaluation of a hospital-based continuing education workshop on death and dying. *Journal of Medical Education*, 1977, *52*(5), 423-424. Described is a continuing education workshop on death for 19 health professionals including tentative results of a program evaluation.

Easson, W. M. *The dying child: The management of the child or adolescent who is dying.* Springfield, IL: Thomas, 1970. Easson considers the child with a prolonged period of dying in terms of developmental stages of the understanding of death, the effects of hospitalization, physiological reactions, symptoms of the disease, changing role relationships, fantasy, and religious factors. The adjustment of the family of the dying child is discussed as well as the role of health care personnel in assisting the family. Throughout the book the need for an atmosphere of love and caring for the dying child is stressed. This is useful reference, particularly for health professionals.

Easson, W. M. The family of the dying child. *Pediatric Clinics of North America*, 1972, *19*(4), 1157-1165. The author, a pediatrician, urges his colleagues to give special attention to a dying child and to work closely with the child as well as the family and provide a bereavement follow-up. Pediatricians have to work through their own grief over the loss of their young patients.

Epley, R. J., & McCaghy, C. H. The stigma of dying: Attitudes toward the terminally ill. *Omega*, 1977-1978, *8*(4), 379-393. The authors found that the dying are viewed in more negative terms than are the healthy or the merely ill. The negative attitudes indicate that the terminally ill are stigmatized.

Evans, A. E., & Edin, S. If a child must die. *The New England Journal of Medicine*, 1968, *278*(3), 138-142. The authors describe how pediatricians can help provide support for the dying child and the family, using the concept of "total care" and involving the entire health care team.

Folck, M. M., & Nie, P. J. Nursing students learn to face death. *Nursing Outlook*, 1959, 7, 510-513. This article suggests incorporating sociological, psychiatric, and religious aspects of death early into nursing students' curriculum, contending that this facilitates working with dying patients and their families.

Furman, R. A. The child's reaction to death in the family. In B. Schoenberg, A. C. Carr, D. Peretz, & A. H. Kutscher (Eds.), *Loss and grief: Psychological management in medical practice.* New York: Columbia University Press, 1970, 70-86. Pediatricians and family physicians are urged to assist parents in educating their small children about death. The article is illustrated with anecdotal material.

Garfield, C. A. The impact of death on the health-care professional. In H. Feifel (Ed.), *New meaning of death.* New York: McGraw-Hill, 1977, 144-151. Through a personal case history of an encounter with a dying patient the author demonstrates the powerful effect of this experience.

Goldfogel, L. Working with the parents of a dying child. *Journal of American Nursing*, 1970, 70, 8, 1676-1679. In assisting the mother during the eight weeks her child was dying, the author was able to assess the mother's various forms of coping behavior and to provide reassurance and support when most needed. The author admits to having had personal difficulties with negative feelings toward death.

Goldstein, E. C. Teaching a social work perspective on the dying patient and his family. In E. R. Prichard, J. Collard, B. A. Orcutt, A. H. Kutscher, I. Seeland, & N. Lefkowitz (Eds.), *Social work with the dying patient and the family.* New York: Columbia University Press, 1977, 301-312. A psychiatric social worker offers a teaching perspective involving a value base, knowledge, and skill components, for teaching a section on death and dying as part of a course on human behavior and the social environment to social work students at the master's level.

Gosselin, J. V., Perez, E. L., & Gagnon, A. Attitudes of psychiatrists toward terminally ill patients. *Psychiatric Journal of the University of Ottawa*, 1977, 2(3), 120-123. The article reports a survey of psychiatrists in Ottawa and Northern Ontario concerning their attitudes toward the terminally ill.

Gramlich, E. P. Recognition and managements of grief in elderly patients, *Geriatrics*, 1968, 23, 87-92. The author urges physicians to view grief as a psychosomatic reaction and to be alert for it especially in elderly patients. Treatment is outlined which prevents grieving from becoming more disabling, or even fatal.

Griffith, W. H. *Confronting death.* Valley Forge, PA: Judson, 1977. The roles of the Christian clergy, physician, lawyer, and funeral director are described from the point of view of a Baptist minister. The book includes case studies, discussion questions and resource suggestions.

Gyulay, J. *The dying child.* New York: McGraw-Hill, 1978. Written for nurses, this 192 page volume treats in a superficial way a large number of subjects from dying children, parents, siblings, significant others, the nursing process to the various phases of dying including the postdeath period.

Hankoff, L. D. Adolescence and the crisis of dying. *Adolescence,* 1975, *10,* 373–389. This article explores the complex processes of adolescence, and their relationship to death and dying. It suggests that the adolescent experience will determine the psychological reaction to dying.

Hopping, B. L. Nursing students' attitudes toward death. *Nursing Research,* 1977, *26*(6), 443–447. Examined are the effects upon their attitudes toward death of nursing students' participation in a clinical course on nursing care of adult patients with malignant neoplastic disease. No significant differences were found between students in this course and a comparable control group.

Howard, E. The effect of work experience in a nursing home on attitudes toward death held by nurses' aides. *The Gerontologist,* 1974, *14*(1), 54–56. It was found that those with the longest work experience were least willing to discuss death with a resident, were less often in favor of telling a resident or friend about impending death, and were less in favor of euthanasia. Work experience increased death avoidance. The author recommends attitude training.

Jaffe, L. The dying professor as death educator. In E. R. Prichard, J. Collard, B. A. Orcutt, A. H. Kutscher, I. Seeland, & N. Lefkowitz (Eds.), *Social work with the dying patient and the family.* New York: Columbia University Press, 1977, 323–344. This article describes the personal odyssey of a dying (now dead) social work professor who sought to provide an intensive thinking and feeling classroom experience in death education for students of various helping professions, utilizing both didactic and experiential learning.

Jaffe, L. Letter to seminar students in "methods of intervention with the dying." *Death Education,* 1977, *1*(3), 325–337. This moving letter was written by Lois Jaffe to her social work students in a death seminar during remission from acute myelogenous leukemia.

Karon, M., & Vernick, J. An approach to the emotional support of fatally ill children. *Clinical Pediatrics,* 1968, *7*(5), 274–280. A program of open discussion about the children's terminality and a close doctor-child relationship on a cancer ward is discussed. None of the 51 children involved had significant adjustment problems. Freed from the energies required for keeping "the secret," the staff could devote themselves more fully to their dying patients' care.

Kliman, G. The child faces his own death. In A. H. Kutscher (Ed.), *Death and bereavement.* Springfield, IL: Thomas, 1969, 20–27. It is suggested that terminal children frequently have an emotional maturity far beyond their years, know long before they are told that they are dying, often shield those around them, and face death with acceptance and serenity.

Kopel, K., O'Connell, W. E., & Paris, J. A didactic experimental death and dying lab. *Newsletter for Research in Mental Health and Behavioral Sciences*, 1973, *15*, 1-2. This article briefly describes a human relations laboratory on death which uses a team approach including nurses, nursing students, and social workers. The laboratory was at the V.A. hospital in Houston, Texas.

Kopel, K., O'Connell, W., Paris, J., & Girardin, P. A human relations laboratory approach to death and dying. *Omega*, 1975, *6*(3), 219-222. Here the authors describe a 1-day laboratory experience focusing on death and dying. The lab consisted of four exercises which are described.

Krant, M. J. *Dying and Dignity.* Springfield, IL: Thomas, 1974. In this book the author includes discussion on helping the families of dying children and offers some proposals for death education.

Krant, M. J., & Sheldon, A. The dying patient: Medicine's responsibility. *Journal of Thanatology*, 1971, *1*(1), 1-24. The authors discuss in detail the role of the health professional with respect to dying patients. Among the conclusions are: 1. Education for terminal care should become part of the curriculum in medical and nursing schools. 2. Interprofessional training and discussion should become a regular part of hospital functions. 3. Physicians and nurses should recognize their important role in terminal care. 4. The aim of terminal care should be pain and symptom control.

Krieger, S. R. Death orientation and the specialty choice and training of physicians. Unpublished doctoral dissertation, University of Florida, 1975. Following up on the previously reported high fear of death among physicians, the author compared the death orientations of 243 medical and law students. He found that medical students did not have more negative death orientations than law students. However, general practitioners tended to be lower on a measure of death threat than other physicians.

Kübler-Ross, E., & Worden, J. W. Attitudes and experiences of death workshop attendees. *Omega*, 1977-1978, *8*(2), 91-106. Attendees of workshops and lectures on death completed questionnaires concerning personal experiences with death, conceptualization of death, anticipated reactions to death, and other aspects. Significant differences with respect to age, sex, religion, and profession are reported.

LaGrand, L. E. Reducing burnout in hospice and the death education movement. Accepted for publication in *Death Education*. The author proposes four techniques for reducing stress and burnout in the helping professions and the death movement.

Lascari, A. D., & Stehbens, J. A. The reactions of families to childhood leukemia. *Clinical Pediatrics*, 1973, *12*(4), 210-214. This is a report of parents' reactions to a program of emotional support that was based on candid and frank information given to parents and child. The authors give an estimate of survival. Parents were positive about this approach, reported few prolonged grieving reactions and few problems with siblings.

Lasagna, L. The doctor and the dying patient. *Journal of Chronic Disease*, 1969, *22*, 65-68. The author points at a common tendency for medical staff to label patients as "good" or "troublesome" and treat them accordingly. Similarly, the "social worth" of patients affects the manner of treatment. The author raises the issues of openness, patients' rights, emotional strain, and the need for a scientific approach to study and dealing with these problems.

Laube, J. Death and dying workshop for nurses: its effect on their death anxiety level. *International Journal of Nursing Studies*, 1977, *14*, 111-120. No significant change in level of death anxiety was found immediately following the death and dying workshop, but a significant decrease was discovered one month later. Additional testing three months later showed that the death anxiety means remained below the pre-workshop level.

LeShan, L. *You can fight for your life: Emotional factors in the causation of cancer.* New York: Evans, 1977. This book offers insights into the influence that emotions are viewed as having in developing cancer. LeShan describes therapeutic approaches to the treatment of cancer patients. This book should be of interest to many.

Lester, D., Getty, C., & Kneisl, C. R. Attitudes of nursing students and nursing faculty toward death. *Nursing Research*, 1974, *23*(1), 50-53. In their study the authors found that fears of death and dying decreased with increased education. Fears of death were not found to be related to choice of clinical specialization.

Lewis, F. M. A time to live and a time to die: An instructional drama. *Nursing Outlook*, 1977, *25*(12), 762-765. The author recounts attempts to deal with the affective dimensions of death in her instruction for nursing students. She developed a dramatic play and suggests ways of using such drama as an instructional device to help health care personnel cope with dying patients' needs.

Lipton, J., & Kutscher, A. H. Student emotional responses to teaching cancer training by a psychological, psychiatric-psychosocial motivational approach. In A. H. Kutscher, & I. K. Goldberg (Eds.), *Oral care of the aging and dying patient.* Springfield, IL: Thomas, 1973, 192-198. A survey of dental students showed that they were able to accept a new psychosocial approach to the care of terminal cancer patients. For most it was the first personal confrontation with terminal patients and stimulated personal evaluation of feelings.

Liston, E. H. Education of death and dying: A survey of American medical schools. *Journal of Medical Education*, 1973, *48*, 577-578. Of 83 responding medical schools, 42 reported that they had no formal educational program on the dying patient. Twelve indicated the subject was dealt with informally, and eight planned a course. The author concludes that death education is probably increasing in medical schools.

Liston, E. H. Education on death and dying: A neglected area in the medical curriculum. *Omega*, 1975, *6*(3), 193-198. The author contends that there is little instruction about psychosocial aspects of life-threatening illness in the medical curriculum. He favors structured courses over informal instruction, and suggests the need for improved communication among death educators.

Livingston, P. B., & Zimet, C. N. Death anxiety, authoritarianism and choice of specialty in medical students. *Journal of Nervous and Mental Disease*, 1965, *140*(3), 222–230. It was found that future surgeons, internists, and pediatricians are significantly more authoritarian than psychiatrists. Surgeons-to-be are less anxious about death than future internists who, in turn, are less anxious than pediatricians. Potential psychiatrists were lower on authoritarianisms and higher on death anxiety when compared to the other three specialties.

Lourie, R. S. The pediatrician and the handling of terminal illness. *Pediatrics*, 1963, *32*, 477–479. In this article the author comments on pediatricians' lack of preparation for handling terminal children and their parents. Literature on grief that may be of help is reviewed.

Martin, L. B., & Collier, P. A. Attitudes toward death: A survey of nursing students. *Journal of Nursing Education*, 1975, *14*(1), 28–35. Results of a 2-year survey of nursing students in a baccalaureate program are presented, including changes in attitude toward death as a result of a death education program.

McGrory, A. *A well model approach to care of the dying client.* New York: McGraw-Hill, 1978, 146–165. Guidelines are offered for a nursing curriculum that is based on the author's philosophy of a "well model" and person-to-person approach to terminal care in which integration and a multidisciplinary model are proposed. Course topics, rationale, methods, and suggested readings are included. Excellent for a nursing instructor seeking specific guidance.

Miller, L. B., & Erwin, E. A study of attitudes and anxiety in medical students. *Journal of Medical Education*, 1959, *34*, 1089–1092. The authors compared sophomore and senior medical students on cynicism, humanitarianism, anxiety, and academic success. There was no significant difference between seniors and sophomores; the highly anxious were also the most cynical. Academic success and anxiety were positively correlated.

Miller, R. S. Teaching death and dying content in the social work curriculum. In E. R. Prichard, J. Collard, B. A. Orcutt, A. H. Kutscher, I. Seeland, & N. Lefkowitz (Eds.), *Social work with the dying patient and the family.* New York: Columbia University Press, 1977, 289–300. The author describes her efforts to introduce death and dying content into a required casework or practice course for first-semester social work students. The emphasis is on the interaction between teacher and student.

Morissey, J. R. Children's adaptation to fatal illness. *Social Work*, 1963, *8*, 81–88. This is a report of a study of death anxiety in terminal children. Some findings are: Half the children, except the very young, had considerable anxiety; children expressed anxiety in different ways; parent participation is helpful; about one third speculated on the significance of their illness.

Mount, B. M., Jones, A., & Patterson, A. Death and dying: Attitudes in a teaching hospital. *Urology*, 1974, *4*(6), 741–747. A survey of the medical and paramedical staff of a general hospital and critically ill patients on attitudes toward death showed that patients want complete openness and honesty, while physicians are reluctant, residents relatively unconcerned, and social workers tend to minimize the problem. The major sources of emotional support for the terminal patients were the family.

Murray, P. Death education and its effects on the death anxiety levels of nurses. *Psychological Reports*, 1974, *35*, 1250. Using Templer's Death Anxiety Scale the author found no significant decrease in death anxiety immediately following the 6-week course but discovered a significant decrease on a post-post test four weeks later.

Nash, M. L., Connors, C., & Gemperle, R. Toward dignity in care: An in-service model. *Death Education*, 1977, *1*(1), 113–130. The authors describe a short-term, in-service training program to assist hospital personnel, including physicians, nurses, nurse's aides, nurse supervisors, social workers, and chaplains to become more sensitive to patients' need for dignity.

O'Connell, W. E., Kopel, K., Paris, J., Girardin, P., & Batsel, W. Thanatology for everyone: Developmental labs and workshops. *Death Education*, 1977, *1*(3), 305–313. This article describes laboratories and workshops on death for nurses in a hospital setting, with the long-term goal of adapting them for death education for the general public.

Oken, D. What to tell cancer patients: A study of medical attitudes. *Journal of the American Medical Association*, 1961, *175*, 1120–1128. This survey of 219 physicians' policies about truth-telling showed that 90 percent of the sample indicated a preference for not telling cancer patients the truth about their illness. No relationship was found between policy and age or experience.

Olin, H. S. A proposed model to teach medical students the care of the dying patient. *Journal of Medical Education*, 1972, *47*, 564–567. It is reported that few medical schools deal adequately with the subject. The author offers a model that would teach medical students about the psychology of death.

Padilla, G. V., Baker, V. E., & Dolan, V. A. *Interacting with patients: An inter-hospital nursing research and nursing education project.* Duarte, CA: City of Hope National Medical Center, 1975. The authors describe carefully and in detail an educational program for nurses who provide terminal care, and present their evaluation of its effectiveness. Useful training materials are included.

Pollack, B. R. A challenge to dental education: Caring for the bereaved and dying. In A. H. Kutscher, & I. K. Goldberg (Eds.), *Oral care of the aging and dying patient.* Springfield, IL: Thomas, 1973, 171–175. This article provides a rationale for including terminal patients as a target group and for adjustments in the curriculum to help the dental practitioner deal with the dying or bereaved client.

Quint, J. C. Obstacles to helping the dying. *American Journal of Nursing*, 1966, *66*, 157-158. The author discusses situations, and patient behavior that is troublesome for health care personnel and that may prevent effective care during the patients' terminal phase.

Quint, J. C. Preparing nurses to care for the fatally ill. *International Journal of Nursing Studies*, 1968, *5*, 53-61. Here the author contends that training nurses to care for the dying is a difficult educational problem. Quint gives reasons for this view, and makes a number of carefully considered recommendations to bring about change.

Quint, J. C., & Strauss, A. L. Nursing students, assignments, and dying patients. *Nursing Outlook*, 1964, *12*, 24-27. The authors report that nursing students have little or no instruction about death, that patient assignments are made on the basis of disease and encounters with death are therefore a matter of chance rather than plan, and that student nurses, although encouraged to talk with terminal patients, are rarely made accountable. The authors caution nursing faculty to give considerable thought and planning to the important but sensitive area of death education.

Rea, M. P., Greenspoon, G., & Spilka, B. Physicians and the terminal patient: Some selected attitudes and behavior. *Omega*, 1975, *6*(4), 291-302. Based on a survey of 151 physicians in 10 medical specialties, the authors conclude that most physicians feel that the patient must be told about terminal illness regardless of physical status, age, and life expectancy, and that few drugs are employed to ease the pain. There is strong opposition to the use of heroic measures. Older physicians are most negative to offering prognosis, and physicians do not perceive terminality as personal failure.

Robinson, L. We have no dying patients. *Nursing Outlook*, 1974, *22*(10), 651-563. A 14-week death course for nursing students, including a relationship with a terminal patient is described. Over 96 percent of the class reported their experience with a dying patient as the most beneficial aspect of the course. Students no longer avoided patients and responded more spontaneously to them.

Schnell, R. Helping parents cope with the dying child with a genetic disorder. *Journal of Clinical Child Psychology*, 1974, *3*(2), 34-35. The author relates experiences, problems, and approaches taken in helping families with children who suffer from Hurler's syndrome, inborn errors of metabolism. Schnell stresses the need for several sessions to help parents understand the course of the disease, to help with their feelings and their tendency toward overprotection.

Schoenberg, B. The nurse's education for death. In A. H. Kutscher, (Ed.), *Death and bereavement.* 1969, Springfield, IL: Thomas, 55-74. This paper discusses factors during training and practice which largely determine how the nurse copes with a terminal patient. Two case histories are included.

Schoenberg, B., & Carr, A. C. Educating the health professional in the psychosocial care of the terminally ill. In B. Schoenberg, Carr, A. C., Peretz, D., & Kutscher, A. H. (Eds.), *Psychosocial aspects of terminal care.* New York: Columbia University Press, 1972, 3-17. The authors state that inadequate education in the care of the terminally ill by health professionals is the greatest failure of professional education. They provide supporting evidence for their charge from results of surveys conducted by the Foundation of Thanatology of departments of medicine, surgery, pediatrics, psychiatry, and schools of nursing.

Schoenberg, B., Carr, A. C., Peretz, D., & Kutscher, A. H. (Eds.), *Loss and grief: Psychological management in medical practice.* New York: Columbia University, 1970. The work of 24 contributors appears in this book, which includes a selected annotated bibliography on grief. The emphasis is on psychological management of patient and family with serious loss. Contents are: Psychological concept central to loss and grief; Loss and grief in childhood; Reaction to and management of partial loss; The dying patient; Humanistic and biological concepts regarding loss and grief.

Schulz, R., & Aderman, D. How the medical staff copes with dying patients: A critical review. *Omega,* 1976, 7(1), 11-21. A comprehensive review of the literature suggests that medical practitioners associate dying patients with failure and tend to avoid them. The authors recommend that psychosocial aspects of medical practice become an important part of the medical curriculum.

Simpson, M. A. Teaching about death and dying. *Nursing Times,* April 1973, *69,* 442-443. The author discusses the need for death education for nurses and medical students, describes a teaching seminar, and reports student support for his seminar.

Simpson, M. A. Teaching about death and dying: An interdisciplinary approach. In R. W. Raven (Ed.), *The dying patient.* London: Pitman Medical, 1975, 92-105. The need for death education for professional and preprofessional students in medicine, nursing, social work, and the ministry is argued. The author describes the conduct of such an interdisciplinary course at McMaster University in Canada.

Simpson, M. A. The do-it-yourself death certificate in evoking and estimating student attitudes toward death. *Journal of Medical Education,* 1975, *50,* 475-478. It is suggested that giving students death certificates inscribed with their names and asking them to complete the certificates is an effective technique for removing emotional distance and giving students a sense of the reality of personal death.

Singher, L. J. The slowly dying child. *Clinical Pediatrics,* 1974, *13*(10), 861-867. A pediatrician urges his colleagues to discuss the prognosis of fatally ill children with their parents, and offers a number of practical suggestions.

Snyder, M., Gertler, R., & Ferneau, E. Changes in nursing students' attitudes toward death and dying—A measurement of curriculum effectiveness. *International Journal of Social Psychiatry*, 1973, *19*, 294–298. First-year curriculum experiences that are found most useful for beginning nursing students in dealing with their fears of failure and their death anxiety are described. The authors recommend consistent presentation of death-related content in the curriculum.

Spinetta, J. J., & Maloney, L. J. Death anxiety in the outpatient leukemic child. *Pediatrics*, 1975, *56*(6), 1034–1037. It is suggested that the leukemic outpatient children in remission display a high level of awareness of the seriousness of their illness and much anxiety. Children need help in coping not only when treated in the hospital, but also when living at home and treated in outpatient clinics.

Spinetta, J. J., Rigler, D., & Karon, M. Anxiety in the dying child. *Pediatrics*, 1973, *52*(6), 841–845. Twenty-five leukemic children aged 6–10 showed significantly more preoccupation with threat to their body integrity and functioning than did a control group with nonfatal chronic illness. The authors conclude that young fatally ill children may understand that they are going to die before they are able to say so in adult terms.

Stillion, J., & Wass, H. Children and death. In H. Wass (Ed.), *Dying: Facing the facts*. Washington, DC: Hemisphere, 1979, 208–235. This chapter includes a discussion on caring for terminally ill children, helping their parents deal with emotions of anxiety, anger, and guilt. (See also pages 90–91.)

Thrush, J. C., Paulus, G. S., & Thrush, P. I. The availability of education on death and dying: A survey of U.S. nursing schools. *Death Education*, 1979, *3*(2), 131–142. This national survey shows that only a small proportion of the nursing schools surveyed require formal instruction on death and dying. An additionally small number of schools offer elective courses in which only a few nursing students enroll.

Vachon, M. L. S., Lyall, A. L., & Freeman, S. J. J. Measurement and management of stress in health professionals working with advanced cancer patients. *Death Education*, 1978, *1*(4), 365–375. This paper reports preliminary results of studies on staff stress in two cancer centers. It describes discussion sessions held to facilitate inter-staff communications and communication with patients, and includes a discussion of stress among physicians.

Vernick, J., & Karon, M. Who's afraid of death on a leukemia ward? *American Journal of Diseases of Children*, 1965, *109*, 393–397. The authors describe a program that provides an atmosphere of freedom on the part of the terminal children to express their concerns, and open and honest answers on the part of the medical staff. As a result, withdrawal and depression occurred very infrequently.

Verwoerdt, A., & Wilson, R. Communication with fatally ill patients: Tacit or explicit? *American Journal of Nursing*, 1967, *67*, 2307–2309. The authors suggest that some patients do not wish to voice their anxiety about death and that nurses should learn to recognize when a patient wants to be explicit or tacit about his or her impending death.

Waechter, E. H. Children's awareness of fatal illness. *American Journal of Nursing*, 1971, *71*(6), 1168-1172. Terminal children aged 6-10 showed up twice as high in death anxiety as a control group. It is suggested that "protection" by adult silence may cause these children not to express their death awareness and fears, but given the opportunity they will, and as a result they feel less lonely and isolated.

Wagner, B. M. Teaching students to work with the dying. *American Journal of Nursing*, 1964, *64*, 128-131. Rationale, content, and methodology for death education for nursing students are discussed, and a death education program carried out at the University of Kansas is evaluated.

Wallace, E., & Townes, B. D. The dual role of comforter and bereaved. *Mental Hygiene*, 1969, *53*(3), 327-332. The authors suggest that medical personnel follow the same triphasic pattern of anticipatory mourning as do parents of a dying child. The article is illustrated with case histories. The conclusion is that it is difficult to be bereaved and to provide comfort at the same time.

Watson, J. M. Death: A necessary concern for nurses. *Nursing Outlook*, 1968, *16*, 47-48. This paper describes a seminar on death and dying offered as part of an integrated course for junior nursing students in medical-surgical and pediatric nursing.

Wiener, J. M. Response of medical personnel to the fatal illness of a child. In B. Schoenberg, A. C. Carr, D. Peretz, & A. H. Kutscher (Eds.), *Loss and grief: Psychological management in medical practice.* New York: Columbia University Press, 1970, 102-115. Results of a survey of 97 pediatricians concerning attitudes and practices of "telling" are presented. The majority felt that terminal children should be informed of the diagnosis only when they ask, and should not be informed of their prognosis. One out of five respondents said parents should "usually" be told their terminal child's diagnosis and only 64 percent of those in practice under 10 years felt parents should be given accurate prognosis upon request.

Wiener, J. M. Reaction of the family to the fatal illness of a child. In B. Schoenberg, A. C. Carr, D. Peretz, & A. H. Kutscher (Eds.), *Loss and grief: Psychological management in medical practice.* New York: Columbia University Press, 1970, 87-101. Physicians are urged to tell parents of their child's terminal illness and to assist them in coping, in helping the child, and the siblings. Included in this article are a number of suggestions about how other health care personnel can be of help.

Williams, H. On a teaching hospital's responsibility to counsel parents concerning their child's death. *Medical Journal of Australia*, 1963, *2*(16), 643-645. Since family physicians are infrequently in charge of seriously ill children, the author feels that the staff of the teaching hospital should adopt the role of personal adviser to parents, and that the hospital institution has a responsibility in helping/counseling the individual.

Wise, D. J. Learning about dying. *Nursing Outlook*, 1974, *22*, 42–44. The author describes a unit on the dying patient for nursing students involving theory and clinical application. Evaluation 2–24 months following the unit showed that 90 percent of the nurses in the unit improved their care of the dying and their own acceptance of death.

Yeaworth, R. C., Kapp, F. T., & Winget, C. Attitudes of nursing students toward the dying patient. *Nursing Research*, 1974, *23*(1), 20-24. This study found senior nursing students to be more open, flexible, and accepting of feeling relative to dying patients than freshmen, and suggested that these differences are due to the influence of the nursing curriculum.

DEATH EDUCATION FOR ADULTS

Aynes, E. A. Education for old age and death. *Archives of the Foundation of Thanatology*, 1978, 7(2), 77. (Abstract) It is recommended that death education begin in youth, but it should occur in the later years if it has not before. It should consist of helping the elderly to accept the inevitable. Concurrently, family and friends should be taught.

Bernstein, B. E. Death and the law. In H. Wass (Ed.), *Dying: Facing the facts*. Washington, DC: Hemisphere, 1979, 282–316. A valuable, practical guide concerning legal matters that affect the dying and the living. The importance of a last will and testament is discussed, as well as the advantage of having a comprehensive estate plan, laws concerning the body, power of attorney, and related matters.

Bertman, S. L. Death education in the face of a taboo. In E. A. Grollman (Ed.), *Concerning death: A practical guide for living*. Boston, Beacon, 1974, 333-361. Deals with questions when should death education begin? What should teachers and parents do and say? and what about parent education in the community?

Bertman, S. L. Workshops in caring: A first module. *Death Education*, 1979, *3*(3), 271-281. The author describes objectives, method, and results of an in-service program designed to sensitize nursing home staff to attitudes, biases, and concerns toward aging, illness, and death.

Bureau of Consumer Protection, Federal Trade Commission. *Funeral industry practices* (Final Staff Report). Washington, DC, June 1978. This report is based on an investigation and analysis of a 45,000-page record of public hearings and written comments on funeral industry practices, funeral director education, and activities of the trade associations. Recommended trade regulations that would eliminate various unfair, deceptive, and illegal practices are described.

Colton, A. E., Gearhart, D. E., & Janaro, R. P. A faculty workshop on death attitudes and life affirmation. *Omega*, 1973, *4*(1), 51–55. The authors report on a faculty workshop on death and life attitudes held at a community college. Included are a list of life-denying characteristics of college teachers, a set of objectives, some strategies, and evaluation. Of the fifty participants 92 percent said they would recommend such a workshop to other colleagues.

Death: The last taboo. *Time Educational Program*, The Classroom Service of Time. A 14-page thanatology unit written by a Time education program staff member offers brief articles on historical and contemporary perspectives on death rituals, discussion questions, a course outline, and an interview with students.

Everett, M. G. Helping parents teach about death. *Health Education*, 1976, 27–29. A lecture/discussion model for telling parents about children and death is presented.

Farmer, J. A. Death education: Adult education in the face of a taboo. *Omega*, 1970, *1*(2), 109–113. This paper describes a death education program for adults consisting of five two-hour sessions. It reports the extent of participation and feedback.

Feifel, H. Religious conviction and fear of death among the elderly and the terminally ill. In R. Fulton (Ed.), *Death and identity*. Bowie, MD: The Charles Press, 1976, 120–130. The author found that religious belief was not significantly associated with strength of the fear of death. Healthy and terminally ill subjects had a co-existing acceptance-avoidance equilibrium toward fear of death.

Glicken, M. D. The child's view of death. *Journal of Marriage and Family Counseling*, 1978, *4*(2), 75–81. See page 47.

Grollman, E. A. *Talking about death.* Boston: Beacon, 1970. This very helpful pamphlet is written for parents to read to small children in a low-keyed manner. It speaks openly, honestly, and directly about death and dying. It includes a parent guide and excellent illustrations by Gisela Héau.

Grollman, E. A. *Talking about death* (New Ed.). Boston: Beacon, 1976. This volume includes a more extensive parent's guide than the 1970 edition, and a bibliography of children's books about death and other resource material. It should be very helpful to parents.

Hardgrove, C., & Warrick, L. How shall we tell the children. *American Journal of Nursing*, 1974, *74*(3), 448–450. The authors present a model for parents to use in telling their children that an expected baby has died.

Harris, A. P. Content and method in a thanatology training program for paraprofessionals. *Death Education*, (in press). A death training program for paraprofessionals in a university teaching hospital is described including objectives, content, organization, and resource materials. Useful particularly for those who wish to develop such training for paraprofessionals.

Jackson, E. N. *Telling a child about death.* New York: Hawthorn Books, Inc., 1965. This is a practical guide for parents to help them know when, how, and why to talk about death with children, and what to say. It includes a discussion of the nature and treatment of children's grief and should be very helpful to parents.

Jackson, E. N. *When someone dies.* Philadelphia: Fortress, 1971. This short booklet written from the Christian viewpoint aims to help the reader who is bereaved. The language is nontechnical. In this context, this is a very useful resource.

Jackson, E. N. Helping children cope with death. In A. H. Kutscher, & L. G. Kutscher (Eds.), *Religion and bereavement.* New York: Health Sciences Publishing Corporation, 1972, 161-164. Practical suggestions are offered about how to deal with children's questions about death in a Christian context.

Jackson, E. N. Bereavement and grief: In H. Wass (Ed.), *Dying: Facing the facts.* Washington, DC: Hemisphere, 1979, 256-281. The nature of the grief experience and its impact and manifestations on the bereaved person are discussed and resources for managing grief. Grief research is critically reviewed and current problems in grief therapy are outlined.

Kalish, R. A., & Reynolds, D. K. The role of age in death attitudes. *Death Education,* 1977, *1*(2), 205-230. This paper reports on one-hour interviews on death, dying, and bereavement of 434 adults equally divided among four ethnic groups, men and women, and three age categories. The role of age was found to be particularly important.

Kastenbaum, R., & Koenig, R. Dying, death, and lethal behavior: An experience in community education. *Omega,* 1970, *1*, 29-36. The development of a death course at Wayne State University's Center for Adult Education is described including the characteristics of the students who enrolled. The authors suggest that such a course has potential as part of community education programs.

Krupp, G. R. Children feel about death. *Parents' Magazine,* 1967, *42*, pp. 55; 89-91. The author reviews some studies that point to the importance of open talk about death with children, and free expression of grief.

Levinson, B. M. The pet and the child's bereavement. *Mental Hygiene,* 1967, *51*, 197-200. It is suggested that the death of a pet may provide valuable preparation for greater losses. When a parent dies, a pet may serve as a crutch that helps fill the void temporarily.

Lichtenwalner, M. E. Children ask about death. *International Journal of Religious Education,* 1964, *40*, 14-16. The author lists a series of questions that children may ask about death, and answers Christian parents should provide.

Lohman, K. D. The student mortician: A survey of occupational socialization. *Colorado Journal of Educational Research,* 1970, *9*, 45-50. In this study of a mortuary school curriculum it was found that, contrary to claims by the trade associations, faculty does not encourage the development of a professional identity and that students see themselves primarily as business entrepreneurs.

Marshall, V. Socialization for impending death in a retirement village. *American Journal of Sociology*, 1975, *80*, 1124-1144. This paper argues that congregate living facilities for the elderly can provide adequate settings for the preparation for death. The author suggests that we can learn from the residents about the conditions favorable for such socialization. Illustrations from a particular retirement village are used.

Maurer, A. Intimations of mortality. *Journal of Clinical Child Psychology*, 1974, *3*(2), 14-17. The author records a conversation between the author and co-op nursery school mothers about how to cope with childrens' questions about death.

Miller, P. G., & Ozga, J. "Mommy, what happens when I die?" *Mental Health*, 1973, *57*, 20. The authors advise parents on what to say and what not to say to their children. Honesty is stressed.

Morgan, E. *A manual of death education and simple burial.* Burnsville, NC: The Celo Press, 1977. This informative pamphlet discusses practical aspects of the topic in a concise manner. It consists of four parts: death education; simple burial and cremation; memorial societies; and how the dead can help the living. Bibliographic and other material is included.

Neale, R. E. Explorations in death education. *Pastoral Psychology*, 1971, *22*, 33-74. This essay is intended for use by clergy who want to explore death with lay persons. It includes description of content and procedures for sessions on denial, fear, grief, belief, and martyrdom.

Nilsen, A. P. Death and dying: Facts, fiction, folklore. *English Journal*, 1973, *62*, 1187-1189. This is an annotated bibliography of contemporary books on death for young adults and their elders. It contains 15 listings.

Ordal, C. C. Treatment of death in selected child care books. *Death Education*, 1979, *3*(2), 121-130. The author reports on an examination of 20 child care books with respect to the presence or absence of information that is potentially helpful to children in coping with death.

Pearlman, J., Stotsky, B. A., & Dominick, J. R. Attitudes toward death among nursing home personnel. *Journal of Genetic Psychology*, 1969, *114*, 63-75. It was found that nursing home personnel avoid discussing dying with a terminal patient. Seventy-three percent of the group reported they did not think of a departed patient for very long.

Peniston, D. H. The importance of death education in family life. *Family Life Coordinator*, 1962, *11*, 15-18. The author points at the importance of open discussion of death with young children, particularly after a death experience within the family.

Pope, B. A., & Raymond, F. B. Dealing with the crisis of death by resolving the crisis of life. *Archives of the Foundation of Thanatology*, 1978, *7*(2), 51. (Abstract) It is suggested that the most feasible way to help the elderly dying patient is to assist him or her in resolving crises of old age in accordance with Erikson's theoretical formulations of these crises.

Rosenthal, N. R. Teaching educators to deal with death. *Death Education*, 1978, *2*(3), 293–306. This article contains a description of a seminar on death conducted for teachers and school counselors. Goals, content, and procedures are outlined. Participants' self-evaluations were positive.

Rudolph, M. The saddest day of my life. *Death Education*, 1978, *2*(3), 281–291. The author argues in straightforward language for the young child's need to be included when a death has occurred in the family, and says that adults need to be attentive to the child's questions and responsive to their feelings.

Rudolph, M. *Should the children know? Encounters with death in the lives of children.* New York: Schocken, 1978. Authored by a seasoned and sensitive educator and writer, this book is based on the sudden death of a 4-year-old girl in the author's nursery school, and the ensuing discussion with the parents. Rudolph shows that very young children can be taught about death at home, at school, directly through a death experience, and vicariously through books.

Samp, R. J., & Curreri, A. R. A questionnaire survey of public cancer education. Obtained from cancer patients and their families. *Cancer*, 1957, *10*, 382–384. Results of a survey of 560 individuals on issues concerning cancer and cancer education are reported. Among the findings are: the majority of the respondents felt that public cancer education aids in earlier diagnosis, lessens fear, and helps save lives, but is not reaching enough people.

Scott, F. G., & Brewer, R. M. (Eds.). *Confrontations of death: A book of readings and a suggested method of instruction.* Corvallis, OR: Continuing Education Publications, 1971. This is a collection of reprinted materials for use in a seminar on death and dying. Literary and analytic pieces are included. There is a course outline in the appendix.

Skelskie, B. An exploratory study of grief in old age. *Smith College Studies in Social Work*, 1975, *45*(2), 158–182. The author describes the grief process in eight elderly subjects who had lost a spouse by death within the preceding three years. It was found that grief in old age lasted longer and tended to be expressed in somatic symptomatology, as well as psychological pain.

Tars, S. E. Death education for the elderly: Facing the inevitable. *Archives of the Foundation of Thanatology*, 1978, *7*(2), 172. (Abstract) From the viewpoint of preventive mental health, the author points at a number of areas in which death education for the elderly and their significant others may be beneficial.

Thorson, J. A. Continuing education in death and dying. *Adult Leadership*, 1974, *23*, 141-144. A continuing education community course on death and dying is described.

Trend Analysis Program (TAP) No. 16. Washington, DC: American Council of Life Insurance, Winter, 1978. A 24-page brochure that discusses topics on public attitudes and values, legal, moral, ethical controversies, projections about death and dying in the future, prolongation of life, etc. Of special interest may be the demographic materials on life expectancy based on actuarial statistics and the implication of these trends for the life insurance business.

Wass, H. Views and opinions of elderly persons concerning death. *Educational Gerontology,* 1977, *2*(4), 15-26. The author reports on a survey that compared views about death of an elderly sample with *Psychology Today* readers who filled out Shneidman's death questionnaire published in the magazine.

Wass, H. Aging and death education for elderly persons. *Archives of the Foundation of Thanatology,* 1978, *7*(2), 6. (Abstract) The position is taken that the subject of death should be an integral part of a human development program made available to elderly persons as part of educational programs. Five subject areas for practical death education are outlined.

Wass, H., Christian, M., Myers, J., & Murphey, M. Similarities and dissimilarities in attitudes toward death in a population of older persons. *Omega,* 1978-1979, *9*(4), 337-354. The authors found significant differences relative to sex, educational level, income level, and type of residence community. Similarities in certain attitudes and views about death were also found. Educational implications are discussed.

Wass, H. Death and the elderly. In H. Wass (Ed.), *Dying: Facing the facts.* Washington, DC: Hemisphere, 1979, 182-207. This chapter includes a section on death education and counseling for elderly persons.

Wass, H., & Sisler, H. H. Death concern and views on various aspects of dying among elderly persons. In A. de Vries and A. Carmi (Eds.), *The dying human,* Ramat Gan, Israel: Turtledove Publishing, 1979, 71-86. Among the findings were that females, widowed persons, rural dwellers, and persons living alone with little formal education were more concerned about death than were males, married, urban persons, those living with family, and those highly educated.

Weber, J. A. *Family centered unit for helping children become aware of death.* Paper read at the National Symposium for Children and Parents, Iowa City, Iowa, April 24-26, 1978. This paper presents a curriculum unit designed to be used by parents to help their children examine and cope with their feelings toward death. The author believes that the family is the major educator in understanding the life cycle.

Wolf, A. W. M. *Helping your child to understand death.* New York: Child Study Press, 1975. This pamphlet offers simple, practical advice and answers parents can give to children's questions about death. The author also suggests answers to some of the questions parents commonly ask professionals.

Wolff, K. Helping elderly patients face the fear of death. *Hospital Community Psychiatry,* 1967, *13*, 142-144. This paper reports that restlessness and insomnia in the elderly are frequently caused by the fear of dying. The author found that 80 percent of geriatric patients in the author's care are very concerned about death, and suggests that the therapist search for and find positive feelings and value in being old, and a purpose for living.

Zeligs, R. Children's attitudes toward death. *Mental Hygiene*, 1967, *51*, 393-396. The author touches briefly upon a variety of topics such as death fear in adults, its effect on children, children's reactions to a death in the family, etc.

Zinner, E., & McMahon, J. D. *How to conduct a one day conference on death education: The do's and don'ts.* New York: Highly specialized promotions publishers (in press). A practical guide to assist planners in organizing a successful conference on death.

DEATH EDUCATION FOR COUNSELORS AND THERAPISTS; SELF-HELP GROUPS

Bascue, L. O., & Krieger, G. W. Death as a counseling concern. *Personnel and Guidance Journal*, 1974, *52*, 587-592. It is suggested that counselors be responsive to the death concerns of those they serve, and become knowledgeable about the field and explore their own beliefs and feelings about death. Approaches to helping children and adolescents are outlined.

Bernardi, J. M., & Sanders, C. M. Self-help groups in illness and bereavement. *Death Education*, 1978, *2*(3), 311-317. The authors describe the reasons for the formation of self-help groups, discuss their functions as support systems, and describe their organization.

Bernstein, B. E. Lawyer and counselor as an interdisciplinary team: Interfacing for the terminally ill. *Death Education*, 1977, *1*(3), 277-291. It is recommended that mental health workers consult with the terminally ill about their need for taking care of legal matters such as will drafting. Counselors and lawyers might work as an interdisciplinary team in serving dying persons.

Bernstein, B. E. Lawyer and therapist as an interdisciplinary team: serving the survivors. *Death Education* (in press). Here the author recommends that lawyers and therapists work together to assist the survivors with personal, financial, and governmental requirements more effectively to avoid additional trauma.

Blazer, J. A. The concept of death as a factor in mental health. *Psychology*, 1978, *15*(1), 68-77. Blazer argues that personal confrontation with death is necessary for mental health. Proposes the creation of a "National Institute of Death" to facilitate program development for community mental health centers.

Bowers, M. K., Jackson, E. N., Knight, J. A., & LeShan, L. *Counseling the dying.* New York: Jason Aronson, 1975. In this very helpful book, the authors provide a rationale for psychotherapy with dying persons, with the basic principle of being honest. They describe problems in working with dying persons. Included are studies and observations of how different persons cope with death and recommendations for enhancing effective communication between caregiver and patient.

Bugen, L. A. Fundamentals of bereavement intervention. In L. A. Bugen (Ed.) *Death and dying: Theory/research/practice.* Dubuque, IA: William C. Brown, 1979, 99-112. A discussion of basic components of a crisis event, reactions to it, and basic approaches to grief management.

Clark, M. A therapeutic approach to treating a grieving two and a half year old. *Journal of American Academy of Child Psychiatry,* 1973, *11*(4), 705-711. Clark reports a case history of the intervention in the life of a mother and her child after the death of her husband.

D'Afflitti, J. G., & Weitz, G. W. Rehabilitating the stroke patient through family-patient groups. *International Journal of Group Psychotherapy,* 1974, *25,* 323-332. Describes the group method, techniques, problems and success for helping patients and family adjust to chronic disability.

DeMuth Berg, C. Cognizance of the death taboo in counseling children. *The School Counselor,* 1973, *21,* 28-32. Counselors are urged to become aware of the death taboo and work through distortions surrounding death to be able to provide an atmosphere in which children feel free to ask questions, share memories, and tell about their concerns and fears.

Dunlop, R. S. Training bereavement therapists. *Death Education* (in press). The preparation of professionals and advanced graduate students in bereavement therapy are described including recruitment, course content, and field experiences.

Garfield, C. A., Clark, R. O. The Shanti Project: A community model. *Death Education,* 1978, *1*(4), 397-408. The Shanti Project in Berkeley, a volunteer counseling service for patients and families facing life-threatening illness, is described, including its origins and aims.

Glicken, M. D. The child's view of death. *Journal of Marriage and Family Counseling,* 1978, *4*(2), 75-81. Ways are discussed in which therapists may help children learn to deal with death. It is suggested that inability to cope with death may have important negative consequences for the child's emotional well-being.

Goddard, H. L., & Leviton, D. Intimacy-sexuality needs of the bereaved: An exploratory study. *Death Education* 1980, *3*(4), 347-358. This study explores the problems of loneliness, isolation, ostracism, and sexual frustrations of a group of widows. The large majority of the sample group suffered increased mental and physical ailments. Includes recommendation for therapists and counselors working with widows.

Heller, B. D., & Schneider, C. D. Interpersonal methods for coping with stress: Helping families of dying children. *Omega,* 1977-1978, *8*(4), 319-331. The authors discuss a hospital-based self-help program designed to help the families of terminally ill children through shared peer counseling. They include evaluation of the program and a set of recommendations for future attempts to organize such groups.

Helmvath, T. A., & Steinitz, E. M. Death of an infant: Parental grieving and the failure of social support. *Journal of Family Practice*, 1978, *6*(4), 785-790. The authors studied white middle-class couples who lost an infant through death and found that society does not provide adequate support for such parents. It is suggested that society's view of the perceived worth of a newborn infant may have undergone a change.

Jackson, E. N. Wisely managing our grief: A pastoral viewpoint, *Death Education*, 1979, *3*(2), 143-155. The author stresses the importance of wisely managing grief and relates a variety of emotional and physical problems that result from unwise management. The issue of grief and its resolution is discussed in the framework of the Christian belief system.

Kopel, K., & Mock. L. A. The use of group sessions for the emotional support of families of terminal patients. *Death Education*, 1978, *1*(4), 409-422. The article describes weekly group sessions held on a cancer unit for family members of terminal patients. The development and goals of this group, established to meet the need for emotional support, are discussed.

Krieger, D. Therapeutic touch: The imprimatur of nursing. *American Journal of Nursing*, 1975, *75*, 784-787. Reports results of a study in which a group of nurses used the laying-on of hands or the method of "therapeutic touch" with patients. The research literature and previous studies by the authors are reviewed as well. It is suggested that the nurse's touch can indeed be therapeutic using changes in the patients' hemoglobin values as the critical variable.

Martinson, I. Parents help each other. *American Journal of Nursing*, 1976, *76*(7), 1120-1122. Martinson provides an account of meetings of parents of leukemic children, and reports on the mutual support provided.

Nelson, R. C. Counselors, teachers, and death education. *The School Counselor*, 1977, *24*(5), 322-329. The author examines various ways in which counselors can help teachers deal with death. Group activities to build death awareness are emphasized.

Nelson, R. C., & Peterson, W. D. Challenging the last great taboo: Death. *The School Counselor*, 1975, *22*, 353-358. Suggestions are made about how counselors and teachers can help young people understand and cope with death.

Robinson, C. M. Developmental counseling approach to death and dying education. *Elementary School Guidance and Counseling*, 1978, *12*, 178-187. A 7½-week required death and dying unit for 96 seventh graders as part of an enrichment and developmental counseling program is described, including objectives, activities, and evaluation. Negative responses to "feeling" words about death decreased from 73 percent prior to the unit to 56 percent following it, whereas the positive responses increased from 27 to 44 percent.

Satterwhile, B. B., Belle-Isle, J., & Conradt, B. Parent groups as an aid in mourning and grief work. In O. J. Z. Sahler (Ed.), *The child* *and death*. St. Louis: Mosby, 1978, 211–218. An informative discussion of the need, development, and effectiveness of parent self-help groups, with emphasis on the Candlelighter's Society and Cure Childhood Cancer Association. Helpful for those who wish to initiate or join such groups.

Schiff, H. S. *The bereaved parent*. New York: Crown, 1977. This book is written by a mother whose son died of a congenital heart defect at the age of 10. The author's intent is to help other parents who experience the death of a child to cope with and accept their reactions, and to offer suggestions for self-help. Topics include guilt, powerlessness, marital relationship during bereavement, effect on siblings, the role of religion, and communication with relatives and friends. The book should be helpful to bereaved parents as well as professionals.

Silverman, P. R. The widow as a care giver in a program of prevention and intervention with other widows. *Mental Hygiene*, 1970, 5(4), 540-547. The author discusses a self-help program using widows to help widows.

Steele, St. *Bereavement outreach network*, Baltimore, MD: Wyman Institute, 1977. This brief manual describes how to initiate and organize self-help groups for bereaved persons.

Temes, R. *Living with an empty chair: A guide through grief*. Amherst, MA: Mandala, 1977. The author, a grief counselor, presents guidelines for bereaved persons, including a section on bereavement counseling and on conducting workshops for widows.

Williams, W. V., Lee, J., & Polak, P. R. Crisis intervention: Effects of crisis intervention on family survivors of sudden death situations. *Community Mental Health Journals*, 1976, *12*(2), 128-136. The effects of short-term crisis service provided for 39 families (60 subjects) who had recently experienced the sudden death of a child are studied. Two control groups existed for comparison purposes. It was found that short-term crisis service had no major impact on family adjustment following bereavement.

Wright, L. An emotional support program for parents of dying children. *Journal of Clinical Child Psychology*, 1974, *3*(2), 37-38. Consultation technique and modelling are suggested as ways of therapeutic interaction for parents who need to improve their skills in raising terminal children. The author reports on ongoing research of psychological profiles of dying children and their parents.

Selected Text
and Reference
Books

In this section, we have assembled descriptive and evaluative information about 28 text and reference books we judge to be among the most prominent in the field of death, dying, and bereavement. In so doing, we intend to achieve several goals simultaneously. First, we believe that by bringing this information together in one convenient place we can save our readers much time and effort. Through an examination of the descriptive data we provide, those who do not have immediate access to these books should be able to tell which of them might suit their needs for personal reading, as a text for some course they are or may be teaching, or for general reference purposes. No doubt the reader will wish to personally examine each likely volume, but we hope that our work will show some of the options that are available and assist in determining the individual books to be investigated further. To that end we have employed a standard format in dealing with each of the following books: (a) we furnish basic data, such as author(s) or editor(s), title of the book, place and date of publication, publisher, number of pages, hard or soft binding,

price(s), and international standard book number(s); (b) we reproduce
the book's table of contents, indicating part and chapter titles, and
(where appropriate) names of contributing authors; and (c) we outline the characteristic features of the work, employing the author's
own descriptions insofar as that is possible. This information should
help the reader in deciding whether to order a copy for individual
inspection or to recommend the book for library acquisition.

Our standard format also includes our evaluation of the
particular book's major strengths and its serviceability for various
uses. We offer these judgments to serve the other two purposes of
this section, that is, we want to provide explicit guidance to the
reader who is seeking advice about which books to adopt for a course
or to select for additional investigation. Our judgments are inevitably
filtered through our own perceptions, understanding, and experiences, and we realize that some readers may not agree with what we
have to say. However, we believe that evaluations are often implicit
in descriptions and that it is only fair to come forward with our own
assessments of the books we have chosen to include here. We have
sought to be evenhanded and constructive in phrasing our evaluations,
and we hope that they may be regarded as in some degree authoritative, at least by those who are new to the field of death education or
those who are unsure of their own powers of judgment at this point.

A broader goal of this section is to help formulate or sharpen
standards of evaluation in the selection of text and reference books
in this field. This goal is consistent with our respect for a growing
individual and collective maturation of judgment in this area, and
with our recognition of the limits of our own evaluations. In effect,
then, our assessments of the books that follow offer a pattern of
judgment based on more or less explicit standards. That is, we
selected books for this section principally in terms of their ability to
serve the needs of a significant audience in our field with both
breadth and depth. Our assessments consider the comprehensiveness
and authoritativeness with which each book's subject matter is
treated, as well as the effectiveness of its organization and presentation and the quality of the insights that it offers to readers. These
criteria are rather basic, but as we have applied them they suggest *a*
way of regarding books in this field. We hope that those who do not
share our evaluations will, by forming their own judgments in contrast to ours, be assisted in the very process of evaluation and assessment. If so, then the descriptive information and normative judgments that we provide will be, as they ultimately should be, but one
element in each individual's own complex of decision making.

It goes without saying that a list of 25 books from a literature of
hundreds or perhaps thousands of volumes must inevitably be
selective and incomplete. We believe, however, that the list that
follows is representative of most of the major comprehensive textbooks in the field, and of at least one example in each of its principal subfields. We began by drawing up a collection of recent anthol-

ogies that seemed to have been designed to serve as textbooks for broad-based introductory courses on death, dying, and bereavement. To those we added a number of works with a similar pedagogical orientation, but with a more limited scope. Among these were books for physicians, nurses, or other caregivers, as well as volumes with a dominant psychological, sociological, or philosophical orientation. Further, we have also included one or two classic volumes that may now be a bit dated, such as Feifel's *The Meaning of Death* or Kübler-Ross's *On Death and Dying*. At one time or another they were the primary textbooks in the field and still merit our attention as reference sources, background reading, and benchmarks by which to measure the evolving sophistication of other books. Finally, we have chosen to include one or two titles that in our judgment do not work well as textbooks, but have some notable value as reference works or for personal reading. A good example of this is Feifel's *New Meanings of Death*. As indicated above, our tendency has been to lean toward anthologies, but we construe that term broadly to encompass both edited collections of previously published articles and volumes of newly written pieces by contributing authors. Also, we have not hesitated to admit the so-called "systematic" text written by a single author, like Kastenbaum's *Death, Society, and Human Experience*, where an important aspect of the book's value is its potential as a classroom text.

An important new resource that does not fit the format of this section but should be brought to the attention of our readers is the *Encyclopedia of Bioethics*, published by The Free Press at the beginning of 1979. Prepared by editor-in-chief Warren T. Reich, eight associate editors, and an editorial advisory board of 80 prominent scholars, this is the first comprehensive encyclopedia in the field of bioethics. Its four volumes, totaling approximately 1900 pages, include 315 articles written by 285 contributors, an Index, and an Appendix containing codes and statements related to medical ethics. There are 15 articles dealing with various perspectives on death, euthanasia, death-related attitudes, and questions related to definition and determination of death. The four-volume set sells for $200.00.

We urge our readers not to be irritated if a favorite or newly published book does not appear below in our short list. Readers can use our format to draw up a general description and evaluation of the volume in question, and then to compare it with those that follow in order to see its relative merits in serving the needs they may have in mind.

Ariès, Philippe. [*Western attitudes toward death: From the middle ages to the present*] (Patricia M. Ranum, trans.). Baltimore: The Johns Hopkins University Press, 1974. Pp. xiv + 111. Hardbound, $7.50. Paperbound, $2.25. ISBN 0-8018-1566-5.

Contents. Preface: Orest Ranum; Chapter I: Tamed Death; Chapter II: One's Own Death; Chapter III: Thy Death; Chapter IV: Forbidden Death; Index.

Features. This book is the printed version of a set of lectures given by Ariès in April 1973 under the sponsorship of the History Department of Johns Hopkins University. Its topic is "a history of changing attitudes toward death in Western societies since the Middle Ages." Chapter I describes a period of approximately 1000 years from the earliest romances. During this time death was a familiar part of human experience. Individuals were usually aware of its imminent arrival, and they faced it with resignation according to a familiar public ritual that they conducted. The living and the dead also co-existed insofar as churches and their graveyards were located in the middle of population centers. Chapter II notes a series of changes beginning around the eleventh or twelfth centuries whose collective import was to heighten the emphasis on death as an occasion for achieving self-awareness. Following increasing dramatization and eroticization of death from the sixteenth to eighteenth centuries, Chapter III observes the growing perception of death as a break with life and the consequent tendency to distance one's self from it by emphasizing the death of the other. In the last chapter Ariès recounts some of the many ways in which, during the past century and especially in the United States, death has become shameful and forbidden. Throughout the text, Ariès's words are supported by a number of photographs and visual illustrations.

Evaluation. Aries is a well-known French cultural historian and this little book has become a minor classic in the field. The style is sweeping and sophisticated, but the book can be read with profit by college-level students. Aries's work can be useful as a supplementary textbook. It is especially valuable for private reading by individuals interested in the history of ideas, and as general background for classroom instructors. Aries's book draws upon and provides a broader framework for Geoffrey Gorer's 1955 essay, "The Pornography of Death."

□   □   □

Barton, David. *Dying and death: A clinical guide for caregivers.* Baltimore: Williams & Wilkins, 1977. Pp. xviii + 238. Paperbound, $14.95. ISBN 0-683-00440-9.

Contents. Foreword: Harry S. Abram; Preface: David Barton; List of Contributors; Part I—An Approach to Caring for Dying Persons, David Barton: 1. Dying, Death, and Bereavement as Health-Care Problems; 2. Dying and Death: Theoretical Considerations; 3. The Dimensions of Caring; 4. The Dying Person; 5. The Family of the Dying Person; 6. The Caregivers; 7. Approaches to the Clinical Care of the Dying Person; 8. The Process of Grief; Part II—Perspectives: 9. Linda Cummings, The Thoughts, Feelings, and Reflections of a Person with a Life-Threatening Illness; 10. John W. Gattis, The Thoughts, Feelings, and Reflections of a Person with a Life-Threatening Illness; 11. Charles E. Scott, Healing and Dying; 12. Robert M.

Veatch, Caring for the Dying Person: Ethical Issues at Stake; 13. John M. Flexner, Dying, Death, and the "Front-Line" Physician; 14. Ann Hamric, Deterrents to Therapeutic Care of the Dying Person: A Nurse's Perspective; 15. Liston O. Mills, Issues for Clergy in the Care of the Dying and Bereaved; 16. Daniel T. Peak, The Elderly Who Face Dying and Death; 17. Jan van Eys, Caring for the Child Who Might Die; Index.

Features. This is a book intended for caregivers of all sorts, professional and lay, who deal with dying and bereavement. Barton describes it in the following way in his Preface:

> This book is based on the idea that in order to develop more effective approaches to caring for dying persons, one need to be able to discern and respond appropriately to the myriad of needs of the person and the members of his or her family, to have a working knowledge of basic theoretical concepts and basic knowledge about the area of dying, death, and bereavement, and to develop the ability to appreciate the perspectives and abilities of a wide variety of health-care and health-care-related personnel. An approach that achieves a synthesis of these dimensions of the care process is felt to be one which will best equip caregivers to provide optimal assistance to all those involved.

The first eight chapters of the book are by Barton. They are "intended to provide an overview of basic material and an approach to caring for dying persons and their families." The review is selective, but "a central theme in this portion of the book is the concept that those problems and conflicts involved in adapting to dying and death are largely related to the problems and conflicts related to living in the context of dying and the threat of death." The last nine chapters consist of "contributions from people representing varying caregiving disciplines, and ... the reflections and thoughts of two dying patients." Part II thus reinforces the concern for a multidisciplinary approach to caring that pervades Part I, and also appears to consist of newly written material.

Evaluation. This book combines the cohesiveness of a systematic text in Part I with the advantages of a plurality of viewpoints in Part II. It maintains a guiding focus on what is necessary to understand and improve interactions among dying persons, their families and relatives, and their caregivers. The book is not designed for a general course on death and dying, but it will serve well as a text for those working as, or studying to become, caregivers of the dying. Barton's own chapters draw on his personal experience as a psychiatrist and on the best available insights in the field to provide the breadth and depth that is needed by his chosen audience. The pieces by his contributors give concrete examples of what dying looks like to patients, a philosopher, an ethician, a nurse, a pastoral counselor, and three physicians. The principal omission, which Barton acknowledges with regret, is the perspective of a social worker. With that limitation, this volume should be highly recommended for being so current and competent in what it has to say.

□   □   □

Brim, Orville G., Jr., Freeman, Howard E., Levine, Sol, & Scotch, Norman A. (Eds.), with the editorial consultation of Greer Williams. *The dying patient.* New York: Russell Sage Foundation, 1970. Pp. xxvi + 390. Hardbound, $10.00 ISBN: 0-87154-155-6.

Contents. Contributors; Preface: Robert S. Morison; Introduction: Howard E. Freeman, Orville G. Brim, Jr., & Greer Williams, New Dimensions of Dying; Part One—The Social Context of Dying: 1. Monroe Lerner, When, Why, and Where People Die; 2. John W. Riley, Jr., What People Think About Death; 3. Andie L. Knutson, Cultural Beliefs on Life and Death; Part Two—How Doctors, Nurses, and Hospitals Cope With Death: 4. Louis Lasagna, The Prognosis of Death; 5. Louis Lasagna, Physicians' Behavior Toward the Dying Patient; 6. Robert J. Glaser, Innovations and Heroic Acts in Prolonging Life; 7. Anselm L. Strauss & Barney G. Glaser, Patterns of Dying; 8. Elisabeth K. Ross, The Dying Patient's Point of View; 9. David L. Rabin with Laurel H. Rabin, Consequences of Death for Physicians, Nurses, and Hospitals; 10. David Sudnow, Dying in a Public Hospital; Part Three—Termination of Life: Social, Ethical, Legal, and Economic Questions: 11. Sol Levine & Norman A. Scotch, Dying as an Emerging Social Problem; 12. Osler L. Peterson, Control of Medical Conduct; 13. Bayless Manning, Legal and Policy Issues in the Allocation of Death; 14. Richard M. Bailey, Economic and Social Costs of Death; Conclusion: Diana Crane, Dying and Its Dilemmas as a Field of Research; Death and Dying, a Briefly Annotated Bibliography: Richard A. Kalish; Name Index; Subject Index.

Features. Robert Morison describes this collection of newly written articles in the Preface:

> It explores the medical, social, economic, and ethical issues raised by man's increasing control over death and dying. In doing so, it incidentally reveals how the pursuit of a "value-free" science and technology brings us to a whole new range of value-loaded questions. It also provides us with another equally interesting paradox: the same science that has knocked many of the supports from the ethical structures of the past now demands a more thorough ethical understanding than could ever have been conceived of when the world operated according to God's will.

The contributors are primarily professors of medicine or of the social sciences. They deal principally with two somewhat different aspects of the dying patient. The first includes the large range of professional analyses and decisions, as well as the intensely personal feelings, involved in determining how and when an individual's death should occur. The second concerns the process of dying: what actually goes on now and what might be done to make the process somewhat less graceless and more acceptable not only to the dying patient but also to those who love and attend him.

By thus contributing to our short-range understanding of the situation of the dying patient, the long-range effect is to bring to the fore important problems of value within our society as a whole.

Evaluation. This is an earlier and influential volume. It is broad-based and thorough, though it tends to focus on physicians and the health care system as a whole, with less attention to nurses and other caregivers. Along with others, this book helped to draw attention to the quality of life in the period preceding death and to show that much could be learned and done about this period by social scientists and health professionals. Many of the articles report valuable data, and research was further stimulated by Crane's concluding essay and Kalish's annotated bibliography. There is a praiseworthy sensitivity throughout to the historical, social, and institutional context of dying, and to the many-sided problems of values and decision making that affect the dying person. Because of its high level of competence, the volume remains useful today both as a textbook for courses on the care of the dying and as a general reference source, although a contemporary student might wish to augment this collection with materials on more recent developments in the care of the dying.

□   □   □

Carse, James P., & Dallery, Arlene B. *Death and society: A book of readings and sources.* New York: Harcourt, 1977. Pp. xx + 472. Paperbound, $6.95. ISBN 0-15-517211-5.

Contents. Preface; Introduction; Section One—Abortion: Introduction; James Carse, Review of the Supreme Court Decisions on Abortion; Eugene F. Diamond, The Humanity of the Unborn Child; Joseph R. Donceel, A Liberal Catholic's View; R. J. Gerber, Abortion: Parameters for Decision; Judith Jarvis Thomson, A Defense of Abortion; Michael Tooley, Abortion and Infanticide; Philip J. Resnick, Murder of the Newborn: A Psychiatric Review of Neonaticide; Section Two—Euthanasia: Introduction; Eliot Slater, The Case for Voluntary Euthanasia; Antony Flew, The Principle of Euthanasia; James Rachels, Active and Passive Euthanasia; Paul Ramsey, The Indignity of "Death with Dignity"; Joseph Sanders, Euthanasia: None Dare Call It Murder; Joseph Fletcher, Ethics and Euthanasia; Anthony Shaw, Dilemmas of "Informed Consent" in Children; Section Three—Suicide: Introduction; Suicide: International Comparisons; Mathew Ross, Suicide Among Physicians; H. L. P. Resnik & Larry H. Dizmang, Suicidal Behavior Among American Indians; Jerome A. Motto, The Right to Suicide: A Psychiatrist's View; James Hillman, Suicide as the Soul's Choice; Section Four—Death and the Law: Introduction; Capital Punishment and the Law; Brendan F. Brown, Individual Liberty and the Common Good; Carol S. Vance, Reinstatement of the Death Penalty; Alexander Morgan Capron & Leon R. Kass, A Statutory Definition of the Standards for Determining Human Death: An Appraisal and a Proposal; Alfred M. Sadler, Jr., Blair L. Sadler & E. Blythe Stason, The Uniform Anatomical Gift Act: A Model for Reform; Section Five—Death and Aging: Introduction; Richard A. Kalish, The Aged and the Dying Process: The Inevitable Decisions; W. R. Bytheway, Aspects of Old Age in Age-Specific Mortality Rates; James O. Carpenter & Charles M. Wylie, On Aging, Dying, and Denying: Delivering Care to Older Dying Patients; Sharon R. Curtin, Social Death and Aging; Section Six—Death and the Caring Institutions: Introduction; Henry K. Beecher, et al., A Definition of Irreversible Coma: Report of the Ad Hoc Committee of the Harvard Medical School to Examine the Definition of Brain Death; Mark Lappe, et al., Refinements in Criteria for the Determination of Death: An Appraisal; Hans Jonas, Against the Stream: Comments on the Definition and Redefinition of Death; Nicholas Rescher, The Allocation of Exotic Medical Lifesaving Therapy; William F. May, Institutions as Symbols of Death; Robert E. Neale, Between the Nipple and the Everlasting Arms; Appendix: Monroe Lerner, When, Why, and Where People Die; Bibliography.

Features. In the Preface to this book the editors suggest a general framework for their work by commenting on the recent discussion of death: "The primary concern in the current literature is not with the fate of the dead but with the process or the experience of dying." They then place this volume more specifically through the following distinction within that interest in dying:

> In the most recent books and articles we can, rather generally, identify two major emphases. There has been, on the one hand, great popular interest in the personal experience of dying. . . . On the other hand, there is an increasing interest in the social context of dying. . . .
> This book is concerned with the latter category: the shared, or social meaning of death.

This is, in other words, a collection of previously published materials on the social—and very often, the moral—aspects of death. Further, the introduction adds the classic intention of the Socratic teacher.

> This book is offered as a provocation for further reflection on the problem of death. Its design is to provide not conclusions but

goads to further thought. Where conclusions do occur in the following essays, they were selected because they are certain to arouse more deliberation than they will quiet.

Finally, "the selection of the pieces gathered in this volume was guided by three philosophical convictions: that the discussion of the issues addressed by the authors of the following pages is inherently resistant to conclusions; it is not possible to speak of death without speaking of life, [i.e., both death and life properly direct attention to a something which lives and dies] ; and life can neither originate nor continue in a social or physical vacuum." Living things (especially persons) are always interdependent, social or communal.

Evaluation. The selections in this book, drawn mainly from journal articles of the early 1970s, generally represent the views of well-known writers in the debates they address. The volume as a whole has a clear topical focus and good breadth of coverage within its intended scope. It should work well as a primary textbook for a college course on social ethics with a topical slant toward death and dying. The emphasis on conceptual and philosophical argumentation might also make it useful as a (rather hefty) supplement to a data-based course on the sociology of death, or to more general courses on death and dying.

□   □   □

Caughill, Rita E. (Ed.). *The dying patient: A supportive approach.* Boston: Little, Brown, 1976. Pp. xii + 228. Paperbound, $6.95. ISBN 0-316-13216-0.

Contents. Contributing Authors; Preface: Rita E. Caughill; Chapter 1: Ruth Gale Elder, Dying and Society; Chapter 2: Carol Ren Kneisl, Griefing: A Response to Loss; Chapter 3: Ruth A. Assell, If You Were Dying; Chapter 4: Clark Hopkins, The Right to Die with Dignity; Chapter 5: Rita E. Caughill, Coping with Death in Acute Care Units; Chapter 6: Carol S. Green-Epner, The Dying Child; Chapter 7: Claudine R. Gartner, Growing Up to Dying: The Child, the Parents, and the Nurse; Chapter 8: Rita E. Caughill, Supportive Care and the Age of the Dying Patient; Index.

Features. In her Preface the editor provides the following description of this volume:

Despite the current proliferation of books dealing with various aspects of death, grief, and bereavement, there is little available for practicing nurses or nursing students, who are at the bedside of dying patients every day, to guide them in recognizing their responsibilities in the care of the dying. It is for such nurses that this book was written. It makes no claim to be a comprehensive text but is, rather, a supplementary book of readings. It is intended as a reference source to assist nursing personnel in developing the knowledge and skills they need in order to give thoughtful, supportive care to dying patients.

In other words, the book emphasizes "the basic psychological needs of the dying" in order to mitigate "the extreme discomfort experienced by most people in the presence of dying and of death" (after all, "few nurses are any better prepared than the lay person to cope with the realities of dying") and to make it possible "for caregivers to improve their relationships with the terminally ill." The contributors include six nursing faculty members from SUNY at Buffalo or the University of Kentucky, Lexington, and one professor emeritus of classical art and archeology from the Univeristy of Michigan. One of the selections is revised from a 1973 journal article; the others all appear to be newly written for this volume.

Evaluation. This book reads easily. Its contributors are heavily dependent on other authors, but they use them to provide a competent review of their topics and of the relevant literature. Nurses who care for dying persons will find many practical suggestions to aid their work, and each chapter supplies bibliographical references for additional reading. The book does not offer depth or comprehensiveness of treatment, but meets its goal as a supplementary text and as a useful starting point for practitioners.

Chapter 4—the only one not written by a nurse—is rather a different kind of piece that deserves a separate word of comment. It recounts the author's work in arguing for living wills and the right to die with dignity and a minimum amount of pain. That is, it advocates voluntary euthanasia in the form of administering lethal drugs to hasten the moment of death. No mention is made here or elsewhere in the volume of hospice programs. Nor is there any discussion of recent developments along the lines of the California Natural Death Act. Finally, the author's treatment of difficult and controversial topics is not balanced by a contrasting viewpoint in any other section of the book.

□   □   □

Choron, Jacques. *Death and western thought.* New York: Macmillan, 1963. Hardbound, $6.95. Paperbound, $3.95. Library of Congress No. 62-17575.

Contents. Foreword; Introduction; Book I—Antiquity: 1. The Pre-Socratic Philosophers; 2. Socrates (469-399 B.C.), Death May Be Better Than Life; 3. Plato (427-347 B.C.), Death Is the Release of the Soul from the Body; 4. Aristotle (384-322 B.C.), The "Immortality" of Reason; 5. Epicurus (341-270 B.C.), Death Is Nothing to Us; 6. Stoicism, Greek and Roman (The Older Stoa; Seneca; Epictetus and Marcus Aurelius); Book II—The Christian Answer to Death: 7. Death in the Old Testament; 8. Death in the New Testament; Book III—The Renaissance: 9. The Crisis of the Christian View of Death; 10. Montaigne (1533-1592), On How to Learn to Die; 11. Giordano Bruno (1548-1600), Death Is Not Possible in the Infinite Universe; Book IV—The Answers to Death in Modern Philosophy: 12. Descartes (1596-1650), Our Souls Outlast Our Bodies; 13. Pascal (1623-1662), The Best in This Life Is the Hope of Another Life; 14. Spinoza (1632-1677), The Human Mind Cannot Be Absolutely Destroyed; 15. Leibniz (1646-1716), No Living Creature Perishes Completely . . . There Is Only Metamorphosis; 16. The Eighteenth Century: The Denial of Immortality; 17. Kant (1724-1804), The "Moral" Argument for Immortality; 18. Hegel (1770-1831), Death Is the Reconciliation of the Spirit with Itself; 19. The Romantics: The Glorification of Death; 20. Schopenhauer (1788-1860), Death Is the True Aim of Life (The World as Will and Idea; The Fear of Death; The Indestructibility of Our "True Nature"; The Denial of the Will); 21. Feuerbach (1804-1872), Life Must Be Lived Fully in Spite of Death; 22. Nietzsche (1844-1900), The Doctrine of the "Eternal Recurrence of the Same"; Book V—Contemporary Philosophy: 23. Bergson, Klages, Simmel, Death and "Philosophies of Life"; 24. Scheler (1874-1928), Survival after Death Is Plausible and Probable; 25. Whitehead (1861-1947), Immortality of Realized Value; 26. Existential Philosophies and the Problem of Death (Jaspers; Heidegger; Sartre; Marcel); Afterword: Death as Motif and Motive of Philosophy; Present-day Philosophers and the Problems of Death; Notes to Chapters; Name Index.

Features. In his Foreword, Choron refers to this book as a "survey of what the great philosophers of the Western world have thought about death," and he expresses the hope that it "will not only be a contribution to the history of ideas but also helpful to those who, at a time when the consolations of religion have lost their force, seek to come to terms with death." Choron's review of history has convinced him that "the discovery of the inevitability of death, measured against man's total presence on earth, is a relatively recent occurrence." And yet, that point alone is incomplete for "we also have to consider the strange—although by now well-established—fact that no one really believes in his own death, even though no one doubts its inevitability." It is to help us deal with these facts in a secularized context that Choron looked back upon the accumulated wisdom of Western philosophy. As he says, "the question of the meaning of human existence in the totality of Being, this fundamental question of philosophy, gains its true and practical importance through man's total discovery of death."

Evaluation. This book is a minor classic, a tour de force on Western philosophy and the history of ideas. Chapters are brief and clear, and the notes give leads for further reading. Those who wish to do personal reading in this area, who seek a text for a course on philosophers and death, or who desire a general reference source on this subject will find this book valuable in many ways. Not everyone will share Choron's personal outlook, which seems to revolve around a central contrast between religion and philosophy, and a specific position within philosophy as to the proper role of philosophizing vis-a-vis death. But we can all agree that the felt need to deal with death has been an important motivation for many Western philosophers. And most of us can profit from a reflection on some of Choron's "immediate conclusions" as stated in his Afterword:

> The survey of the answers which Western philosophers have given throughout the ages to the problems of the fear of death and the nature of death made it obvious that any answer to death that an individual seeks and finds satisfactory depends, in the last resort, on the individual's attitude to life, the intensity of his fear of death, and the particular kind of his death-fear. It is obvious, too, however, that such an answer cannot be merely speculative, but must actually be accepted, made one's own. And it must be added that an answer to death found satisfactory at one time may not be so at another. Thus there can be no universal answer, least of all a universally valid one. A genuine reconciliation with death may not in fact be possible for some; for others almost any argument may modify their apprehension of death and free them from despair at its inevitability and apparent absurdity.

□   □   □

Davidson, Glen W. *The hospice: Development and administration.* Washington, DC: Hemisphere, 1978. Pp. vii + 232. Hardbound, $14.95. ISBN 0-89116-103-1.

Contents. Preface: Glen W. Davidson; Models of Care: Dottie C. Wilson, Ina Ajemian, and Balfor M. Mount, Montreal (1975)—The Royal Victoria Hospital Palliative Care Service; Norman A. Wylie, Halifax (1976)—Victoria General Hospital: A Nursing Model; Sylvia Lack, New Haven (1974)—Characteristics of A Hospice Program of Care; William M. Lamers, Jr., Marin County (1976)—Development of Hospice of Marin; John A. Hackley, William C. Farr & Sr. Teresa Marie McIntier, Tucson (1977)—Hillhaven Hospice; James Fox, Springfield (1978)—St. John's Hospice; Problems When Caring: Sr. M. Simone Roach, The Experience of an Academic as Caregiver: Implications for Education; Mary L. Vachon, Motivation and Stress Experienced by Staff Working with the Terminally Ill; Barry LeGrove Rogers, Using the Creative Process with the Terminally Ill; Robert W. Buckingham III & Susan H. Foley, A Guide to Evaluation Research in Terminal Care Programs; Issues In Caring: Glen A. Davidson, In Search of Models for Care; George J. Agich, The Ethics of Terminal Care; Theodore Raymond LeBlang, Death With Dignity: A Tripartite Legal Response; Annotations: The Literature—Annotated

Bibliography; The Media; A Directory of Hospice Programs in the United States; Contributors; Index.

Features. In his preface Davidson states: "So far as can be determined, this is the first attempt to bring together in one volume a report on the hospice movement in North America." This book deals both with what has been done so far and what is being planned for improving the institutional care of the terminally ill. The six hospice programs described are not the first historically, and they do not represent all the many possible ways that institutional terminal care can be organized. However, Davidson hopes that from the description of these programs—at different phases of development—one can see how the hospice movement is taking shape in North America. Another feature of this book is the sections dealing with problems and issues of hospice care. It is all too easy to begin new ventures and approaches without careful consideration of issues involved and problems to be resolved. Davidson stresses that this volume is only a beginning on how the dying, their families, and caregivers "wrestle with questions of care, competence, and compassion."

Evaluation. This is a timely volume that should be of great interest and help to all those involved in hospice programs already in operation, and most particularly to those who are planning such programs. The authors contributing to this book are intimately involved in their programs and write not only with pride but also from a solid base of experience. Of special value are the discussions of problems and issues of hospice care particularly for the novice, who may have much enthusiasm and compassion but may be naive about the complexity of terminal care alternatives. This volume is an excellent reference resource and guide for caregivers, health care administrators, and death educators for preservice and in-service education including workshops and seminars, and other short-term training programs.

□ □ □

Earle, Ann M., Argondizzo, Nina T., & Kutscher, Austin H. (Eds.), with the editorial assistance of Lillian G. Kutscher. *The nurse as caregiver for the terminal patient and his family.* New York: Columbia University Press, 1976. Pp. x + 255. Hardbound, $17.50. ISBN 0-231-04020-2.

Contents. Introduction: Eileen M. Jacobi, Nursing and the Therapeutic Relationship; Chapter 1: Jeanne Quint Benoliel, Overview: Care, Cure, and the Challenge of Choice; Part One—Living, Dying, and Those Who Care: 2. Shirley L. Williams, The Nurse as Crisis Intervener; 3. Lucy Warren, The Terminally Ill Child, His Parents, and the Nurse; 4. A. Barbara Coyne, The Nurse's Responsibilities; 5. Yvonne Singletary, Case Report; 6. Kenneth A. Chandler, Continuing and Discontinuing Care; 7. Joan M. Liaschenko & Richard J. Torpie,

A Case Review on Death, from Two Perspectives; 8. Pauline M. Seitz, The Deadborn Infant: Supportive Care for Patients; 9. Joy Rogers & M. L. S. Vachon, Therapeutic Intervention with the Bereaved; Part Two—Coping Problems of Professionals: 10. June S. Lowenberg, Working Through Feelings Around Death; 11. James S. Eaton, Jr., Coping with Staff Grief; 12. John E. Schowalter, Pediatric Nurses Dream of Death; 13. Liberty Kovacs, A Personal Perspective of Death and Dying; 14. Joseph F. Fennelly, Female Chauvinism in Nursing; 15. M. L. S. Vachon, W. A. L. Lyall & J. Rogers, The Nurse in Thanatology: What She Can Learn from the Women's Liberation Movement; 16. Nancy Proctor Greenleaf, Stereotyped Sex-Role Ranking of Caregivers and Quality Care for Dying Patients; 17. Peter Koestenbaum, The Existential Meaning of Death; Part Three—Education: 18. Beverly Capaccio Fineman, Teaching to Individual Differences; 19. Joseph R. Proulx, Let the Teacher Beware!; 20. Eleanor C. Friedenberg, Continuing Education in Aging and Long-Term Care; Appendix: Jeanne Quint Benoliel, Death Influence in Clinical Practice: A Course Outline for the Nursing School Curriculum; Index; Contributors.

Features. Sponsored by the Foundation of Thanatology, this volume is a collection of papers dealing broadly with the nurse's role in caring for dying patients and bereaved survivors. The book also considers problems nurses experience in coping with this kind of work, and some questions concerning educational techniques designed to improve care and minimize problems. In essence, this is an appeal for more concern and better conduct in education and practice, and for a humane approach to all of these topics. A brief Introduction by Eileen Jacobi and a prefatory chapter by Jeanne Quint Benoliel attempt to provide context for the volume, and an Appendix by Benoliel offers a course outline for the nursing school curriculum. The editors provide no introductory material of their own to aid the reader in understanding the aims of the volume as a whole or the character of its components, whether in themselves or in their interconnections. Apparently only one of the chapters has previously been published. Of the 23 contributors, 14 are nurses, 5 are physicians.

Evaluation. This volume is not so large or theory-laden as to be intimidating. It reads well and contains a roughly equal balance between case studies or personal reports and interpretive analyses. The contributors are knowledgeable in their respective subjects and frequently draw on experiences from their work with those who are coping with dying. The book is useful as personal reading for those interested in its range of issues, and it might serve as a supplementary text for a course in nursing, drawing on the more important primary contributions in the field and applying them to practice.

□   □   □

Feifel, Herman. *New meanings of death.* New York: McGraw-Hill, 1977. Pp. xvi + 367. Hardbound, $11.95. Paperbound $7.95. ISBN 0-07-020350-4 hardbound; 0-07-020349-0 paperbound.

Contents. List of Contributors; Preface; Part One—Introduction: 1. Herman Feifel, Death in Contemporary America; Part Two—Developmental Orientations: 2. Robert Kastenbaum, Death and Development Through the Lifespan; 3. Myra Bluebond-Langner, Meanings of Death to Children; 4. Edwin S. Shneidman, The College Student and Death; Part Three—Clinical Management: 5. Laurens P. White, Death and the Physician: Mortuis Vivos Docent; 6. Avery D. Weisman, The Psychiatrist and the Inexorable; 7. Jeanne Quint Benoliel, Nurses and the Human Experience of Dying; 8. Charles A. Garfield; Impact of Death on the Health-Care Professional; 9. Cicely Saunders, Dying They Live: St. Christopher's Hospice; 10. Orville E. Kelly, Make Today Count; 11. Lois and Arthur Jaffe, Terminal Candor and the Coda Syndrome: A Tandem; Part Four—The Survivors: 12. Richard A. Kalish, Dying and Preparing for Death: A View of Families; 13. Howard C. Raether & Robert C. Slater, Immediate Postdeath Activities in the United States; Part Five—Responses to Death: 14. Daniel Leviton, Death Education; 15. Robert J. Lifton, The Sense of Immortality: On Death and the Continuity of Life; 16. Thomas L. Shaffer & Robert E. Rodes, Jr., Law For Those Who Are to Die; 17. Michael A. Simpson, Death and Modern Poetry; 18. David L. Gutmann, Dying to Power: Death and the Search for Self-Esteem; Part Six—Epilogue: 19. Herman Feifel, Epilogue; Name Index; Subject Index.

Features. Feifel says in his Preface that he updated his earlier work because of "my increasing understanding that knowledge tends to be dynamic and ever-changing, that information is filtered and re-translated as it moves through time." And surely the state of our understanding of death, dying, and bereavement has changed greatly in the nearly two decades since the appearance of *The Meaning of Death* (1959). But another factor was even more significant in inspiring this new book. "Most overriding for me, however, was the conviction that in the last analysis all human behavior of consequence is a response to the problem of death. . . . Life's ultimate meaning remains obscure unless it is reflected upon in the countenance of death." *New Meanings of Death* seeks to aid our reflective response to death by providing a collection of newly written essays containing the insights and viewpoints of many prominent authors. Because Feifel adds no connecting materials beyond a Preface and his introductory and concluding chapters, the volume naturally reflects the interests and strengths of its contributors. In this, there is no effort to be comprehensive. As Feifel says, "since the book does not attempt to encompass the panoramic realm of thanatology, such sectors as religion, philosophy, epidemiology, economics, and the humanities are touched only glancingly."

Evaluation. The principal feature that commends this volume is the strength of many of its individual selections. Among the more notable are the pieces by Kastenbaum, Kalish, Bluebond-Langner, Weisman, White, Lifton, Quint Benoliel, Saunders, Kelly, L. and R. Jaffe, Leviton, and Simpson. And of course Feifel's own essays are authoritative and helpful. *New Meanings of Death* is a valuable book that could serve as a resource and as supplemental reading for a course on death and dying.

□   □   □

Feifel, Herman. *The meaning of death.* New York: McGraw-Hill, 1959. Pp. xvi + 351. Paperbound, $2.95. ISBN 0-07-020347-4.

Contents. Contributors; Preface; Introduction; Part I—Theoretical Outlooks on Death: 1. Carl G. Jung, The Soul and Death; 2. Charles W. Wahl, The Fear of Death; 3. Paul Tillich, The Eternal Now; 4. Walter Kaufmann, Existentialism and Death; 5. Herbert Marcuse, The Ideology of Death; Part II—Developmental Orientation Toward Death: 6. Maria H. Nagy, The Child's View of Death; 7. Robert Kastenbaum, Time and Death in Adolescence; 8. Herman Feifel, Attitudes toward Death in Some Normal and Mentally Ill Populations; Part III—Death Concept in Cultural and Religious Fields: 9. Frederick J. Hoffman, Mortality and Modern Literature; 10. Carla Gottlieb, Modern Art and Death; 11. David G. Mandelbaum, Social Uses of Funeral Rites; 12. Edgar N. Jackson, Grief and Religion; Part IV—Clinical and Experimental Studies: 13. Arnold A. Hutschnecker, Personality Factors in Dying Patients; 14. Gerald J. Aronson, Treatment of the Dying Person; 15. August M. Kasper, The Doctor and Death; 16. Irving E. Alexander & Arthur M. Adlerstein, Death and Religion; 17. Edwin S. Shneidman & Norman L. Farberow, Suicide and Death; 18. Curt P. Richter, The Phenomenon of Unexplained Sudden Death in Animals and Man; Part V—Discussion: 19. Gardner Murphy, Discussion; Name Index; Subject Index.

Features. This book is one outcome of a symposium on the psychology of death and dying that Herman Feifel organized for the 1956 convention of the American Psychological Association. It deals with a subject largely regarded as "taboo" in the late 1950s. Feifel knew this and was fully aware of the deficiencies characterizing previous work in this field. "Even after looking hard in the literature, it is surprising how slim is the systematized knowledge about death. . . . There is no book on the American scene which offers a multi-faceted approach to its problems." Feifel's collection sought to fill that void, but it too has limitations, as he openly admits. It is "a first attempt, . . . not an organized text but rather a series of spotlights beamed on a common area," and it makes "no pretense of providing definitive answers." But Feifel knew what needed to be done and his overall assessment of this anthology has been validated over the years: "We do perceive the book, however, as providing a groundwork of reflection and information that will illuminate issues and stimulate fresh insights, suggest therapeutic and practical possibilities, and direct the way toward future research requirements."

Evaluation. This book is now a classic, considered a cornerstone in the evolution of the study of death and dying. Many of its selections are still valuable and worthwhile reading. It remains a convenient source for personal study. Even though some of its selections are uneven, and its organization is rudimentary, it can serve as a valuable work of reference.

　　　　　□　　　□　　　□

Fulton, Robert (Ed.), in collaboration with Robert Bendiksen. *Death and identity* (Rev. ed.). Bowie, MD: The Charles Press, 1976. Pp. xvi + 448. Hardbound, $15.95. ISBN 0-913486-78-7.

Contents. Contributors; Preface to the Revised Edition; Section I—Theoretical Discussions on Death: Introduction; 1. David Sudnow, Dead on Arrival; 2. Robert J. Lifton, The Sense of Immortality: On Death and the Continuity of Life; 3. Robert Blauner, Death and Social Structure; 4. Robert Bendiksen, The Sociology of Death; Section II—Attitudes and Responses toward Death: Introduction; 5. Irving E. Alexander, Randolph S. Colley & Arthur M. Adlerstein, Is Death a Matter of Indifference?; 6. Wendell M. Swenson, Attitudes toward Death among the Aged; 7. Irving E. Alexander & Arthur M. Adlerstein, Affective Responses to the Concept of Death in a Population of Children and Early Adolescents; 8. Paul J. Rhudick & Andrew S. Dibner, Age, Personality, and Health Correlates of Death Concerns in Normal Aged Individuals; 9. Herman Feifel, Religious Conviction and Fear of Death among the Healthy and the Terminally Ill; 10. Donald I. Templer, The Construction and Validation of a Death Anxiety Scale; 11. Barney G. Glaser & Anselm L. Strauss, Awareness Contexts and Social Interaction; 12. Robert Fulton, The Sacred and the Secular: Attitudes of the American Public toward Death, Funerals, and Funeral Directors; Section III—Grief and Mourning: The Reaction to Death: Introduction; 13. Robert J. Lifton, Psychological Effects of the Atomic Bomb in Hiroshima: The Theme of Death; 14. Erich Lindemann, Symptomatology and Management of Acute Grief; 15. Paula Clayton, Lynn Desmarais & George Winokur, A Study of Normal Bereavement; 16. Edmund H. Volkart with the collaboration of Stanley T. Michael, Bereavement and Mental Health; 17. Mervyn Shoor & Mary H. Speed, Death, Delinquency, and the Mourning Process; 18. Josephine R. Hilgard, Martha F. Newman & Fern Fisk, Strength of Adult Ego Following Childhood Bereavement; 19. Robert Bendiksen & Robert Fulton, Death and the Child: An Anterospective Test of the Childhood Bereavement and Later Behavior Disorder Hypothesis; 20. Avery D.

Weisman & Thomas P. Hackett, Predilection to Death; 21. Richard Schulz & David Aderman, Effect of Residential Change on the Temporal Distance to Death of Terminal Cancer Patients; 22. Robert Fulton & Julie Fulton, A Psychosocial Aspect of Terminal Care: Anticipatory Grief; Section IV—Ceremony, Social Organization, and Society: Introduction; 23. David G. Mandelbaum, Social Uses of Funeral Rites; 24. W. Lloyd Warner, The City of the Dead; 25. Talcott Parsons, Renée C. Fox & Victor M. Lidz, The Gift of Life and Its Reciprocation; 26. Felix Berardo, Widowhood Status in the United States: Perspective on a Neglected Aspect of the Family Life Cycle; 27. Vanderlyn R. Pine & Derek L. Phillips, The Cost of Dying: A Sociological Analysis of Funeral Expenditures; Bibliography; Index.

Features. The first edition of *Death and Identity* appeared in 1965. "This edition," we are told in the Preface, "has been revised in response to the growing need for a new compendium of the sociological and sociopsychological literature on death." The volume, in other words, is a collection of previously published, recent examples of clinical and experimental research, expository articles, and theoretical interpretations. Its contributors are almost exclusively sociologists, psychologists, and psychiatrists. The principal criteria for inclusion of selections seem to have been the following:

> Among the experimental or clinical studies, primary consideration was given to those recent studies that reflected, tested, or extended the work of the pioneers in this field whose writings, although important theoretically and historically, have but limited value for modern contemporary research. . . . Selection of the theoretical or expository essays and the articles on ritual and ceremony was based on a desire to place the experimental reports within a framework that not only would provide perspective for the research reported, but also would expose speculative statements to the hard glare of empirical evidence.

The editors share a combined sense of incompleteness or limitation and achievement in their work: "It would require a volume several times this size to include all the material currently available. We believe, however, that the items included are representative of the major work that has been and is being done in the area of death."

Evaluation. The strength of this volume rests on the competence of its editors and contributors, its unifying perspective, and its breadth of coverage within that perspective. Fulton and his colleagues have produced knowledgeable and effective introductions and they have assembled a good collection of articles, a number of them by recognized writers who share their sociological and sociopsychological interests. The result is a fine reference source and a textbook suited to courses emphasizing this particular aspect of death and dying.

□ □ □

Fulton, Robert, Markusen, Eric, Owen, Greg, & Scheiber, Jane L. (Eds.). *Death and dying: Challenge and change.* Reading, MA: Addison-Wesley, 1978. Pp. xviii + 428. Hardbound, $12.00. Paperbound, $5.95. ISBN 0-201-07724-8 hardbound; 0-201-07723-X paperbound.

Contents. Acknowledgments; Preface; Prologue; Part One— Changing Meanings of Death and Dying; Section 1. Death and Dying: The Issues Today: Robert L. Fulton, On the Dying of Death; Melvin Maddocks, Life and Death in the USA; Edwin S. Shneidman, National Survey of Attitudes toward Death; Samuel Vaisrub, Dying is Worked to Death; Ronald Jay Cohen, Is Dying Being Worked to Death?; Section 2. Historical Perspectives on Death: David E. Stannard, The Puritan Way of Death; Stanley French, The Cemetery as Cultural Institution; Philippe Ariès, The Reversal of Death; Section 3. Death in Popular Culture: Michael J. Arlen, The Air: The Cold, Bright Charms of Immortality; Alexander Walker, The Case of the Vanishing Bloodstains; Geoffrey Gorer, The Pornography of Death; Section 4. Demography of Death: Monroe Lerner, When, Why, and Where People Die; Robert Blauner, Death and Social Structure; Calvin Goldscheider, The Social Inequality of Death; Section 5. Death and Social Change: Stanislav Grof, The Changing Face of Death; Ivan Illich, Death against Death; Eric J. Cassell, Dying in a Technological Society; Section 6. Life after Death: Old and New Meanings: Eric Markusen, Religious Conceptions of Afterlife; Rosalind Heywood, Death and Psychical Research; Raymond Moody, Cities of Light; Peggy Taylor & Rick Ingrasci, Out of the Body: An Interview with Elisabeth Kübler-Ross; Samuel Vaisrub, Afterthoughts on Afterlife; Bertrand Russell, Do We Survive Death?; Part Two—The Experience of Death; Section 7. The Dying Patient: Claire F. Ryder & Diane M. Ross, Terminal Care: Issues and Alternatives; Roberta Lyder Paige & Jane Finkbiner Looney, Hospice Care for the Adult; Cicely Saunders, Should a Patient Know?; Thomas Powers, Learning to Die; Edwin S. Shneidman, Death Work and the Stages of Dying; Elisabeth Kübler-Ross, Interview with a Seventeen-Year-Old Girl; Stewart Alsop, Stay of Execution; Avery Weisman, An Appropriate Death; Section 8. Death and the Child: Edgar Jackson, When to Talk About Death; Robert Kastenbaum, The Kingdom Where Nobody Dies; Earl Grollman, How Does a Child Experience Grief?; Part Three—Survivors of Death; Section 9. Grief: Erich Lindemann, Symptomatology and Management of Acute Grief; Philippe Aries, The Denial of Mourning; Geoffrey Gorer, Death, Grief, and Mourning; Colin Murray Parkes, The Broken Heart; Robert L. Fulton, Anticipatory Grief, Stress, and the Surrogate Griever; Section 10. Widowhood: Helena Z. Lopata, Living through Widowhood; Lynn Caine, Widow; Arnold Toynbee, Man's Concern with Death: Epilogue; Section 11. The Funeral: Vanderlyn Pine, The Care of the Dead: A Historical Portrait; Ruth Mulvey Harmer, Funerals, Fantasy, and Flight; Howard C. Raether, The Place of the Funeral: The Role of the Funeral Director in Contemporary Society; Part Four—Dilemmas of Death; Section 12. Morality and Mortality in Modern Society: Elizabeth Hall with Paul Cameron, Our Failing Reverence for Life; Daniel C. Maguire, Death, Legal and Illegal; Robert M. Veatch, The Legislative Options; Sonya Rudikoff, The Problems of Euthanasia; Robert White & H. Tristram Engelhardt, Jr., A Demand to Die; Julie Fulton, Robert Fulton & Roberta Simmons, The Cadaver Donor and the Gift of Life; Section 13. Suicide: Alex D. Pokorny, Myths about Suicide; Edwin S. Shneidman, Ambivalence and Subintention; Dean Schuyler, Counseling Suicide Survivors; Lael Wertenbaker, Death of a Man; Section 14. Death, War, and the Human Condition: Arnold Toynbee, Death in War; Edwin S. Shneidman, Megadeath: Children of the Nuclear Family; Robert Jay Lifton, Witnessing Survival; Bernard T. Feld, The Consequences of Nuclear War; Section 15. The Death System: Review and Prospectus: Willard Gaylin, Harvesting the Death; Hans Morgenthau, Death in the Nuclear Age; Ignace Lepp, The Experience of Death; Epilogue; Further Reading; Notes about the Authors.

Features. As the editors tell us in their Preface:

This is the tenth in a series of books developed for Courses by Newspaper (CbN). A national program originated and administered by University Extension, University of California, San Diego, and funded by the National Endowment for the Humanities, Courses by Newspaper develops materials for college-level courses that are presented to the general public through the nationwide cooperation of newspapers and participating colleges and universities.

The present volume is the reader, or supplementary anthology for the course. It is a broad collection of previously published materials by well-known authors, interspersed with poems, black and white photographs, and other illustrations. The book is available alone in paperback or hardbound editions, or bound together with a study guide in a single paperback volume (ISBN 0-201-07722-1). According to the editors,

Four objectives have guided the organization of this book and the selection of articles. First, we wanted to cover a broad time spectrum, thereby examining present realities in the light of past circumstances and future possibilities. Second, we have considered death and dying from a variety of perspectives, including the individual, the family, and the society. Third, we have included diverse academic disciplines, from history and sociology through medicine and psychology to literature and ethics. Fourth, we have presented several points of view on such controversial topics as life after death, care of the dying patient, funerals, and moral and ethical dilemmas.

To save space, many of the original articles have been abbreviated for inclusion in this volume. The editors note that they have added "extensive editorial commentary—in the prologue and epilogue, introductions to the major parts, introductory essays for each section, and headnotes for each article" as an integral part of the book, supplementing and highlighting its selections. An annotated bibliography offers suggestions for further reading organized according to the fifteen sections of the text.

Evaluation. We have already indicated that this book is primarily intended to function as the backup reader for the course by newspaper project, which defines its structure. It serves that purpose well. Its size, the effective use of editorial summaries and linking passages, a careful mixture of older and more recent articles, and the counterpoint of poetry and art work all make this quite a satisfying supplementary anthology. The book is also useful as a convenient collection of articles by many well-known authors, i.e., for personal reading or as a reference source. Finally, this book could also be used as a text quite independently of the course by newspaper project.

□   □   □

Garfield, Charles A. *Psychosocial care of the dying patient.* New York: McGraw-Hill, 1978. Pp. xviii + 430. Hardbound, $13.95. ISBN 0-07-022860-4.

Contents. List of Major Contributors; Preface: Charles A. Garfield; Part One—Introduction: 1. Charles A. Garfield, On Caring, Doctors, and Death; Part Two—Guidelines for Terminal Patient Care: 2. Arthur H. Schmale & W. Bradford Patterson, Comfort Care Only: Treatment Guidelines for the Terminal Patient; 3. Cicely Saunders, Terminal Care; 4. Jeanne Quint Benoliel, Care, Communication, and Human Dignity; 5. S. Malkin, Care of the Terminally Ill at Home; 6. Bernard Isaacs, Treatment of the "Irremediable" Elderly Patient; Part Three—Patients and Families Facing Life-threatening Illness: 7. Orville Eugene Kelly, Living with a Life-threatening Illness; 8. Sandra L. Barger, Personal-Professional Support: From a Patient's Point of View; 9. Caroline Driver, What a Dying Man Taught Doctors about Caring; 10. Nancy Harjan, One Family's Experience with Death; 11. Walter Hollander, Jr., & T. Franklin Williams, Dr. Strauss' Last Teaching Session; Part Four—Doctor-Patient Relationships: Emotional Impact: 12. Eric J. Cassell, Treating the Dying: The Doctor vs. the Man Within the Doctor; 13. Morris D. Kerstein, Help for the Young

Physician with Death and Grieving; 14. Charles A. Garfield, Elements of Psychosocial Oncology: Doctor-Patient Relationships in Terminal Illness; 15. Michael A. Friedman, The Changing Relationship Between Cancer Patient and Oncologist; 16. G. W. Milton, Self-willed Death or the Bone-pointing Syndrome; 17. Howard P. Hogshead, The Art of Delivering Bad News; Part Five—Psychological Needs: Recognition and Action; 18. E. Mansell Pattison, The Living-Dying Process; 19. Ernest H. Rosenbaum, Oncology/Hematology and Psychosocial Support of the Cancer Patient; 20. Avery D. Weisman, Misgivings and Misconceptions in the Psychiatric Care of Terminal Patients; 21. Edwin S. Shneidman, Some Aspects of Psychotherapy with Dying Persons; 22. Richard A. Kalish, A Little Myth Is a Dangerous Thing: Research in the Service of the Dying; 23. Robert Kastenbaum, In Control; Part Six—Counseling the Patient's Family: 24. David M. Kaplan, Aaron Smith, Rose Grobstein & Stanley E. Fishman, Family Mediation of Stress; 25. Robert E. Taubman, The Physician and the Dying Patient and His Family; 26. Abraham B. Bergman, Psychological Aspects of Sudden Unexpected Death in Infants and Children; 27. J. Fischhoff & N. O'Brien, After the Child Dies; Part Seven— Specific Issues: 28. Lewis Thomas, Notes of a Biology Watcher: The Long Habit; 29. Ernlé W. D. Young, Reflections on Life and Death; 30. Milton D. Heifetz, Ethics in Human Biology; 31. Mona Wasow, Human Sexuality and Serious Illness; 32. Harry S. Abram, Adaptation to Open Heart Surgery: A Psychiatric Study of Response to the Threat of Death; 33. Harry S. Abram, Survival by Machine: The Psychological Stress of Chronic Hemodialysis; Part Eight—Care of the Dying Patient: Recent Developments: 34. Charles A. Garfield & Rachel Ogren Clark, A Community Model of Psychosocial Support for Patients and Families Facing Life-threatening Illness: The SHANTI Project; 35. Robert Woodson, Hospice Care in Terminal Illness; 36. R. Melzack, J. G. Ofiesh & B. M. Mount, The Brompton Mixture: Effects on Pain in Cancer Patients; 37. Balfour M. Mount, I. Ajemian & J. F. Scott, Use of the Brompton Mixture in Treating the Chronic Pain of Malignant Disease; 38. Balfour M. Mount, The Problem of Caring for the Dying in a General Hospital: The Palliative Care Unit as a Possible Solution; 39. David Barton, John M. Flexner, Jan van Eys & Charles E. Scott, Death and Dying: A Course for Medical Students; Epilogue: Charles A. Garfield; Name Index; Subject Index.

Features. This is a very large collection. Many of the articles have been published elsewhere during the early and middle years of this decade, though several appear to have been newly written for this volume. This list of contributors is studded with well-known names and their contributions address many central issues, though they differ greatly in length and character. The editor speaks of this book as "the definitive (and perhaps only) resource text primarily for physicians on psychosocial care of the dying patient." Further, he states that its purpose "is as much to inspire as to provide information." By that, he means that he wants to overcome "the single greatest obstacle to providing adequate emotional support to dying patients and their families," i.e., "the professional distinction between 'us' and 'them'" with all the inequities of status and technological mastery that that distinction implies.

Evaluation. The principal advantage of this volume is that it brings together a large number of recent articles on this important subject by respected writers. The disadvantage is that these pieces are merely set alongside one another in terms of topical similarity. Beyond his brief introduction to the book as a whole, Garfield provides no further introductory or linking materials for the remaining parts or chapters. One could not easily sit down and read through a volume of this sort, but it is a rich and convenient source for reference purposes and background reading. At the same time, too much bulk can be a disadvantage, especially when one has in mind busy physicians and medical students. However, where sufficient time is available or when used selectively, this volume can serve as a good textbook for such audiences. In the final analysis, instructors will have to weigh its virtues and deficiencies against those of other texts in its field and the needs of their students.

□   □   □

Grollman, Earl A. (Ed.). *Concerning death: A practical guide for the living.* Boston: Beacon, 1974. Pp. xviii + 365. Hardbound, $9.95. Paperbound, $3.95. ISBN 0-8070-2764-2 hardbound; 0-8070-2765-0 paperbound.

Contents. Introduction: Earl A. Grollman; Chapter 1: Edgar N. Jackson, Grief; Chapter 2: N. H. Cassem, Care of the Dying Person; Chapter 3: Melvin J. Krant, The Doctor, Fatal Illness, and the Family; Chapter 4: Earl A. Grollman, Children and Death; Chapter 5: Merle R. Jordan, The Protestant Way in Death and Mourning; Chapter 6: Richard J. Butler, The Roman Catholic Way in Death and Mourning; Chapter 7: Earl A. Grollman, The Jewish Way in Death and Mourning; Chapter 8: Matthew H. Ross, The Law and Death; Chapter 9: Andrew J. Lyons, Insurance and Death; Chapter 10: Cyril H. Wecht, The Coroner and Death; Chapter 11: Howard C. Raether & Robert C. Slater, The Funeral and the Funeral Director; Chapter 12: William Morgan, How to Select a Cemetery; Chapter 13: Ian R. Winters, Choosing a Memorial; Chapter 14: Paul Irion, To Cremate or Not; Chapter 15: Benjamin A. Barnes, Organ Donation and Transplantation; Chapter 16: Regina Flesch, The Condolence or Sympathy Call; Chapter 17: Edgar N. Jackson, The Condolence Letter; Chapter 18: Robert L. Buchanan, The Widow and Widower; Chapter 19: Earl A. Grollman, What You Should Know About Suicide; Chapter 20: Sandra L. Bertman, Death Education in the Face of a Taboo; Index.

Features. In his introduction Grollman bases this book on a now-familiar litany of comments regarding our society and death: It is a forbidden topic, denied because of lack of experience (resulting from new mortality rates, institutionalization, and various demographic alterations) and because of our difficulties in coping with it as a personal threat in a context of shifting conceptualizations and values. Nevertheless, he notes a recent broadening of interest in death and dying, and he asserts that we can no longer avoid these subjects: "There can be no death without life, and, conversely, no life without death." Our viewpoint should be one of interpersonal community and mutual assistance: "In helping others to solve the inexplicability of non-existence, we strengthen ourselves in the realization that dying and death are phases of life and living. Each one of us is a helper." This book, then, is a collection of newly published materials intended as "a practical guide for the living," i.e., for all of us in our roles as helpers of self and of neighbor. Its emphasis on practicality and counsel defines its distinctive approach to death education.

One need not wait for tragedy before confronting these fundamental and inevitable questions. This book should encourage the reader to share thoughts, perceptions, and knowledge with the living and to plan as rationally and meaningfully for that unavoidable moment of separation. And when the crisis does come, this volume can be used as a guide for the emotion-laden, death-related situations. The adequacy of your counsel may be the monumental factor in your future well-being as well as for loved ones who remain. The book is then dedicated to the inevitability of death and the preparation for life.

Evaluation. This is a helpful book that will work for personal use, for discussion groups, and for courses emphasizing practical assistance for lay persons. Its contributors—many of whom are well-known and many of whom come from the Massachusetts area or nearby—write clearly and effectively. The text employs a general question-and-answer format with frequent thematic or topical headings. Quite often, additional readings are suggested and specialized vocabulary is defined. It is perhaps notable that some of the topics treated in this volume are hardly mentioned in other texts, e.g., the coroner, selecting cemeteries and memorials, and condolence calls or letters. In short, this book does not emphasize clinical and experimental data or theoretical interpretations, but it fulfills its promise as a practical guide to the facts and feelings surrounding death.

□   □   □

Kastenbaum, Robert. *Death, society, and human experience.* St. Louis, MO: C. V. Mosby Co., 1977. Pp. xii + 328. Paperbound, $7.95. ISBN 0-8016-2617-X.

Contents. Preface; Chapter 1: Introduction; Chapter 2: Death Happens; Chapter 3: Death Is; Chapter 4: Death Is Like; Chapter 5: Death Means; Chapter 6: The Individual in the Death System: Two Perspectives; Chapter 7: A Larger Perspective: The Death System; Chapter 8: Disaster and the Death System; Chapter 9: Intimations of Mortality: In Childhood's Hour; Chapter 10: Death as Life's Companion: The Adult Years; Chapter 11: Dying: Transition From Life; Chapter 12: Dying: Reflection on Life; Chapter 13: Dying: Innovations in Care; Chapter 14: Bereavement, Grief, Mourning; Chapter 15: Suicide; Chapter 16: Between Life and Death; Chapter 17: Death Will Be; Suggested Readings; Index.

Features. The focus of this book is on what Kastenbaum calls "the interplay between the individual and the *death system*." By "death system"—a notion that he had proposed several years earlier, but one that only reaches maturity in this volume—Kastenbaum means a "socio-physical network by which the relationship to mortality is mediated and expressed." Hence, this is a book centering on psychosocial dimensions of death and their manifestations, one in which the many ramifications of death are considered from the standpoint of "the individual *in* society." Kastenbaum's work is intended both as a textbook for a course, and "for the person of any age who is willing to be his or her own instructor and student combined." For either situation, the author gives us all some useful advice.

> I would encourage an approach in which both emotional and intellectual, both individual and socially oriented, both experiential and scholarly facets of the educational process are welcomed. A book or a course in "death education" can make its most significant contribution if it helps us to integrate our total selves rather than lead us to either "emotional trips" on the one hand, or aloof intellectual analysis on the other. There is no better area in which to bring our thoughts, skills, and feelings together.

We are counseled to be tolerant and patient in exploring these subjects, to listen carefully to ourselves and to others, to respect our own thoughts and feelings as well as those of everyone who shares our quest, and to seek to integrate what we learn into a responsible whole. With this in mind, we might restate the main topics that Kastenbaum addresses in somewhat less cryptic language than that of the Table of Contents: the many ways death appears in our lives both as an event and as a state; the items it is commonly said to resemble or to signify; individual perspectives concerning one's own death as contrasted with the death of the other, and the larger viewpoint of the death system; disaster and its social implications; lifespan perspectives from childhood and from adulthood; dying as a many-sided process, one that grows out of our present modes of living, and an experience that can be made easier by new forms of care like hospices, by better education, and by simple human presence; bereavement and the situation of survivors; an overview of suicide; the difficult case of Karen Ann Quinlan; and an orientation for the future.

Chapters are not too long, there are occasional exercises, and each chapter usually ends with a summary section.

Evaluation. Kastenbaum is one of the few people who can do a good job in a survey of this breadth. He knows his material and is well organized. In this book he makes the most of his particular areas of expertise. However, like all single-author, "systematic" texts, this volume does sacrifice a certain comprehensiveness and the competition of diverse viewpoints. Kastenbaum's broad scope partly compensates for this. But restrictions are evident when one seeks treatments of such specialized topics as euthanasia, definition of death, war, and "unnatural" death, or for the broad framework of history and religious or philosophical values. However, these are limitations, not failings. Throughout the book the manner is gentle and sensitive, and the writing style clear and readable. Within its acknowledged parameters, this is a useful book for personal reading or for classroom use at many levels.

□   □   □

Kübler-Ross, Elisabeth. *On death and dying.* New York: Macmillan, 1969. Pp. xii + 289. Hardbound, $6.95. Paperbound, $1.95. Library of Congress Catalog Card No. 69-11789.

Contents. Preface; I—On the Fear of Death; II—Attitudes Toward Death and Dying; III—First Stage: Denial and Isolation; IV—Second Stage: Anger; V—Third Stage: Bargaining; VI—Fourth Stage: Depression; VII—Fifth Stage: Acceptance; VIII—Hope; IX—The Patient's Family; X—Some Interviews with Terminally Ill Patients; XI—Reactions to the Seminar on Death and Dying; XII—Therapy with the Terminally Ill; Bibliography.

Features. This is a classic in the field and has probably introduced more people to the area of death and dying than any other work. In her Preface, Elisabeth Kübler-Ross states:

> I have worked with dying patients for the past two and a half years and this book will tell about the beginning of this experiment, which turned out to be a meaningful and instructive experience for all participants. It is not meant to be a textbook on how to manage dying patients, nor is it intended as a complete study of the psychology of the dying. It is simply an account of a new and challenging opportunity to refocus on the patient as a human being, to include him in dialogues, to learn from him the strengths and weaknesses of our hospital manage-

ment of the patient. We have asked him to be our teacher so that we may learn more about the final stages of life with all its anxieties, fears, and hopes. I am simply telling the stories of my patients who shared their agonies, their expectations, and their frustrations with us. It is hoped that it will encourage others not to shy away from the "hopelessly" sick but to get closer to them, as they can help them much during their final hours.

Included in this book are the five stages of dying the author has identified and which have become widely known though often misunderstood. Each stage is discussed in a separate chapter, followed by an excellent chapter on hope.

Evaluation. This extremely readable book (a large bulk is organized around interviews with patients) aims to sensitize the reader to the lonely and inhumane treatment of the dying patient. As Elisabeth Kübler-Ross says

If this book serves no other purpose but to sensitize family members of terminally ill patients and hospital personnel to the implicit communications of dying patients, then it has fulfilled its task. [If it] can help the patient and his family to get 'in tune' to each other's needs and come to an acceptance of an unavoidable reality together, we can help to avoid much unnecessary agony and suffering on the part of the dying and even more so on the part of the family that is left behind.

Elisabeth Küber-Ross states in the Preface that this work is not designed to be a textbook on the management of dying patients but instead an opportunity to refocus on the patient as a human being. Taken in this light, it can be highly recommended as supplemental reading for an introductory experience in a death and dying course.

□ □ □

Mills, Liston O. (Ed.). *Perspective on death.* Nashville: Abingdon, 1969. Pp. 288. Hardbound, $6.50. ISBN 0-687-30824-0. Paperbound 1974, $4.95. ISBN 0-687-30825-9.

Contents. Introduction: Liston O. Mills; Chapter I: Lou H. Silberman, Death in the Hebrew Bible and Apocalyptic Literature; Chapter II: Leander E. Keck, New Testament Views of Death; Chapter III: Milton McC. Gatch, Some Theological Reflections on Death From the Early Church Through the Reformation; Chapter IV: John Killinger, Death and Transcendence in Contemporary Literature; Chapter V: William May, The Sacral Power of Death in Contemporary Experience; Chapter VI: Lloyd C. Elam, A Psychiatric Perspective on Death; Chapter VII: Ernest Q. Campbell, Death as a Social Practice; Chapter VIII: James T. Laney, Ethics and Death; Chapter IX: Liston O. Mills, Pastoral Care of the Dying and the Bereaved; Index

Features. "Until recently," says Mills in the Introduction to this book, "death has been largely the domain of the Christian church in the Western world." One could face death and life with hope stemming from belief in God and an eternal life. However, "over the past decade numerous books and essays have appeared describing a transition in the Western—and particularly the American—view of death. A break with the tradition is said to be in process." Religious conviction is undermined, we opt for life, and death is avoided or denied. Many agree that "the results of the present stance have been to rob life of much of its depth and meaning;" this volume is an effort to test the necessity or the appropriateness of that stance. It results from a course offered at the Vanderbilt Divinity School in 1967.

> A fourfold purpose guided our decisions to offer the course and to publish the results. First, we wanted to make available the biblical teachings on death and their subsequent development and interpretation by the church. Second, we wanted to investigate current concepts of death as these are reflected in contemporary literature and contemporary theology. Third, we sought to include material which would help the students and the reader to appreciate the meanings of death as a psychological and a social event. Finally, we wanted to present some of the pressing ethical and pastoral problems associated with the care of the dying and the bereaved.

In short, this book represents an intersection of psychosocial, theological and pastoral, and biblico-historical perspectives on death and dying. But Mills adds an important disclaimer: "At no time have we considered these statements to constitute the Christian view of death. We have simply desired to raise issues arising out of Christian faith which appear pertinent to our current situation."

Evaluation. This book reports some modulations of death concepts and their development in the Judeo-Christian tradition. It then includes contemporary viewpoints from literature, theology, psychiatry, and social science to affirm the power of death and the value of developing ways to acknowledge it in the context of a larger commitment to life. Finally, these themes are illustrated in applications to ethical and pastoral problems. The book will be of greatest interest to students of the Christian tradition and to those who assume that it is monolithic, or that it cannot speak to contemporary issues in death and dying. The book might also serve as a text for a course in pastoral theology.

□   □   □

Neale, Robert E. *The art of dying.* New York: Harper & Row, 1973. Pp. xiv + 158. Hardbound, $5.95. ISBN 0-06-066090-2.

Contents. Preface; Death; Exercise 1, In the Midst of Life: Intimacy with Death; Possibility of Awareness; Usefulness of Awareness; Exercise 2, Fear of Death and Life: Universality of Fear; Fears of Death; Fears of Life; Gestation; Exercise 3, Death in Life: Prevalence of Suicide; Suicide as a Problem; Prevention by Permission; Exercise 4, Transformation by Grief: Task of the Bereaved; Task of the Dying; Task of Everyman; Rebirth; Exercise 5, Life in Death: Images of Death; Concepts of Death; Beliefs about Death; Exercise 6, In the Midst of Death: Witness Through Death; Consummation of Life; Wonder; Notes; Selected Bibliography.

Features. In his Preface, Neale says that "the purpose of these exercises is to facilitate our own movement from death to life." In other words, "although the focus of the exercises is our own death, the intent is exploration of our own living." In short, this little book is a reflection on death and life conducted on the basis of a series of mental exercises. The exercises are linked by the author's text, which provides background information, explanation, analysis, and comment. The book as a whole is intended to facilitate a process of personal confrontation and exploration, with the goal of making it easier to face the prospect of one's own death. Neale adds the following advice to the reader, which helps to describe the sort of process that he has in mind:

> The exercises are constructed to help you explore yourself. Mechanically all you need bring to them are pencil and paper. But no exercise is self-working. I hope you will not read all the exercises in one evening, seek only information and opinion from the authorities, or reflect only on the dying and living of others. To do so would severely limit the possibility of genuine wonder. Rather you should do one exercise a week in the company of one or more persons. Taking time, reflecting on yourself and sharing with others, will help the process rule over the content.

The exercises are mainly questionnaires or other forms of paper and pencil probes. There is also an annotated bibliography correlated to the appropriate sections of the text.

Evaluation. This is an insightful book that might be used most profitably for personal reading or as the basis for a class or discussion group emphasizing affective concerns and self-exploration. The text is elegant in its simplicity and gracefulness. Neale knows his subject and he draws on resources from his own experiences with death and from his work as a pastor, chaplain, and professor at Union Theological Seminary in New York. He realizes that there are personal resolutions regarding mortality, but no universal "answers" for everyone. And he is aware that an adequate accommodation with death entails a balance of elements that is rarely achieved by a one-sided insistence on any single coping mechanism.

□   □   □

Parkes, Colin Murray. *Bereavement: Studies of grief in adult life.* New York: International Universities Press, 1972. Pp. 233. Hardbound, $12.50. ISBN 0-8236-2230-40.

Contents. Foreword by John Bowlby; Acknowledgments; Introduction; 1. The Cost of Commitment; 2. The Broken Heart; 3. Alarm; 4. Searching; 5. Mitigation; 6. Anger and Guilt; 7. Gaining a New Identity; 8. Atpical Grief; 9. Determinants of Grief; 10. Helping the Bereaved; 11. Reactions to Other Types of Loss; Appendix; Some National UK and US Organizations Offering Help to the Bereaved; References; Index.

Features. There have been few books to date on bereavement which are derived from empirical research. This is one of the few, and a welcome addition to the literature. Based on the author's and others' research studies over a 12-year span and a biological theory of bereavement, the book describes in successive chapters "the nature of the principal components of the reaction of bereavement, the effects of bereavement upon physical and mental health, the non-specific reaction to stress in general, the highly specific 'search' component that characterizes grieving, the ways in which we attempt to avoid or postpone grief, the part played by feelings of anger and self-reproach, and the gradual build-up of a fresh identity. Also discussed are the morbid or atypical directions that grief can sometimes take, and what factors tend to exacerbate the grief phenomenon. The author treats bereavement as an enormous change, a psychosocial transition, when individuals must reassess their world and the part they play in it.

The book discusses a number of important bereavement studies, and the Appendix includes statistical information for those readers who wish to avail themselves of it. Other types of loss, such as of a home or of a limb, are discussed as well. Parkes believes that a basic understanding of grief can provide the basis for comprehending human behavior in a variety of crises. He says that "times of transition are times of opportunity and any confrontation with an unfamiliar world is both an opportunity for autonomous mastery and a threat to one's established adjustment to life."

Evaluation. This is a most valuable treatment of bereavement. Parkes has surveyed the literature and presented the principal research studies and his own work, indicating that grief has a potentially detrimental effect on physical and mental health. Written with clarity, understanding and conviction, this book is recommended as a resource for students and researchers in this particular area, as well as for other professionals. The interested lay person could find it helpful as well.

◻   ◻   ◻

Prichard, Elizabeth R., Collard, Jean, Orcutt, Ben A., Kutscher, Austin H., Seeland, Irene, & Lefkowitz, Nathan (Eds.), with the editorial assistance of Lillian G. Kutscher. *Social work with the dying patient and the family.* New York: Columbia University Press, 1977. Pp. xiv + 350. Hardbound, $17.50. ISBN 0-231-04021-0.

Contents. Acknowledgment; Preface: Elizabeth R. Prichard; Part I—Introduction: 1. Leon H. Ginsberg, The Social Worker's Role; 2. Gary A. Lloyd, The Expression of Grief as Deviant Behavior in American Culture; Part II—The Family and Death: 3. Ben A. Orcutt, Stress in Family Interaction When a Member is Dying; 4. Hilda C. M. Arndt & Mittie Gruber, Helping Families Cope with Acute Grief and Anticipatory Grief; 5. C. Murray Parkes, Evaluation of Family Care in Terminal Illness; 6. Delia Battin, Irwin Gerber, Alfred Wiener & Arthur Arkin, Clinical Observations on Bereaved Individuals; 7. Marion Wijnberg & Mary C. Schwartz, Competence or Crisis; Part III—Facing Death in Childhood, Adolescence, Middle- and Old-Age: 8. Erna Furman, Bereavement in Childhood; 9. Grace Fields, The Dying Child and His Family; 10. Rachel Rustow Aubrey, Adolescents and Death; 11. Mary K. Parent, The Losses of Middle-Age and Related Developmental Tasks; 12. Jordan I. Kosberg, Social Work with Geriatric Patients and Their Families; Part IV—Interdisciplinary Resources in the Community: 13. Barbara McNulty, Home Care for the Terminal Patient and His Family; 14. Jean Markham & Sylvia Lack, The Social Worker and Terminal Illness; 15. Lee H. Suszycki, Effective Nursing Home Placement for the Elderly Dying Patient; 16. Sharol Cannon, Program Development for Problems Associated with Death; 17. John Freund, When Should the Clergyman Be Called?; 18. Larry Lister, Cultural Perspectives on Death as Viewed from within a Selected Nursing Facility; Part V—Therapeutic Approaches and Concepts: 19. Phyllis Mervis, Talking About the Unmentionable; 20. Clelia P. Goodyear, Group Therapy with Advanced Cancer Patients: What Are the Issues?; 21. Ruth R. Boyd, Developing New Norms for Parents of Fatally Ill Children to Facilitate Coping; 22. Phyllis R. Silverman, Bereavement as a Normal Life Transition; 23. Burton Gummer & Diane M. Simpson, Private Troubles or Public Issues; Part VI—The Education of the Social Worker: 24. Rosalind S. Miller, Teaching Death and Dying Content in the Social Work Curriculum; 25. Eda C. Goldstein, Teaching a Social Work Perspective on the Dying Patient and His Family; 26. Helen Cassidy, Helping the Social Work Student Deal with Death and Dying; 27. Lois Jaffe, The Dying Professor as Death Educator; Index: Compiled by Lucia Bove.

Features. This volume, sponsored by the Foundation of Thanatology, is a collection of papers that appear to be published here for the first time. In her Preface, Elizabeth Prichard describes the book in the following way:

> The contributors to this book present a view of social work's thanatological tasks, reviewing these from the historical perspective of social work as a profession. In their papers are discussions of the impact of death on the family in its fullest consequences; interventive techniques and practice modalities; preparation methods and aims of research. These are presented also with the hope that the need for further understanding of the dimensions of loss and grief will be highlighted for all allied health practitioners, academicians, and researchers.

The contributors represent diverse backgrounds and interests; their papers include case reports, theoretical analyses, and guidelines for practical intervention. The editors have assembled these papers in broad topical groupings without further introductory or linking materials.

Evaluation. The distinctive characteristic of this volume is its emphasis on the field of social work. Social workers have historically been concerned with situations of interpersonal separation and loss, but until recently they—like many other professional groups—have perhaps not always paid as much overt attention as was rightly due to problems associated with death, dying, and bereavement. However, as this book demonstrates, social workers are an important group of professionals with natural routes of access as counselors and caregivers before, during, and after death. We cannot afford to ignore the resources of a profession that is capable of providing valuable assistance during both the dying trajectory and the period of bereavement, that can intervene throughout the lifespan, and that can operate in a variety of institutional or noninstitutional settings. Practicing social workers who are interested in the special focus of this volume will find it a readable and useful resource. It can also serve, either alone or with some thoughtful supplementation, as a textbook for the education of social workers in this particular area.

□   □   □

Quint, Jeanne C. *The nurse and the dying patient.* New York: Macmillan, 1967. Pp. vii + 307. Paperbound, $6.25. Library of Congress Catalog Card No. 67-14418.

Contents. Foreword: Helen Nahm; Preface; 1. The Student, The School, and the Problem of Death: Development of Identity Educational Socialization, Bereavement; Nurses and the Problem of Death; Social Change and the Education of Nurses; 2. Dying Patients, Death, and the Curriculum: The Curriculum Emphasis on Life-Saving Goals; Assignment Characteristics and Standardized Teaching Practices; The Influence of Hospital Locale; Assignment Purpose; Accountability, as

Student and as Nurse; In Summary; 3. Teacher Perspectives on Death: Conditions Affecting the Teacher's Work World; Conditions Affecting Perspectives on Dying; Types of Perspectives; Reactions to Teaching About Death; The Faculty as Models; A Resume; 4. Conversations with Dying Patients: Rules Governing Professional Conversation; The Assignment Context and Recognition of Dying; Awareness and Non-difficult Conversation; Conversations Described as Difficult; Conditions Further Maximizing Difficulties; The Management of Conversations with Dying Patients; Some Conversational Consequences for Students; 5. Encounters with Death: Death in the Hospital; First Encounters and the Unfamiliar; Adequate and Inadequate Performance; Reactions to Death and Dying; The Significance of Unassigned Events; The Aftermath of Encounters with Death; 6. Nurse Identity and Care of Dying Patients: Conditions Which Contribute to Identity Stresses; The Basic Student in Nursing; The Beginning Staff Nurse; The Graduate Student in Nursing; Rewards, Gratification, and the Nurse Identity; In Summary; 7. Some Consequences for Dying Patients: The Influence of Assignment Length; The Unreported Events in Patient Assignments; Nurse Responsibility and Accountable Assignments; The Use of the Clergy as a Resource; Some Results of the Teachers' Psychiatric Emphasis; Additional Effects of Inexperience; A Proviso; 8. Implications for Change: Cultural Values and Nursing Practices; Some Proposals for Change; In Conclusion; Appendix A: Study Background and Methods; Appendix B: Some Assignment Policies; Index.

Features. This book is part of a larger study carried out at the University of California School of Nursing that examined the question of how nursing and medical personnel give care to dying patients. As such, its unique quality rests in its empirical underpinnings and objective approach. In the Foreword, Helen Nahm states: "The theme of Miss Quint's book may be stated as follows: The dying patient's behavior is a function of his interactions with significant persons around him. If these interactions are such that the patient is enabled to live each moment as it comes, he will gain the added psychological strength he needs to face the approach of death."

Quint identifies and discusses many difficult problems concerning care of dying patients, such as the lack of common agreement about what is good in caring for the patient, the frequent failure in medical personnel to live up to unrealistic expectations, the problem of the registered nurse who returns to school and is threatened by her or his own insecurity in learning new methods of functioning.

The final chapter offers concrete suggestions for change in nursing curricula, and broader experiences for nurses. Among the suggestions are: a planned and coordinated teaching program during the first year which focuses specifically on nursing care of the dying patient; assistance of sensitive, perceptive nurse teachers who know what happens to patients in hospitals; better communication among hospital personnel; and provision for support to nurses involved in care. The author feels that innovativeness in teaching and practice of nursing is essential, including the need to break old, established patterns in dealing with physicians and to encourage the nurse to speak out for the patient.

This book reports on what happens to students of nursing when they must interact with terminal patients. Nurses are systematically prepared to take care of the dying patient's body but are rarely given preparation for dealing with psychosocial support. Miss Quint says: "The general taboo about death has resulted in nursing curricula which have given minimal attention to many serious issues and difficult decisions which nurses face in providing care for dying patients and their families. Phrased somewhat differently, cultural values concerning death have led to a gap in the education of nurses and, in turn, to a gap in the nursing services available to patients who are dying. Undoubtedly the curricula in medical school shows a similar gap."

Evaluation. This book is a classic in its field. Published in 1967, it reflects an early concern and desire on the part of the author and her colleagues to correct the deficits in nurses' training and experience. Despite its age, the material is still as relevant as it was when newly published. Because the data are based on empirical study, the work carries authenticity and credibility. The book is a valuable resource for pre- and in-service education for health care personnel, particularly nurses.

□   □   □

Schoenberg, Bernard, Gerber, Irwin, Wiener, Alfred, Kutscher, Austin H., Peretz, David, & Carr, Arthur C. (Eds.), with the editorial assistance of Lillian G. Kutscher. *Bereavement: Its psychosocial aspects.* New York: Columbia University Press, 1975. Pp. xx + 380. Hardbound, $15.00. ISBN 0-231-03974-3.

Contents. Acknowledgment; Foreword: Victor W. Sidel, Services for the Bereaved: A Social-Medicine Perspective; Preface: Austin H. Kutscher & Lillian G. Kutscher; Part One—Fundamental Concepts: 1. Arthur C. Carr, Bereavement as a Relative Experience; 2. Ned H. Cassem, Bereavement as Indispensable for Growth; 3. Joseph H. Smith, On the Work of Mourning; 4. David Maddison & Beverley Raphael, Conjugal Bereavement and the Social Network; 5. Paul C. Rosenblatt, Uses of Ethnography in Understanding Grief and Mourning; Part Two—The Bereavement Process: 6. Alfred Wiener, Irwin Gerber, Delia Battin & Arthur M. Arkin, The Process and Phenomenology of Bereavement; 7. W. Dewi Rees, The Bereaved and Their Hallucinations; 8. Paula J. Clayton, Weight Loss and Sleep Disturbance in Bereavement; 9. John J. Schwab, Jean M. Chalmers, Shirley J. Conroy, Patricia B. Farris, & Robert E. Markush, Studies in Grief: A Preliminary Report; Part Three—The Bereaved Family: 10. Jeffrey C. Lerner, Changes in Attitudes Toward Death: The Widow in Great Britain in the Early Twentieth Century; 11. C. Murray Parkes, Unexpected and Untimely Bereavement: A Statistical Study of Young Boston Widows and Widowers; 12. Thomas C. Welu, Pathological Bereavement: A Plan for Its Prevention; 13. Bruce L. Danto, Bereavement and the Widows of Slain Police Officers; 14. Margot Tallmer, Sexual and Age Factors in Childhood Bereavement; 15. John E. Schowalter, Parent Death and Child Bereavement; 16. Rose Wolfson, A Time to Speak; 17. John W. Bedell, The Maternal Orphan: Paternal Perceptions of Mother Loss; 18. Phyllis R. Silverman & Sam M. Silverman, Withdrawal in Bereaved Children; Part Four—The Health Professional: 19. Melvin J. Krant, The Health Professional; 20. Alan Lyall & Mary Vachon, Professional Roles in Thanatology; 21. Phyllis Caroff & Rose Dobrof, The Helping Process with Bereaved Families; 22. Marta Ochoa, Elizabeth R. Prichard & Ellen L. Shwartzer, Social Work and the Bereaved; 23. Clara L. Adams & Joseph R. Proulx, The Role of the Nurse in the Maintenance and Restoration of Hope; 24. Elsa Poslusny & Margaret Kelley Arroyo, Bereavement and the Nursing Student; Part Five—Therapeutic Intervention: 25. Gerald Adler, Morton Beiser, Rosanne Cole, Lee Johnston & Melvin J. Krant, Approaches to Intervention with Dying Patients and Their Families: A Case Discussion; 26. Delia Battin, Arthur M. Arkin, Irwin Gerber & Alfred Wiener, Coping and Vulnerability Among the Aged Bereaved; 27. Irwin Gerber, Alfred Wiener, Delia Battin & Arthur M. Arkin, Grief Therapy to the Aged Bereaved; 28. Vamik D. Volkan, "Re-Grief" Therapy; 29. Arthur W. Arkin & Delia Battin, A Technical Device for the Psychotherapy of Pathological Bereavement; 30. Glen W. Davidson, The "Waiting Vulture Syndrome"; 31. Bernard Schoenberg, Arthur C. Carr, David Peretz, Austin H. Kutscher & Daniel J. Cherico, Advice of the Bereaved for the Bereaved; Index: Compiled by Lucia Bove.

Features. This is one of many similar volumes sponsored by Austin H. Kutscher and his colleagues at The Foundation of Thanatology. Its orgin is indicated by the following comment from Austin and Lillian Kutscher in their Preface: "Caring for the dying is a response to a necessary professional commitment; but there is also a more dimly recognized but not necessarily less urgent call for attention to the problems of those who are being exposed to anticipatory grief, acute grief, and bereavement." Put this baldly the point is obvious, just as it is obvious that for each person who dies many are normally left bereaved. But "the literature, to date, seems to indicate that for every dozen professionals involved with the dying patient, only a few are involved in the continuing problems of the bereaved-to-be and the bereaved." This book aims to help correct that imbalance, addressing (as Victor Sidel says in the Foreword) health services planning, community organization, and the training and role of health workers, among other topics. Or, as the Kutschers say:

> In this collection of essays, the multidisciplinary approach (always implicit in our endeavors) has been taken. The contributors have examined the psychosocial aspects of bereavement and have formed insights from sociological research; clinical studies based on psychiatric, psychological, and physiological determinations; and theoretical designs that have been augmented by anecdotal information. The value of interdisciplinary health support systems, the usefulness of self-help groups, and the prospects of methods of crisis intervention with all age groups are a few among the significant topics considered.

Evaluation. There is always a certain unevenness and repetition in books of this sort, but this volume is generally well-designed and draws on good contributors. It brings together case histories, clinical materials, research data, guidelines for caregivers, theoretical interpretation, and humanistic concern. It is a useful reference source and would serve as a good general textbook for courses studying bereavement and the care of those who are grieving.

□   □   □

Schulz, Richard. *The psychology of death, dying, and bereavement.* Reading, MA: Addison-Wesley, 1978. Pp. xiv + 197. Paperbound, $7.95. ISBN 0-201-07328-5.

Contents. Preface; Acknowledgments; Chapter 1: Introduction: General Issues and Research Strategies; Chapter 2: Thinking About Death; Chapter 3: The Demography of Death; Chapter 4: The Terminal Phase of Life; Chapter 5: Lengthening Life; Chapter 6: Surviving Death: Grief and Bereavement; Chapter 7: Death Education; Bibliography; Index.

Features. Schulz provides a succinct characterization of this volume in the opening paragraph of his Preface.

> This book is designed to fill an existing gap in the literature on death and dying. It presents a comprehensive review and analysis of the available empirical findings on death, dying, and bereavement. Such an analysis is possible because of the large quantities of systematic empirical data that have been collected on this topic in the last two decades. However, the usefulness of these data have in the past been limited because of the absence of an integrative review.

In short, "the primary focus of this book is a critical analysis and synthesis of available data." The aim is not so much to break new trails as to define the present state of our knowledge about psychological aspects of major death-related issues, and to point the way for future research. Schulz envisions a broad readership for his text: "audiences ranging in sophistication from freshmen to graduate students in psychology and professional schools." Neophytes and college students are introduced to the psychological perspective as distinct from personal, humanistic, and philosophical viewpoints; practitioners are brought up to date on current knowledge and given practical guidance; and graduate students or researchers are guided toward future research directions.

Evaluation. This book is essentially an introductory guide to a certain set of topics in the field of death, dying, and bereavement. The subject does not easily lend itself to disciplinary compartmentalization, but Schulz consistently emphasizes issues that might seem to be of greatest interest to professional psychologists. More importantly, he always tries to draw upon or lead discussions towards quantitative data and empirical research. The effect is to provide a handy but fairly brief review of recent research on a large number of questions. A work of this sort lacks the scope and depth of a book as Kastenbaum's *Death, Society, and Human Experience* (q.v), but it can be useful as a supplementary text or as an overview for beginners.

□   □   □

Shneidman, Edwin S. *Death: Current Perspectives.* Palo Alto, CA: Mayfield Publishing Co., 1976. Pp. xxiv + 547. Hardbound, $12.95. Paperbound, $7.95. ISBN 0-87484-333-2 hardbound; 0-87484-332-4 paperbound.

Contents. Preface; Introduction; Epigrammatic Prologue: John Fowles, Human Dissatisfactions; Part One—Cultural Perspectives on Death; Chapter 1: Concepts of Death: Arnold Toynbee, Various Ways in Which Human Beings Have Sought to Reconcile Themselves to the Face of Death; Milton McC. Gatch, The Biblical Tradition; Rosalind Heywood, Death and Psychical Research: The Present Position Regarding the Evidence of Survival; Bertrand Russell, Do We Survive Death?; Chapter 2: Death as a Social Disease: Geoffrey Gorer, The Pornography of Death; Philippe Ariès, Forbidden Death; Jonathan Baird, The Funeral Industry in Boston; Joel Baruch, Combat Death; Robert Jay Lifton & Eric Olson, The Nuclear Age; Gil Elliot, Agents of Death; Part Two—Societal Perspectives on Death; Chapter 3: The Demography of Death: Monroe Lerner, When, Why, and Where People Die; Calvin Goldscheider, The Mortality Revolution; David Sudnow, Death, Uses of a Corpse, and Social Worth; Calvin Goldscheider, The Social Inequality of Death; Chapter 4: The Determination of Death: Barner G. Glaser & Anselm L. Strauss, Initial Definitions of Dying Trajectory; A. Keith Mant, The Medical Definition of Death; Robert M. Veatch, Brain Death; Edwin S. Shneidman, The Death Certificate; Thomas L. Shaffer, Psychological Autopsies in

Judicial Opinions; Part Three—Interpersonal Perspectives on Death; Chapter 5: The Participants of Death: Barney G. Glaser & Anselm L. Strauss, The Ritual Drama of Mutual Pretense; Elisabeth Kübler-Ross, Coping with the Reality of Terminal Illness in the Family; John Hinton, Speaking of Death with the Dying; Elisabeth Kübler-Ross, Therapy with the Terminally Ill; Chapter 6: The Survivors of Death: Arnold Toynbee, The Relation Between Life and Death, Living and Dying; Colin Murray Parkes, The Broken Heart; Edwin S. Shneidman, Postvention and the Survivor-Victim; Phyllis Rolfe Silverman, The Widow-to-Widow Program: An Experiment in Preventive Intervention; Part Four—Personal Perspectives on Death; Chapter 7: Psychological Aspects of Death: Robert Kastenbaum & Ruth Aisenberg, Death as a Thought; Herman Feifel, Attitudes toward Death: A Psychological Perspective; Samuel L. Feder, Attitudes of Patients with Advanced Malignancy; Avery D. Weisman, Common Fallacies about Dying Patients; Edwin S. Shneidman, Death Work and Stages of Dying; Avery D. Weisman, Denial and Middle Knowledge; Chapter 8: Death and Dignity: Victor Richards, Death and Cancer; George P. Fletcher, Prolonging Life: Some Legal Considerations; W. R. Matthews, Voluntary Euthanasia: The Ethical Aspect; Avery D. Weisman, Appropriate and Appropriated Death; Lauren E. Trombley, A Psychiatrist's Response to a Life-Threatening Illness; Cicely Saunders, St. Christopher's Hospice; Simone de Beauvoir, Epilogue to *A Very Easy Death;* Poetic Epilogue: Ted Rosenthal, How Could I Not Be Among You?; Name Index; Subject Index.

Features. In the Preface to this book, the editor states: "My essential aim in assembling this volume was to provide a representative sample of recent and contemporary writings on the myriad aspects of death and dying." This is, then, a collection of previously published materials, selected with an eye to both significance and timeliness. With regard to the latter criterion, Shneidman chose (with one exception) "to limit the selections entirely to those written in the last decade, 1965-1975 . . . I needed some criterion for restraint, and *recency* seemed to be an especially relevant one. Also, I chose mostly from books rather than items from the periodical literature, believing that the latter, in general, tend to be more ephemeral and to become dated more quickly." Another feature of this book is its pedagogic focus. "My principal goal was to create a set of materials which would serve as either a primary or a supplementary text for a college undergraduate course relating to death." This end is served both by the structure of the volume—which works through cultural and social, to interpersonal and personal perspectives—and by the added framing provided in the introduction to the book and the Prefaces to each chapter. An idea of the range of Shneidman's ambition for this book may be gathered from the following comment: "Though it is intended for use as a college text, I would hope that this book will also be useful to professionals in medicine, nursing, theology, law, public health and mortuary science, in police academies, and in the social and behavioral sciences in general, especially in the disciplines of psychology and sociology."

Evaluation. This volume exemplifies many good features of a college text-anthology. Its special strengths are its size, breadth of coverage, recency of selections, and representation from many leading authors. It will be particularly suited to advanced college students with good verbal abilities, and to a course stressing intellectual comprehension. As a reference source, it provides a good one-volume sampler of pieces by major authors taken from their own books, journals, or other anthologies that appeared during the late 1960s and early 1970s.

□ □ □

Toynbee, Arnold, et al. *Man's concern with death.* New York: McGraw-Hill, 1968. Pp. 280. Hardbound, $7.95. ISBN 0-07-065126-4.

Contents. Contributors; Foreword: Robin Denniston, Hodder & Stoughton Ltd.; Part One—Death and Dying: 1. A. Keith Mant, The Medical Definition of Death; 2. Ninian Smart, Philosophical Concepts of Death; 3. John Hinton, The Dying and the Doctor; 4. Simon Yudkin, Death and the Young; Part Two—Attitudes Toward Death: 1. Arnold Toynbee, Traditional Attitudes Towards Death; 2. Ninian Smart, Attitudes Towards Death in Eastern Religions; 3. Ninian Smart, Death in the Judeo-Christian Tradition; 4. Arnold Toynbee, Changing Attitudes Towards Death in the Modern Western World; 5. Ninian Smart, Some Inadequacies of Recent Christian Thought About Death; 6. Ninian Smart, Death and the Decline of Religion in Western Society; 7. Arnold Toynbee, Death in War; 8. Arnold Toynbee, Increased Longevity and the Decline of Infant Mortality; 9. Eric Rhode, Death in Twentieth-Century Fiction; Part Three—Frontiers of Speculation: 1. Arnold Toynbee, Perspectives From Time, Space and Nature; 2. Rosalind Heywood, Attitudes to Death in the Light of Dreams and Other Out-of-the-Body Experience; 3. Rosalind Heywood, Death and Psychical Research; 4. H. H. Price, What Kind of Next World?; Epilogue: Arnold Toynbee, The Relation Between Life and Death, Living and Dying; Index.

Features. This is the U.S. edition of a book first published in London in 1968, and apparently first conceived some 5 years earlier. It is somewhat unusual in that it appears to have been proposed and assembled by its British publisher. Robin Denniston gives us the following historical comment in the Foreword:

> The form of *Man's Concern With Death* was dictated by a proposed plan of contents which we sent to a number of writers and thinkers whom we hoped would express interest. Several did.

One, Professor Arnold Toynbee, was so interested that he proposed writing a substantial section of the book himself. Our other distinguished contributors ranged themselves conveniently and co-operatively at his side, thus preserving the initial contents plan with a few small changes.

Toynbee is the principal contributor to this volume, offering 5 chapters and the epilogue for a total of over 80 pages. Ninian Smart is the other major contributor, with 5 chapters totalling 50 pages. All of the contributors are well-known British writers and scholars, their chapters apparently freshly written for this book, and the result does "show a common mind and spirit and an organic unity" as hoped by its publisher. The authors' perspectives are diverse, but the most prominent feature is an emphasis on large-scale concepts and attitudes, especially those with religious or cosmic significance.

Evaluation. This book is well known and some of its chapters have been reprinted elsewhere. Its contributors are articulate and distinguished in their fields. The overall range is impressive: from ancient Greeks to contemporary existentialists, from East to West, and from medicine to parapsychology. The book as a whole is a good general reference source and might usefully be read or used as a text especially by those with historical, philosophical, or religious interests.

□   □   □

Wass, Hannelore (Ed.). *Dying: Facing the facts.* Washington, DC: Hemisphere, 1979. Pp. xvi + 426. Hardbound, $19.95. Paperbound, $10.95. ISBN 0-07-068438-3 hardbound; 0-07-068437-5 paperbound.

Contents. Contributors; Preface: Hannelore Wass; Part One—The Problem: Denial and Ambivalence Toward Death; Chapter One: Charles A. Corr, Reconstructing the Changing Face of Death; Chapter Two: Charles A. Corr, Living With the Changing Face of Death; Part Two—The Data: The Facts of Death; Chapter 3: Ralph A. Redding, Physiology of Dying; Chapter Four: Michael A. Simpson, Social and Psychological Aspects of Dying; Chapter Five: Jeanne Quint Benoliel, Dying in an Institution; Chapter Six: Glen W. Davidson, Hospice Care for the Dying; Chapter Seven: Hannelore Wass, Death and the Elderly; Chapter Eight: Judith M. Stillion & Hannelore Wass, Children and Death; Chapter Nine: Robert Fulton, Death and the Funeral in Contemporary Society; Chapter Ten: Edgar N. Jackson, Bereavement and Grief; Chapter Eleven: Barton E. Bernstein, Death and the Law; Part Three—The Challenge: Meeting the Issues of Death; Chapter Twelve: Robert M. Veatch, Defining Death Anew: Technical and Ethical Problems; Policy Options; Chapter Thirteen: Ronald A. Carson, Euthanasia or the Right to Die; Chapter Fourteen: Carol Taylor, The Funeral Industry; Chapter Fifteen: J. Eugene Knott, Death Education For All; Author Index; Subject Index.

Features. In the Preface to this book, the editor describes the aim in assembling this volume as follows: "In designing this volume, I envisioned it to become a *comprehensive basic text* for the serious student whether he or she be an undergraduate student, a professional in the field, a parent, or simply an interested person." The result is a book that presents the fundamental facts and issues of death in a systematic manner. The contributors represent a broad spectrum of relevant fields such as philosophy, psychology, medicine, nursing, sociology, anthropology, law, and education. The book is organized to delineate the problems related to dying and death that confront individuals and society as a whole, then to present the facts of death as we now know them, and to describe the main issues and controversies that emerge from these facts. Several contributors suggest ways to clarify or resolve these issues. This volume is intended to impart information, but beyond that it ambitiously aims to assist the reader who seeks his or her own confrontation with death in order to be better able to define life purposes and goals. It should help the reader achieve a clearer sense of self within a larger order of things.

Evaluation. This volume is designed to serve as a college textbook, a professional reference book, or a volume for anyone interested in the subject. It offers comprehensive coverage of basic and essential materials. Its chapters are written by leading authors in a relatively nontechnical manner, but they maintain high standards of scholarship. A special strength is the *recency* of the material covered. For example, Chapter 6 offers an excellent overview of the development and administration of hospice programs. Chapter 3 is a unique contribution in which a physician describes for the nonmedical reader the physiological facts of dying, death, and decomposition. The chapter on death and the law offers valuable practical information to the reader; another chapter deals specially with the elderly; a third with children and death. This volume presents valuable new material from various fields in a compact and highly readable manner. Continuity is provided through introductions to each major part and editorial introductions of each chapter.

□　　□　　□

Weisman, Avery D. *On dying and denying: A psychiatric study of terminality.* New York: Behavioral Publications, 1972. Pp. xviii + 247. Hardbound, $14.95. ISBN 0-87705-068-6.

Contents. Foreword by Herman Feifel; Preface; Chapter 1: The Practical Significance of Mortality; Chapter 2: Basic Concepts and Assumptions; Chapter 3: Common Misconceptions about Death and Denial; Chapter 4: Case Material and Methods; Chapter 5: Denial and Middle Knowledge; Chapter 6: Denial and Acceptance in Myocardial Infarction and Cancer; Chapter 7: Death from a Fatal Illness: Cancer;

Chapter 8: The Terminal Stage; Chapter 9: Death from Terminal Old
Age; Chapter 10: Indications of Impending Death; Chapter 11:
Counterparts of Death; Chapter 12: Death and Responsibility;
Chapter 13: Illusion and Incipient Death; Bibliography; Index.

Features. Herman Feifel in writing the Foreword of this book
states that "American culture, confronting death, has attempted to
cope by disguising it, pretending that it is not a basic condition of all
life. The health professional responsible for care of the dying has also
been captured by this orientation." At least in the U.S. the result is a
widespread attempt to deny death. Health professionals tend to subscribe to curative treatment even beyond the time when it can
benefit the patient. When response is poor and death imminent, too
often the dying patient is left to die emotionally and spiritually alone.

On the basis of his work with terminal patients at Massachusetts
General Hospital, Weisman has gathered together here a rich collection of material that deals with the subject of denial and death. As he
states, "... no detailed study of death in its specific relation to denial
has yet appeared. Instead, the process of denial is still discussed as if it
were an independent, unambiguous, self-contained mental mechanism
that everyone understood. While the study of denial as a psycho-
dynamic process is common enough in psychiatric literature, its con-
figurations with respect to death have not been explored." Herman
Feifel adds that Weisman "views denial as a total process and specifies
how it can serve to negate reality and also to nullify threat in order
to help one participate in reality." The author provides guidelines for
enhancing self-knowledge and acknowledgment of death and presents philosophical and practical direction for promoting a dignified
and appropriate death. Many clinical interviews with individuals
facing death from heart disease, cancer, and advanced age illustrate
his research findings.

Evaluation. This book investigates an area which is debated by
many but understood by few. Its position is that dying and denying
are basic counterparts and that both have their place in the psychosocial phases of terminal illness. For those trying to understand the
subtle nuances of the terminal condition, this book is an invaluable
reference. It is sophisticated, well written, enriched with a wealth of
illustrations, and offers new methods and concepts for recognizing
and dealing with impending death.

□   □   □

Wilcox, Sandra Galdieri, & Sutton, Marilyn (Eds.). *Understanding
death and dying: An interdisciplinary approach.* Port Washington,
NY: Alfred, 1977. Pp. xviii + 474. Paperbound, $8.95. ISBN 0-88284-
052-5.

Contents. Preface; Note to the Instructor: The Use of Structured
Exercises in the Classroom; Chapter One: The Definition and Mean-

ing of Death: Introduction; Encounter: Confronting Your Death; Plato, *Phaedo*: The Death Scene; Talcott Parsons & Victor Lidz, selection from *Death in American Society;* Dylan Thomas, "Do Not Go Gentle Into That Good Night"; William Carlos Williams, "To Waken An Old Lady"; Robert J. Lifton, "The Struggle for Cultural Rebirth"; Mary Shelley, selections from *Frankenstein*; Task Force on Death and Dying of the Institute of Society, Ethics and the Life Sciences, Refinements in Criteria for the Determination of Death: An Appraisal; Life and Death: Definitions (Legal, Medical and Common Usage); R. A. Kalish, "Life and Death: Dividing the Indivisible"; Questions; Projects for Further Study; Structured Exercises; For Further Reading; Chapter Two: The Experience of Dying: Introduction; Encounter: Return from Clinical Death; E. Mansell Pattison, "Help in the Dying Process"; Elisabeth Kübler-Ross, "What Is It Like to Be Dying?"; Emily Dickinson, "I Heard a Fly Buzz When I Died" [and] "Exultation Is the Going"; Harvey Bluestone & Carl L. McGahee, "Reaction to Extreme Stress: Impending Death by Execution"; Horace, "Carpe Diem"; John Donne, "Death Be Not Proud"; Anselm L. Strauss & Barney G. Glaser, "Awareness of Dying"; Robert Kastenbaum, "The Foreshortened Life Perspective"; Questions; Projects for Further Study; Structured Exercises; For Further Reading; Chapter Three: Grief, Mourning, and Social Functions: Introduction; Encounter: The Experience of Grief; Erich Lindemann, "Symptomatology and Management of Acute Grief"; Leroy Bowman, "Group Behavior at Funeral Gatherings"; Edmund H. Volkhart & Stanley T. Michael, "Bereavement and Mental Health"; Sigmund Freud, "Thoughts for the Times on War and Death: Our Attitudes Toward Death"; Albert C. Cain, "Survivors of Suicide"; Sylvia Plath, "Daddy"; Rex L. Jones, "Religious Symbolism in Limbu Death-by-Violence"; Questions; Projects for Further Study; Structured Exercises; For Further Reading; Chapter Four: Death and the Child: Introduction; Encounter: The First Time Somebody You Knew Died; Maria Nagy, "The Child's Theories Concerning Death"; James Agee, selection from *A Death in the Family;* Simon Yudkin, selection from "Children and Death"; Joan Fassler, *My Grandpa Died Today*; C. M. Binger, A. R. Ablin, R. C. Feuerstein, J. H. Kushner, S. Zoger & C. Mikkelsen, "Childhood Leukemia: Emotional Impact on Patient and Family"; Eugenia H. Waechter, "Children's Awareness of Fatal Illness"; Questions; Projects for Further Study; Structured Exercises; For Further Reading; Chapter Five: Choices and Decisions in Death: Introduction; Joseph Fletcher, "Elective Death"; Michael L. Peck & Carl I. Wold, "The Suicidal Patient: Adolescent Suicide"; Anne Sexton, "Suicide Note"; Edwin S. Shneidman, "The Enemy"; Jon Nordheimer, "From Dakto to Detroit: Death of a Troubled Hero"; Studs Terkel, selection from *Working*: "Bob Patrick"; Questions; Projects for Further Study; Structured Exercises; For Further Reading Epilogue: Robert A. Becker, "Then Suddenly, It Was Jennifer's Last Day"; Appendices: A. Additional Materials for Structured Exercises; B. Physical Facts of Death; C. Additional Teaching Resources; Index.

Features. In their Preface Wilcox and Sutton note that a study of death and dying may have relevance for many personal, professional, and disciplinary interests, and that it may take place in a variety of formats. Their claim is that *"Understanding Death and Dying* can be adapted to any of these interests and uses." They observe that "the chapters in the text have been arranged to lead the student through a studied progression from initial definition to active choice," and that "each chapter proceeds through a somewhat analogous pattern, opening with an encounter followed by multi-disciplinary academic readings and closing with one or more structured exercises." As the Table of Contents shows, the chapters also contain a series of suggested questions, projects, and items for further reading. The editors offer short introductions to each chapter and brief headlines to describe and link together each selection. Two comments describe the pieces that have been gathered here. "The readings from many fields collected in this introductory survey include experience-based pieces that ground the discussion of death and dying to realistic situations, theoretical statements that develop cognitive skills and analyses that suggest guides for intervention"; and "The readings present key concepts in the social sciences (psychology, sociology) and medicine (psychiatry and nursing) as well as in gerontology and social welfare. They outline the germinal concepts in a study of death and dying and embed these concepts in a context provided by the history of ideas." Finally, the three appendices provide a variety of teaching aids in the form of materials to support the structured exercises, data tables on mortality rates and copies of sample documents (e.g., a death certificate and a living will), and three items to guide teachers: a schema linking readings in the text to specific disciplines, a set of topical suggestions for curricular planning, and audiovisual recommendations keyed to chapters in the text. In short, this is an anthology of previously published materials of various sorts framed by a set of practical aids for teaching and self-study.

Evaluation. This volume reads easily in its own right and displays a clear set of organizing principles. It is obviously designed primarily as a textbook for a course or workshop, particularly of an introductory or fairly elementary sort. It will be especially useful for an inexperienced instructor or for one seeking lots of help for students and for his or her own work. Because a good deal of space is devoted to individual or group exercises and other teaching aids, the selections tend to rely on brief poems, short items, and selections from longer works. For similar reasons, the editors prefer older "classical" selections to more recent items with less of a freestanding character. Many will find this unsatisfying in timeliness and depth, which militates against recommending this book as a reference work. However, since its readings are broadly diverse in character and sophistication, the book as a whole does provide a many-hued overview of several key topics in what some like to call "contemporary thanatology."

Bibliographies

An examination of the available bibliographies, mediagraphies, and other guides that are concerned with death, dying, and bereavement offers interesting perspectives on the development and current character of this field. Clearly, all bibliographies indicate a felt need on the part of those who prepare and those who use them. A bibliography comes into existence because someone begins to gather information about the literature on a given subject. It may be a matter of idle curiosity or of dedicated purpose, a project to satisfy oneself or a service for others. In any case, it is a labor of detail and accuracy. Where the work extends beyond the mere collection of data, it requires the development of principles of inclusion, order, and internal allocation. As this continues, techniques of descriptive summary and critical evaluation begin to emerge. The creation of a bibliography is usually regarded as a kind of ancillary activity, although a few people take it on as a primary task. These last are the professional cataloguers, whose comprehensive volumes and ongoing supplements refine the bibliographical art to its highest state. We believe that such a state of the art has recently been reached in the area of death, dying, and bereavement, and we hope to represent it throughout our resource guide and especially in this section on bibliographies.

The sheer length of our list of bibliographies is ample evidence of the felt need for organization and guidance in the literature and other resources on death, dying, and bereavement. There are, of course, rather large bodies of literature and extensive traditions of concern regarding particular aspects of these topics. For example, discussions of the meaning of death and the possibilities of some sort of afterlife trace back beyond the history of the written word. Similarly, fiction and other forms of imaginative literature have long dealt with themes still current in this area. But it is only in the last 20 years or so that these relatively narrow streams have been transformed into a torrent of investigation, dialogue, and publication. Theologians and philosophers were joined—and in many ways overshadowed—by social scientists, clinical researchers, and caregivers who seemed suddenly to discover that their methods were appropriate to the study of many pre- and postdeath activities, and that these activities could no longer legitimately be ignored or set aside as taboo. A spate of biographical and autobiographical books tell first-person stories of facing death and its aftermath in our times, while creative writers have made extensive use of the novel and short story forms to explore similar subjects. In short, the volume of available literature and other materials has grown—and continues to do so—beyond all expectation. That fact alone justifies the many efforts to bring bibliographical organization to exhuberant publication, and it helps to explain the changing nature of the bibliographies we will be studying.

Several features of the expanding materials on death, dying, and bereavement reinforce the special urgency of the need for bibliographic assistance in this area. The first such feature is *the breadth of these topics* and their many ramifications. Death, dying, and bereavement have to do with children as well as the elderly, with those who die and those who survive, with the way we face life and the way we dispose of the dead. They are not isolated topics of inquiry or curiosity for specialists, but broad and fundamental features of human existence, subject to many kinds of interests and concerns. Thus, the topical breadth of these subjects is matched by the *multiplicity of perspectives* from which they can be considered. This is the second interesting feature about discussions in our field. Those who write or otherwise make a statement about these subjects do so from a wide range of professional and nonprofessional backgrounds. Educators, counselors, and caregivers are joined in front of the typewriter, at the podium, and behind the camera by behavioral researchers, artists, novelists, and members of the general public. Each has something important to say and does so in his or her own particular way. As a result, our transdisciplinary topics are presented in *a variety of formats*, which is the third feature of significance in appreciating the need for resource guides on death, dying, and bereavement. Valuable material can be found outside a narrow range of specialized journals, a certain kind of book, or a particular sort of vehicle such as the printed word itself. Short stories, biographies, novels, and films can all be appropriate places for us to learn about these topics. Hence, students in this field need assistance that gathers together an unusual combination of materials and that provides access to the resulting accumulation in a way that is helpful to their particular needs.

In a diverse and wide-ranging field, one finds a variety of workers laboring at tasks that we are here grouping under the adjective "bibliographical." Perhaps it will help if we briefly note some of the different types of bibliographies that result. Most familiar are those appended to the text of a book, monograph, or article as a list of references or sources. Usually, the compilers of such *appended bibliographies* have little more in common than the desire to give credit to their sources. Sometimes they also have in mind their own readers, who may wish to follow up a seminal idea in its original setting or to study some specific area in greater depth. The sort of bibliography offered by such authors is typically quite rudimentary. Some books contain no bibliography at all, even where one might be expected. Those that do appear are often fairly *general* in nature, consisting of no more than an alphabetical list of authors, titles, and publication data. It is hardly worthwhile to attempt to differentiate such bibliographies in terms of length or breadth of coverage. Our collection of these general bibliographies cannot be expected to be complete, though we have sought to make it represent both well-known and more obscure entries. For example, Kübler-Ross's *On Death and Dying* is one of the most widely read books in the field, though its bibliography may not receive proportional attention, while Richard G. Dumont and Dennis C. Foss's *The American View of Death: Acceptance or Denial?* is an interesting book deserving attention, with a useful bibliography for its scope and time.

We have also included in our list a number of books whose textual and bibliographical focus is on some *specialized* topic. For example, the list includes books that have appended bibliographies concerning the dying child (Easson), childhood bereavement (Furman), death and the law (Shaffer), interaction strategies (Epstein), theology (Hick), and hospices (Stoddard). The fact that the study of suicide and suicidal behavior has a longer history than the recent interest in death and dying is evident in the large, specialized appended bibliography in Farberow and Shneidman's early work, *The Cry for Help*. This bibliography introduces two additional features, that of subdivision and of possibly becoming an independent entity (which it later did under Farberow's direction). We must again remind the reader that our coverage of books containing specialized bibliographies makes no claim to completeness. That would be an impossible achievement and besides, our primary interest is in the field of death, dying, and bereavement as a whole. We acknowledge the principal subdivisions of our field, but the reader whose concerns are only tangential to these subjects or whose range of interest is limited may prefer to find sources in books and articles on particular subtopics. Alternatively, certain researchers interested in rapidly evolving and changing topics may be better served by instruments providing ongoing access to journals and other publications with a short lead time. We consider this latter sort of bibliographical assistance below in our discussion of ongoing guides.

Occasionally, an appended bibliography is *subdivided* in some significant way. Often the bibliography itself is little more than a list of books and articles, but the introduction of subdivisions may help to make it more manageable for the user. This can be accomplished by organizing the bibliography according to the section or chapter headings of its supporting text (e.g., Hendin or Veatch's two books), or by introducing some other set of divisions (see Jackson for a three-part arrangement, Pattison who employs 21 separate topical headings for a moderately sized bibliography, or Pearson who developed a rather complex schema of headings and subheadings for a much larger bibliography).

Subdivisions do not necessarily improve a bibliography; some are helpful, others appear little more than idiosyncratic. And the effort to impose a set of topical headings on a bibliography may raise problems for the compiler that are not fully apparent to a naive user. For example, does a given book or article fall only into a single category? Should the same title be listed in more than one category? When guided, by such questions, those who seek to provide an appended bibliography sometimes switch from topical headings to direct *annotation* of individual entries. For reasons of space, this usually means that the number of items to be included must be sharply curtailed, even when the annotations consist only of a short sentence or two. But many feel that an abbreviated list of significant items, accompanied by a brief description, summary, or comment, is preferable to a longer list of unexplained titles. Three examples of the short, appended, annotated bibliography are provided by Irion, Neale, and Kohl (whose bibliography was prepared by Thomas Harvey).

The bibliographies mentioned thus far are all more or less incidental to a text (usually a book), though some are perhaps noteworthy in one respect or another.[1] However, as the literature developed many bibliographies expanded proportionately. This introduced what might be called the *independent* bibliographies of death, dying, and bereavement, self-contained entities without a primary text. The work of Richard Kalish is a good model for these developing directions in the late 1960s. Interested in psychosocial or behavioral aspects of the field, he has made important contributions

---

[1] *The longest appended bibliography that has come to our attention is the unannotated, alphabetical list of over 1,300 entries in Warren Shibles' somewhat idiosyncratic text,* Death: An Interdisciplinary Analysis.

to its growth, and helped launch the journal *Omega*. In 1965—several years before the appearance of Kübler-Ross's *On Death and Dying*—Kalish published a bibliographical article on death and bereavement growing out of his reading over the previous 5 years or so, and an earlier mimeographed list that he had circulated privately. It was no more than a numbered, alphabetical list of titles without comment, but it consisted of 370 items, which suggests that allegations of previous disinterest in these topics are not wholly well-founded. Kalish subsequently contributed "selected" or "briefly annotated" bibliographies to three books published in 1969 and 1970. For *Death and Bereavement*, one of the first of Austin Kutscher's many anthologies, Kalish offered a bibliographical appendix of 57 entries on grief and bereavement, with descriptive and critical annotations. In *Loss and Grief*, edited by Bernard Schoenberg, et al. (including Kutscher), he produced 47 annotated entries, over half of which did not appear in the previous list. And for *The Dying Patient*, edited by Orville Brim, et al., Kalish provided 239 annotated entries on death and dying. Throughout these bibliographies, the emphasis is on crisp summaries and brief evaluations of English-language literature drawn especially from the fields of psychology, sociology, and psychiatry. Although a list of 239 entries can hardly be called short, it is through the annotations and the initiation of independent bibliographies that Kalish has provided a major service.

The history of independent bibliographies during the last 10 years is a bewildering tale of rapid change and independent initiative. We need only sketch the broad outlines of these events by considering in turn four different types of such bibliographies: 1) an arbitrary grouping of annotated and unannotated bibliographies on particular subjects, called here "special-topic" bibliographies; 2) comprehensive or broad-scale bibliographies; 3) mediagraphies; and 4) continuing or cumulative bibliographical guides. The first of these, the *special-topic bibliographies*, like their counterparts the specialized appended bibliographies, developed in a variety of ways. They range from review articles on various subjects in journals (e.g., Pine or Griggs), pamphlets (e.g., those published by the Celo Press), brochures sponsored by the federal government (e.g., those on Sudden Infant Death Syndrome) or private groups (e.g., Clouser & Zucker or Trautmann & Pollard), and the computerized literature searches of the National Library of Medicine, to sections of books (e.g., Bernstein and Fassler) and independent volumes (e.g., Floyd's annual volumes, Strugnell's book, and the work of the Harrahs or the Triches).

Among the more or less *comprehensive bibliographies* undertaken by individuals or groups in the field, there are discernible variations depending upon the way the basic task is construed and perhaps also upon the way the aim has been modified as the work becomes increasingly formidable. We can set the general pattern and illustrate these differences by looking at one of the earliest (and still among the least expensive), and at one of the most recent. Joel Vernick's

Selected Bibliography in Death and Dying (1970) is a bit dated and offers no annotations. But it covers 1494 entries, has an author/ subject index, and costs under $1.00. This bibliography arose from an interest in dying children and it maintains a focus on terminal illness, though it is intended for parents and relatives as well as physicians and educators. Despite its broad title, Irene Sell's *Dying and Death: An Annotated Bibliography* (1977) works in a similar direction by emphasizing what will be useful for nursing practitioners, educators, and students. Sell includes only 71 books and 382 articles, but her paragraph-length annotations, author and subject indexes, and annotations of 53 audiovisual items are quite helpful. Nurses and those with related interests might happily settle for Sell's book if they want to purchase only one recent guide.

For breadth and/or volume of coverage, Vernick and Sell are surpassed by half a dozen other books in the category of comprehensive bibliographies. The first of these to appear was Austin Kutscher's *A Bibliography of Books on Death, Bereavement, Loss and Grief: 1935-1968* (1969), which lists 1191 items without annotations under various topical headings and subheadings. A 1974 supplement offers 470 additional citations from the period 1968-1972, listed in a similar way. In 1975 the Foundation of Thanatology sponsored the publication of *A Comprehensive Bibliography of the Thanatology Literature* under the editorship of Martin Kutscher and others (including Austin Kutscher). This book makes a quantitative generational leap to encompass 4844 items. The entries are again numbered and unannotated, but they are supported by a 40-page index organizing them according to 423 subject headings.

Another important figure in bibliographies of death, dying, and bereavement is Robert Fulton, who exchanged information with Kalish during the 1960s, and who published an appended bibliography of 427 items in the original edition (1965) of his textbook, *Death and Identity*.[2] During the early 1970s the University of Minnesota Center for Death Education made available a series of unpublished bibliographies,[3] and in 1977 Arno Press published the latest of these as *Death, Grief, and Bereavement: A Bibliography, 1845-1975*. Containing a numbered, unannotated alphabetical list of 3856 items, the book also offers an author index and an extensive subject index with 214 headings and subheadings. The emphasis is on references with an empirical perspective.

---

[2] *In the revised edition of this book (1976), Fulton subdivided the bibliography according to the following four-part division of the text: theoretical discussions on death; attitudes and responses toward death; grief and mourning: the reaction to death; and ceremony, social organizations, and society. He also reduced its length to 206 items.*

[3] *Unpublished or privately circulated bibliographies are among the most difficult to identify and locate. They also vary greatly in character and scope. Our list includes Bernardo's very extensive unannotated bibliography on death, bereavement, and widowhood, and Katz's much shorter annotated bibliography on self-help and rehabilitation.*

The last two comprehensive bibliographies that we want to mention are G. Howard Poteet's *Death and Dying: A Bibliography (1950–1974)*,[4] and Albert J. Miller and Michael J. Acri's *Death: A Bibliographical Guide*. Both include references appearing through 1974 and early 1975; hence, they are roughly contemporaneous in coverage with Martin Kutscher's and Fulton's guides. Poteet's book emphasizes literature on the psychology of death, listing 153 books and 2146 articles, with the latter arranged according to 213 subject headings. Miller and Acri's coverage of 3905 items has three special virtues: First, its numbered entries are listed alphabetically under seven headings; second, many of its entries have brief annotations; and third, it includes a separate section listing 182 audiovisual items. These qualities, together with a list of audiovisual sources and the usual author and subject indexes, make Miller and Acri's book a helpful single-volume guide for general use.

The third kind of comprehensive bibliography that we want to consider is the *mediagraphy*, the guide to the "audiovisual literature" on death, dying, and bereavement. We have already mentioned that audiovisual items are included in some other sorts of bibliographies, but mediagraphies devote themselves exclusively to the audiovisual arena. They range from brief pamphlets and mimeographed lists (e.g., those by Mason and the American Cancer Society), to a larger article (Duke), brochures (e.g., Duke, Berg & Daugherty), and a recent paperbound volume (Prince). Nearly all of these lists are annotated, as they must be in order to be of much use to readers. However, the nature of the annotations differs, as does the range of coverage in the lists. The shorter mediagraphies tend to settle for brief summaries of content and data on format, length, and producer. Others limit themselves to a specific sort of material. Duke successively broadens the scope of coverage, while Berg & Daugherty venture a bit beyond mere description. But Prince achieves the broadest coverage (309 items), provides descriptive summaries for each of her entries, and adds full-scale review (synopsis, critical evaluation, and suggestions for use) for one third of them. Her indexes by title, subject, and distributor complement the usual alphabetical list of distributors which one needs to determine availability and changing rental or purchase cost.

Our final type of guide provides *continuing* or *cumulative* bibliographical information, attempting in some measure to include new publications as they appear. To some extent, this service is included in the more general abstracts that serve particular disciplines or professions, e.g., psychological, sociological, and nursing abstracts, as well as the *Index Medicus*. For bioethics, Walter's multivolume *Bibliography of Bioethics* is impressive, the *Bioethics Digest* is quite helpful, and Sollitto & Veatch have published an annual *Bibliography*

---

[4] *As indicated below, this bibliography has now been supplemented by a second volume containing references to suicide, and there is the promise of a third volume yet to come.*

of Society, Ethics and the Life Sciences from the Hastings Center since 1974 which includes a brief, partly annotated section on death and dying. However, the most effective service to the field as a whole comes from Roberta Halporn, a private book dealer, and the journal, *Death Education*. Halporn operates Highly Specialized Promotions and arranges book displays for various meetings in the field. In 1976 she prepared a pamphlet entitled "The Thanatology Library," which, for $1.00, provides capsule descriptions of 225 books, audiovisual, and other materials. Her quarterly newsletter, "The Thanatology Librarian," offers supplementary information on new and backlist items to subscribers for $3.50 per year. As a merchant, Halporn is concerned with books and audiovisual materials rather than journal articles, but her service is current and facilitates purchases for those who are so inclined. Since the spring of 1977, another major source of information has been provided by the "Media Exchange" section of *Death Education*. Here are both the usual journal-type professional reviews of books and audiovisual materials—which are normally fuller and more helpful than other forms of bibliographical annotation— together with an ongoing bibliography containing short annotations for 40–50 items per issue. *Death Education* appears to be developing into the broadest journal in the field, serving educators, counselors, and caregivers alike, and its bibliographical service should be a valuable guide for the future.

In the following list, we have striven for completeness especially in the areas of comprehensive bibliographies and mediagraphies. Where omissions are most likely, e.g., in the area of appended and special-topic bibliographies, we have sought to provide a representative sampling that includes the best known and most useful guides. We will be grateful to readers who bring to our attention bibliographies that do not appear in our list. In the few instances in which we have not actually seen a bibliography ourselves, we give the reference as it is known to us without comment of any kind. Wherever the bibliography is no more than an unannotated, alphabetical list of references, we simply cite the source, give the appropriate page references, and provide an item count of its entries. In all other cases, we add an annotation proportioned to the complexity or distinctive qualities of the bibliography, and to its potential usefulness to readers.

The Allied Memorial Council catalogue of media resources. (Available from the Allied Memorial Council, P.O. Box 30112, Seattle, WA 98103). This 4-page mimeographed brochure describes 10 films, 8 videotapes, and 13 slide or filmstrip presentations (all with brief content summaries), as well as 24 brochures and 18 books.

American Cancer Society. See *Audiovisual materials for professional education*.

An annotated, select bibliography of books and materials relating to the cemetery industry. Compiled and written by the Young

Executives Committee of the National Association of Cemeteries, 1976. (Available from and published by the National Association of Cemeteries, 1911 North Fort Myer Drive, Suite 409, Arlington, VA 22209.) This 16-page brochure provides bibliographical data, brief summaries of content, and evaluations for 22 books, articles, and other documents. An unannotated supplemental bibliography for the years 1970–1975 adds 83 general books, 19 books emphasizing psychological aspects, 73 articles (arranged by year), and 3 bibliographies.

Aradine, C. R. Books for children about death. *Pediatrics*, 1976, *57*(3), 372–378. This review article surveys and describes 12 books for preschool and school-aged children.

Attitude towards death. National Library of Medicine, Literature Search No. 76-13, January 1974 through February 1976. (Available without cost from Literature Search Program, National Library of Medicine, 8600 Rockville Pike, Bethesda, MD 20014.) Prepared by Linda W. Kudrick, this computer-generated bibliography contains 156 citations in English listed alphabetically, each with major and minor topical headings for computer indexing.

Audiovisual materials for professional education. (Available from the National Headquarters of the American Cancer Society, 777 Third Avenue, New York, NY 10017, and from all of its state and regional offices.) February 1977. This is a mimeographed list, with descriptive annotations, of items available for free loan or lease/purchase from the American Cancer Society. It identifies 32 motion pictures and 7 audiotapes for professional education, as well as 9 motion pictures and 5 audiotapes designated "especially for nurses" (though in both cases some items may be useful for more general audiences).

Baler, L. A., & Golde, P. Bibliography on bereavement. In *Working papers in community mental health.* (Vol. 2, No. 1). Boston: Department of Public Health Practice, Harvard School of Public Health, Spring 1964.

Bedau, H. A. (Ed.). *The death penalty in America: An anthology.* Chicago: Aldine, 1964. Pages 565–574 of this book contain a bibliography divided in the following way: 7 bibliographies and collections; 24 public documents; 128 items under the heading "general"; 8 items on classical capital cases; and 8 unpublished sources. There are no annotations.

Berardo, F. *Death, bereavement, and widowhood: A selected bibliography.* (Available from Department of Sociology, University of Florida, Gainesville, FL 32611). This long list of references is a good example of an unannotated, privately circulated, typed bibliography. The work, dated March 1971 with supplements through October 1974, now comprises 159 pages and 2132 entries.

Berg, D. W., & Daugherty, G. G. *Death education: Audio-visual source book.* DeKalb, IL: Educational Perspectives Associates, 1976. The authors have prepared an annotated list of 118 films, filmstrips, videotapes, audiocassettes, and records on a variety of death-related topics. Each entry provides bibliographic data, descriptive summary, and recommendations for use. Titles are indexed according to type of media, suggested level of use, and subject matter content.

Berg, D. W., & Daugherty, G. G. *Perspectives on death: Student activity book* and *Teacher's resource book.* DeKalb, IL: Perspectives on Death, 1972. Both of these handbooks (pp. 50–53 and 65–69, respectively) contain the same bibliography, consisting of 36 articles with one- or two-sentence annotations and a list of 31 books.

Berger, Sr. M. F. L. Books about death for children, young adults, and parents. In O. J. Sahler (Ed.), *The child and death,* 259–278. St. Louis: Mosby, 1978. An annotated bibliography of 95 fiction and 30 nonfiction books mainly published since 1970. Each entry is categorized as representing one or more of Kübler-Ross's five stages and/or fear, grief, or hope. Titles recommended for the young child are marked with an asterisk.

Bernstein, J. E. *Books to help children cope with separation and loss.* New York: R. R. Bowker, 1977. This useful volume contains 100 paragraph-length annotations of selected books for children about death (pp. 84–131), plus a bibliography for adults on separation and loss (pp. 215–226). It is the most extensive and detailed analysis of children's literature in this area now available.

Bernstein, J. E. *Helping children cope with death and separation: Resources for teachers.* (Available from the Publications Office/ICBD, College of Education, University of Illinois, 805 West Pennsylvania Avenue, Urbana, IL 61801.) May 1976. This 38-page pamphlet lists 21 children's books on death and 43 on separation, 18 books or chapters in books on bibliotherapy, 35 films, filmstrips and cassettes on death and separation (with information regarding sources), and 41 references, each with annotations at least one or two sentences long. The treatment of printed materials is superceded by the author's book (q.v.).

Bernstein, J. E. Literature for young people: Nonfiction books about death. *Death Education,* 1979, *3*(2), 111–119. This article reviews 20 recent nonfiction books on death that are suitable for young people.

Bernstein, J. E. *Loss: And how to cope with it.* New York: Seabury, 1977. Pages 121–143 contain: a list with one-sentence annotations of 16 nonfiction and 55 fiction books for children concerning death; an alphabetical list without annotations of 78 books for adult "advanced study"; a list of 13 films about death with brief annotations; and a list with short descriptions of 34 service organizations and sources for information.

Bernstein, J. E. Suicide in literature for young people. *The Alan Review,* 1979, *6*(5), 12–13. A short review article describing 20 fiction and 10 nonfiction books that deal with suicide and are suitable for young people.

Bibliography of society, ethics and the life sciences. See *S. Solitto & R. M. Veatch.*

A bibliography on death education. Burnsville, NC: Celo Press, 1977. The publishers describe this 20-page pamphlet as "intended as a basic reference guide for students, teachers, and serious laypersons. Little has been included in the way of fiction, periodicals, peripheral specialties, and highly technical works." It contains a list of 235 books, many with brief annotations; a separate list of 13 books under the heading "juveniles," also mostly with brief annotations; and an annotated list of 19 audiovisual items.

A bibliography on euthanasia. (Available without cost from Concern for Dying, An Educational Council (formerly, Euthanasia Educational Council), 250 West 57th Street, New York, NY 10019.) This is described as "a list of the most significant books on euthanasia which have been published in the United States during the period 1954-1977." It consists of a two-sided mimeographed sheet listing 25 items with brief annotated descriptions.

The Bioethics Digest. Published by Information Planning Associates, Inc., 2 Research Court, Rockville, MD 20850. A monthly publication, this journal provides approximately 150 abstracts per issue, grouped according to nine major topical headings (one of which is "death and dying"). See page 125 for a fuller description.

Bowers, M. K., Jackson, E. N., Knight, J. A., & LeShan, L. *Counseling the dying*. New York: Thomas Nelson, 1964. Pages 173–183 list 120 items on death and dying, plus 31 on mourning and grief.

Carmody, J. *Ethical issues in health services: A report and annotated bibliography* (United States Department of Health, Education, and Welfare; Public Health Service; Health Services and Mental Health Administration; National Center for Health Services Research and Development; Report HSDR 70-32, November 1970). This 43-page brochure contains a selective, annotated bibliography of literature published between January 1967 and December 1969, with some additional literature from 1970. The 145 entries are arranged alphabetically under five topical headings: the right to health care, death and euthanasia, human experimentation, genetic engineering, and abortion.

Carr, R. L. Death as presented in children's books. *Elementary English*, 1973, *50*, 701–705. This review article contains 20 annotated references.

Celo Press. See *A bibliography on death education*. Also see R. M. Harmer, *A consumer bibliography on funerals*.

Choron, J. *Death and modern man*. New York: Collier, 1972. (Originally published by Macmillan in 1964 as *Modern man and mortality*.) Pages 245–269 list 465 items without annotation, plus a 12-item supplement with brief comments. The author emphasizes historical, philosophic, and psychological materials; literary items are omitted.

Clouser, K. D., & Zucker, A. *Abortion and euthanasia: An annotated bibliography*. Philadelphia: Society for Health and Human Values, 1974. This 32-page brochure lists 240 items on abortion and

118 on euthanasia. In each case the entries are given in alphabetical order. They focus on ethical arguments or factual accounts that might contribute to such arguments, and they include short descriptive and critical annotations. (This bibliography is no longer available from its publisher.)

Concern for Dying (formerly, Euthanasia Educational Council.) See *A bibliography on euthanasia.*

Cook, S. S. *Children and dying: An exploration and selective bibliographies* (Rev. ed.). New York: Health Sciences Publishing Corporation, 1974. In this uneven collection of articles four have brief bibliographies (pp. 16-19; 27; 78; 92-96), only the last of which is annotated.

Davidson, G. (Ed.). *The hospice: Development and administration.* Washington, DC: Hemisphere, 1978. (Originally published as a special double issue of *Death Education,* [Spring-Summer, 1978] *2,* 1-2.) Pages 189-203 contain an annotated bibliography edited by Parimala Desai listing 126 entries on hospice and care of the dying. There are also reviews of 3 films and 2 videotapes, plus an annotated list of 16 other audiovisual items, prepared by Richard Dayringer (pp. 205-214), and a directory of 25 hospice programs in the United States (pp. 215-223).

Death education (Pedagogy—Counseling—Care, An international Quarterly), (Spring, 1977)-, *1*(1)-. The "Media Exchange" section offers reviews of books and audiovisual materials, together with an ongoing annotated bibliography. See page 126 for a fuller description.

Death, dying, and bereavement: A selected bibliography. (Available from Hagemeyer Learning Resources Center, Central Piedmont Community College, Charlotte, NC 28204.) The reference staff of the Center has prepared this unannotated, mimeographed list of 83 books, films, and audiotapes. The most recent fourth edition is dated October 1977.

Dollen, C. *Abortion in context: A select bibliography.* Metuchen, NJ: Scarecrow, 1970. This volume contains 1,405 entries listed alphabetically by both author and title. Entries are identified by letter and number; there are no annotations. The book focuses on publications in English from about 1967 to 1969. There is a subject index and a source index.

Duke, P. Media guide on death and dying. *Omega,* 1975, *6,* 275-287. This article consists of "an annotated list of films, tapes and other instructional aids appropriate for death education courses." It includes 80 items.

Duke, P. *Media guide on death and dying.* New York: Biomedical Communications, 1978. This 32-page brochure offers "a descriptive bibliography of more than 200 film, slide, filmstrip, audio and video programs." It provides capsule descriptions of each item, sources, and rental/sale information.

Dumont, R. G., & Foss, D. C. *The American view of death: Acceptance or denial?* Cambridge, MA: Schenkman, 1972. Pages 111-117 list 160 items.

Easson, W. M. *The dying child: The management of the child or adolescent who is dying.* Springfield, IL: Thomas, 1970. Pages 97-100 list 98 entries.

Epstein, C. *Nursing the dying patient: Learning processes for interaction.* Reston, VA: Reston Publishing Co., 1975. Pages 200-207 list 157 items.

Euthanasia and the right to die. National Library of Medicine, Literature Search No. 77-13, January 1975 through August 1977. (Available without cost from Literature Search Program, National Library of Medicine, 8600 Rockville Pike, Bethesda, MD 20014.) This computer-generated bibliography prepared by Leonard J. Nahlman & Geraldine D. Nowak contains 207 citations in English listed alphabetically, each with major and minor topical headings for computer indexing.

Euthanasia Educational Council. See *A bibliography on euthanasia.*

Farberow, N. L. *Bibliography on suicide and suicide prevention: 1897-1957, 1958-1967* (Department of Health, Education, and Welfare; Public Health Service, Publication No. 1970.) Rockville, MD: National Institute of Mental Health, 1969. A revised edition of 1972 (DHEW, Publication No. [HSM] 72-9080) extends coverage through 1970. Part I is the original bibliography from *The cry for help* (q.v.), expanded from 1437 to 2202 items. Part II adds 1267 items from the period 1958-1967, enlarged in the revised edition to 2542 items. This bibliography focuses on medical, psychological, sociological, and biological literature, though medical items intended exclusively for physicians and surgeons are omitted. For each part there is an author and a subject index.

Farberow, N. L., & Shneidman, E. S. (Eds.). *The cry for help.* New York: McGraw-Hill, 1961. Pages 325-388 offer a "Bibliography on Suicide, 1897-1957"—1437 items presented in four categories: psychological-general (732 items); sociological (318 items); medical-legal (362 items); and religious-philosophical (25 items). Foreign-language titles are translated into English.

Fassler, J. *Helping children cope.* New York: The Free Press, 1978. Chapter One (pp. 1-25) describes 28 recommended books for children about death.

Filstrup, J. M. Children's books confront death and divorce: A reading guide. *Harvard Magazine*, 1979, *81*, 64-68. A brief review article that offers a short historical sketch and gives special emphasis to 17 recent titles.

Floyd, M. K. *Abortion bibliography for 1970.* Troy, NY: Whitston, 1972. Subsequent volumes have appeared for the years 1971-1976. Each volume included separate listings for books and periodical literature, as well as an author index. Periodical literature is listed alphabetically by title and by a series of subject headings.

Fulton, R. *Death and identity.* New York: Wiley, 1965. Pages 397–415 list 427 items.

Fulton, R. *Death and identity* (Rev. ed., in collaboration with R. Bendiksen). Bowie, MD: The Charles Press, 1976. Pages 434–441 list 206 items, organized according to the four-part division of the text.

Fulton, R., Carlson, J., Krohn, K., Markusen, E., & Owen, G. *Death, grief, and bereavement: A bibliography, 1845–1975.* New York: Arno Press, 1977. This is the first published edition of this bibliography, reprinting a 1976 edition prepared by the Center for Death Education and Research at the University of Minnesota. It lists 3806 items (with another 50 in an addendum), arranged alphabetically without annotation. The volume includes a subject index with 214 headings and subheadings. According to the editors, "Generally, in preparing the bibliography, only references that treat the subject from an empirical perspective have been considered. Except in those instances in which a book or article has particular historical significance or relevance, no journalistic, literary or theological works have been included." Also this bibliography mainly omits suicide, and no special effort has been made to include foreign references though some do appear.

Fulton, R., Markusen, E., Owen, G., & Scheiber, J. L. *Death and dying: Challenge and change.* Reading, MA: Addison-Wesley, 1978. This volume is the reader for the course-by-newspaper project of the same title developed by the University of California, San Diego, and funded by the National Endowment for the Humanities. (See Part IV for a further description of this volume and of the course-by-newspaper project.) Pages 411–425 contain an annotated bibliography of 180 items, arranged alphabetically according to the 15 section headings of the text.

Furman, E. *A child's parent dies: Studies in childhood bereavement.* New Haven: Yale University Press, 1974. Pages 297–308 list 185 items.

Green, B. R., & Irish, D. P. *Death education: Preparation for living.* Cambridge, MA: Schenkman, 1971. The selected bibliography (pp. 125–143, 255 items) emphasizes recent behavioral or empirical approaches to death education and to normal socialization for natural death within the American scene, especially for children and youth. Literary, journalistic, theological, and psychoanalytic perspectives are excluded.

Griffith, W. H. *Confronting death.* Valley Forge, PA: Judson, 1977. Pages 55–64 contain a brief, descriptive list of a variety of religious publications, school publications, audiovisual materials, pamphlets, booklets, and organizations providing further resources for those planning educational programs on the subject of death.

Griggs, S. A. Annotated bibliography of books on death, dying, and bereavement. *The School Counselor,* 1977, *24,* 362–371. This review article lists 55 items with paragraph-length annotations.

Grollman, E. *Talking about death: A dialogue between parent and child* (Rev. ed.). Boston: Beacon, 1976. Pages 73-98 briefly describe community resources for assistance, books for children about death, books for adults about children and death, an audio-cassette series, and recommended films.

Gruman, G. J. An historical introduction to ideas about voluntary euthanasia: with a bibliographical survey and guide for inter-disciplinary studies. *Omega*, 1973, *4*, 87-138. The bibliography on pp. 130-138 of this historically oriented review article lists 271 items.

Hall, J. H., & Swenson, D. D. *Psychological and social aspects of human tissue transplantation: An annotated bibliography* (United States Department of Health, Education, and Welfare; Public Health Service; Health Services and Mental Health Administration; National Institute of Mental Health; Public Health Service Publication No. 1838). Washington, DC: U.S. Government Printing Office, 1968. This is a 57-page brochure containing 176 annotated entries arranged alphabetically under 11 topical headings. Most references are from two decades prior to the date of publication. The topical focus is on "psychological, psychiatric, ethical, moral, social, and legal matters in the use of human tissue and in the artificial maintenance of life."

Hall, J. H., & Swenson, D. D. *Psychological and social aspects of human tissue transplantation, supplement no. 1.* (United States Department of Health, Education, and Welfare; Public Health Service; Health Services and Mental Health Administration; National Institute of Mental Health; Public Health Service Publication No. 1838-1). Washington, DC: U.S. Government Printing Office, 1969. This 48-page brochure contains 112 additional entries, arranged alphabetically under 10 topical headings.

Halporn, R. *The thanatology library.* (Available from Highly Specialized Promotions, 228 Clinton St., Brooklyn, NY 11201.) June 1976. Here is a 32-page pamphlet that provides capsule descriptions of books, audiovisuals, and other materials, and is supplemented by *The Thanatology Librarian*, a quarterly newsletter.

Harmer, R. M. *A consumer bibliography on funerals.* Burnsville, NC: Celo Press, 1977. This annotated bibliography of 22 books, 14 pamphlets and government documents, and 72 articles was assembled and prepared by a leading critic of the American funeral industry. The selections and annotations strongly favor cremation and the viewpoint of the memorial society movement.

Harrah, B. K., & Harrah, D. F. *Funeral service: A bibliography of literature on its past, present, and future, the various means of disposition, and memorialization.* Metuchen, NJ: Scarecrow, 1976. According to its compilers, this extensive bibliography was prepared "to assist librarians, students, and those professionally interested in researching funeral service, the means of final disposition, and the memorializing of the dead" (p. ix). The work itself covers 1982 items, many of which are annotated with a brief description or summary of contents. Entries are numbered for convenience and arranged alphabetically in three primary sections: funeral service; interment and other means of disposition; and memorialization. A short fourth section cites some audiovisual materials and 11 appendixes give a brief glossary of funeral terminology, acronyms of professional organizations, information about professional funeral organizations, cemetery and monument associations, trade journals, memorial societies, co-op funeral homes, body donation associations, accredited funeral service colleges, state embalming requirements, and industry codes of ethics and practices. There are also separate author, title, and subject indices.

Harshbarger, D., & Moran, G. A selective bibliography on disaster and human ecology. *Omega*, 1974, *5*, 89-95. This is an alphabetical listing of 101 items without annotations.

Harvey, T. Bibliography. In M. Kohl (Ed.), *Beneficient euthanasia.* Buffalo, NY: Prometheus, 1975. On pages 247-251 appear 14 titles with paragraph-length annotations.

Hendin, D. *Death as a fact of life.* New York: Warner, 1973. Organized according to chapter titles in the text, 264 entries are found on pages 195-209.

Hick, J. *Death and eternal life.* New York: Harper & Row, 1976. Pages 467-481 list 359 works cited.

Hinton, J. *Dying.* Baltimore, MD: Penguin, 1967. Pages 198-209 list 219 items.

Hunt, G. J., & Mondell, A. S. *Social factors in health care: An evaluation of selected films and videotapes.* Baltimore, MD: University of Maryland, School of Medicine, Department of Psychiatry, The Institute of Psychiatry and Human Behavior (645 West Redwood St., 21201), 1972. This 68-page brochure grew out of a medical sociology course and reviews "selected films and videotapes which illustrate the relationship between social factors and health care." It lists 17 items under the heading "Delivery of Health Services" and 23 items under the heading "Problem Areas in Medical Care"; for each item we are given appropriate data, a synopsis, and a general evaluation.

Irion, P. E. *Cremation.* Philadelphia: Fortress, 1968. Pages 141-149 list, with brief annotations, 44 books, articles, pamphlets, and journals dealing with cremation and funeral practices.

Jackson, E. N. *Understanding grief: Its roots, dynamics, and treatment.* Nashville, TN: Abingdon, 1957. Pages 243-247 contain a selected bibliography (108 items) on personality dynamics, grief, and pastoral care.

Kalish, R. A. Death and bereavement: A bibliography. *Journal of Human Relations*, 1965, *13*, 118-141. This bibliographic article provides 370 numbered entries arranged alphabetically.

Kalish, R. A. *Death and bereavement: An annotated social science bibliography.* Philadelphia: Smith, Kline and French Laboratories, 1965. One of the earliest general bibliographies in the field, this annotated list of 408 items is reproduced and distributed by the well-known drug company.

Kalish, R. A. Death and dying: A briefly annotated bibliography. In O. G. Brim, H. W. Freeman, S. Levine, & N. A. Scotch (Eds.), *The dying patient.* New York: Russell Sage Foundation, 1970. Pages 327–380 list 239 annotated entries arranged alphabetically. The compiler says that he tried to be as thorough as possible in psychology, sociology, and psychiatry; that he included items from nursing, general medicine, pastoral counseling, theology, hospital administration, and anthropology; that he only included items published in English and available in libraries; and that he ordinarily omitted items on mourning and grief, suicide, abortion, cryonics, birth control, and homicide.

Kalish, R. A. Grief and bereavement: A selected annotated bibliography of behavioral science and psychiatric writings. In Austin H. Kutscher (Ed.), *Death and bereavement.* Springfield, IL: Thomas, 1969. Pages 343–358 list 57 entries with descriptive and critical annotations, restricted to English-language publications in psychology, sociology, and psychiatry. Two pages of "additional references" by Dorothy Howard and Lee M. Olson list 29 entries (without annotations) under five topical headings.

Kalish, R. A. Loss and grief: A selected bibliography. In B. Schoenberg, A. C. Carr, D. Peretz, & A. H. Kutscher (Eds.), *Loss and grief: Psychological management in medical practice.* New York: Columbia University Press, 1970. The 47 entries on pages 373–385 are annotated descriptively and critically.

Katz, A. H. *Self-help and rehabilitation: An annotated bibliography.* Los Angeles: UCLA School of Public Health, September 1967. This is a 41-page, typed, privately circulated bibliography listing and annotating 98 items under the following six headings: social theory and methods; community and family aspects; institutions (hospitals, prisons, schools); self-help organizations; self-help groups and professional workers; and self-help and community development. It is a selective bibliography drawn from social science literatures and intended for professional workers, social scientists, and students. Now admittedly out of date, this bibliography lacks entries on recent groups concerned with dying or bereavement (except for Parents Without Partners), but it may be useful for its broader context and theoretical suggestions.

Kohn, J. B., & Kohn, W. K. *The widower.* Boston: Beacon, 1978. Pages 157–166 contain a selected, unannotated bibliography of 156 items arranged alphabetically under eight topical headings corresponding to the chapter titles of the book's text.

Kruzas, A. T. *Medical and health information directory.* Detroit: Gale Research Co., 1977. This volume offers a 680-page, double-column "guide to state, national and international organizations, government agencies, educational institutions, hospitals, grant-award sources, health care delivery agencies, journals, newsletters, review serials, abstracting services, publishers, research centers, computerized data banks, audiovisual services, and libraries and information centers."

Kübler-Ross, E. *Death: The final stage of growth.* Englewood Cliffs, NJ: Prentice-Hall, 1975. Pages 169–175 list 150 items.

Kübler-Ross, E. *On death and dying.* New York: Macmillan, 1969. Pages 279–289 list 183 items.

Kutscher, A. H., Jr., & Kutscher, A. H. *A bibliography of books on death, bereavement, loss and grief: 1935–1968.* New York: Health Sciences Publishing Corporation, 1969. A supplement (1974) in the form of a 68-page brochure includes citations from 1968–1972. The editors describe this work as "a comprehensive, uncritical bibliography of . . . [English-language] books published in the United States or the British Commonwealth . . . intended to be used by the layman, ministers, and health science personnel including professionals in the fields of psychiatry, psychology, nursing, sociology, and social work." It includes 1191 items without annotations, listed alphabetically under 42 primary subject headings and many subheadings. The supplement adds another 470 items listed in a similar way. Entries are identified by the letter(s) assigned to the primary subject headings and by their numbered position thereunder. There is also a 10-page triple-column author index in the original, and a similar 7-page double-column author index in the supplement.

Kutscher, M. L., Cherico, D. J., Kutscher, A. H., Hanninen, A. E., & Peretz, D. *A comprehensive bibliography of the thanatology literature.* New York: MSS Information Corporation, 1975. This volume contains 4844 numbered entries without annotation, listed alphabetically by author. A 40-page index organizes these entries according to 423 subject headings in a deliberate attempt to improve breadth and accuracy of indexing in this field. The book represents a massive attempt to reflect and organize a burgeoning, many-sided literature. The editors acknowledge reliance on previous bibliographies, express concern for obsolescence in the literature over time, and mention the eventual need for supplementation.

Langer, M. *Learning to live as a widow.* New York: Julian Messner, 1957. Pages 236–255 contain a resource appendix listing various services available for widows.

Marks, Renée U. *The sociology of death: A selected bibliography.* Department of Epidemiology, School of Public Health, The University of Michigan, Ann Arbor, MI, 1965. This is an early mimeographed list of 59 items that represent sociological work on death at the time, excluding specialized topics, fields, and nonsociological perspectives. It is no longer available.

Marshall, J. G., & Marshall, V. W. The treatment of death in children's books. *Omega,* 1971, *2,* 36–45. This article contains (pp. 41–45) an "Annotated bibliography: A selected list of children's books relating to death" compiled by the first author—57 books divided into general age categories (preschool to age 7; ages 8 to 11; age 12 and over) with one- or two-sentence annotations, plus 8 books that discuss how to explain death to children.

Mason, E. A. *Films on death and dying.* 1973. (Available for $.75 prepaid from the Educational Film Library Association, 43 West 61st Street, New York, NY 10023.) This 4-page pamphlet contains a 2-page narrative with brief summaries and evaluations of a variety of films, followed by a listing of 40 films, together with source information and other useful data for each.

McCormick, R. A. Notes on moral theology: April-September, 1972. *Theological Studies,* 1973, *34,* 53-103. This bibliographical essay deals in part (pp. 65-77) with literature on ethical aspects of death and dying.

Meyer, J. E. *[Death and neurosis.]* (M. Nunberg, trans.). New York: International Universities Press, 1975. Pages 135-147 list 203 items.

Miller, A. J., & Acri, M. J. *Death: A bibliographical guide.* Metuchen, NJ: Scarecrow, 1977. This volume offers a comprehensive listing of 3905 items from "ancient beginnings" through 1974+. Entries are numbered (though additions and omissions render the apparent total of 3,848 inaccurate) and listed alphabetically in an eight-part arrangement. Printed materials appear under the following headings: general works; education; humanities; medical profession and nursing experiences; religion and theology; science; and social sciences. The final part (audiovisual media) lists 192 items. Many entries also have annotations. There are author and subject indices.

Mills, G. C. Books to help children understand death. *American Journal of Nursing,* 1979, *79,* 291-295. A short review article with brief comments about 67 books.

Mills, G. C., Reisler, R., Jr., Robinson, A. E., & Vermilye, G. *Discussing death: A guide to death education.* Homewood, IL: ETC Publications, 1976. The unannotated bibliographies in this book list 23 items for 5-6-year-olds (pp. 25-26), 9 items for 7-9-year-olds (p. 34), 34 items for 10-12-year-olds (pp. 43-44), and 129 items for 13-18-year-olds (pp. 116-122). Some of these items, as well as films and other audiovisual materials, are also described in the book's text.

Morgan, J. H. *Death and dying: A resource bibliography for clergy and chaplains (1960-1976).* Wichita, KS: Institute on Ministry and the Elderly (3100 McCormick Avenue, 67213), 1977. This 30-page brochure contains an alphabetical listing of 128 books and 379 articles without annotations. Articles are arranged under the following headings: care of the dying; attitudes; death; bereavement; children; and religion, ethics, and the law.

Moss, W. G. (Principal Ed.). *Humanistic perspectives on aging: An annotated bibliography and essay.* Ann Arbor, MI: Institute of Gerontology, The University of Michigan-Wayne State University, 1976. This 82-page brochure contains: an essay on "Aging in Humanistic Perspectives"; annotated bibliographies on "Aging Around the World—Nonfiction, Past and Present," "Reflections on the Aging—Autobiographies by Older Authors," "Literature on Aging and the

Aged" (subdivided into drama, essays, novels, poetry, and short stories), and "Reflections on Death" (43 entries); and additional annotated resources in the form of "Films and Videotapes" and "Other Explorations."

Munson, R. *Intervention and reflection: Basic issues in medical ethics.* Belmont, CA: Wadsworth, 1979. Pages 493–506 list 366 items, organized generally according to the part and chapter divisions of the text.

Neale, R. E. *The art of dying.* New York: Harper & Row, 1973. Pages 151–158 offer a selected, annotated bibliography of 44 items.

Neale, R. E. Explorations in death education. *Pastoral Psychology,* Nov. 1971, *22,* 33–74. According to the author, "the purpose of this essay is to provide material for clergy who desire to explore the subject of death with their laymen." The unannotated bibliography (pp. 71–74) lists 158 items alphabetically under the headings "literature," "science," and "religion."

Nevins, M. *Annotated bibliography of bioethics: Selected 1976 titles.* Rockville, MD: Information Planning Associates, 1977. This 96-page brochure contains 1268 entries representing articles and books on bioethics published during 1976. Entries are categorized according to the nine subject areas used by *The Bioethics Digest* (q.v.): general works; mental health; death and dying; medical research; professional/patient relationship; genetics, fertilization, and pregnancy; population control; medical technology; and health care. Within each of these categories, the entries are arranged alphabetically by title under topical headings and subheadings. Each entry includes a brief descriptive annotation. There is also an author index.

Nevins, M. *A bioethical perspective on death and dying: Summaries of the literature.* Rockville, MD: Information Planning Associates, 1977. Another 96-page brochure, this was published as a special supplement to *The Bioethics Digest* (q. v.) and contains all of the abstracts from the first 12 issues of the *Digest.* The 218 entries with paragraph-length annotations are arranged alphabetically by title under the following eight primary headings: attitudes toward death; death education; definition and determination of death; euthanasia (subdivided into ethical and philosophical considerations, and policy and legislation); involuntary euthanasia (subdivided into children, and the Quinlan case); care of the dying; bereavement; and suicide. There is also a list of 86 unannotated references and an author index.

Nilsen, A. P. Death and dying: Facts, fiction, folklore, *English Journal,* 1973, *62,* 1187–1189. This article consists of an annotated bibliography of 15 recent books on death for young adults.

Parad, H. J., Resnik, H. L. P., & Parad, L. G. (Eds.). *Emergency and disaster management: A mental health sourcebook.* Bowie, MD: The Charles Press, 1976. Pages 475–497 of this book contain an unannotated, numbered bibliography of 470 items on this specialized subject listed in alphabetical order.

Pattison, E. M. *The experience of dying.* Englewood Cliffs, NJ: Prentice-Hall, 1977. Pages 329–335 list 128 items organized topically.

Pearson, L. (Ed.) *Death and dying: Current issues in the treatment of the dying person.* Cleveland: Case Western Reserve University Press, 1969. Pages 133–235 offer an annotated bibliography of 760 items organized by subject.

Pine, V. R. A socio-historical portrait of death education. *Death Education*, 1977, *1*, 57–84. This article reviews the evolution of formal death education over the last 50 years, largely through a survey of the most significant sociological literature.

Poteet, G. H. *Death and dying: A bibliography (1950–1974).* Troy, NY: Whitson, 1976. This volume contains an unannotated bibliography listing 153 books and 2146 articles, the latter arranged alphabetically according to 213 subject headings. There is also an author index. According to the editor, "the listings generally have little to do with euthanasia, nothing to do with legal interpretations of death and life, and do not include suicide. Instead, the central point of the work is almost exclusively the psychology of death. In this rather specific area, this volume attempts to be a near complete world bibliography for the years 1950 through 1974" (p. i).

Poteet, G. H., & Santora, J. C. *Death and dying: A bibliography (1950–1974)—Supplement, Volume I: Suicide.* Troy, NY: Whitston, 1978. This book is an unannotated bibliography listing 102 books and 1847 articles, the latter arranged alphabetically according to 234 subject headings, with an author index. The selective bibliography on the literature of suicide for 1950–1974 emphasizes the psychology of self-destruction. As a whole, the work is intended to accompany Poteet's 1976 bibliography on death and dying (q.v.), but it does not duplicate the listings there. A third volume designed as a sequel and supplement to both previous works and covering the years 1975–1977 is planned for publication in late 1979.

Prentice, A. E. *Suicide: A selective bibliography of more than 2,200 items.* Metuchen, NJ: Scarecrow, 1974. This volume lists 2218 items in English, excluding literary works and those of a highly technical sort, published approximately from 1960–1973. The list is without annotations and is intended for the general researcher. It includes: books; theses and dissertations; articles in books, from the popular press, from religious journals, and from legal journals; suicide and state legislation (a two-page essay); articles from medical and other scientific journals (the largest section, containing 1472 items); literary works; and films, tapes, and recordings. There are also author and subject indices.

Prince, A. *Death and dying: A mediagraphy. An annotated listing of audiovisual materials.* Seattle, WA: University of Washington and Allied Memorial Council, 1977. This paperback volume, the largest mediagraphy available in the field until now, is one result of a "media festival on death and dying" emphasizing health care education held in Seattle in June 1974. It contains: full-scale reviews (data, synopsis, evaluation, and suggested use) of 41 films, 19 videotapes (some here and below are multi-unit series), 11 filmstrips, and 36 audiotapes and records; a listing giving only data and brief summaries of an additional 37 films, 80 videotapes, 22 filmstrips, and 63 audiotapes and records; a list of distributors; appendices reproducing the program of the Seattle meeting, its media evaluation form, and a follow-up assessment form; and indices by title, subject, and distributor.

Prouty, D. Read about death? Not me! *Language Arts*, 1976, *53*(6), 679-683. Appendix B to this article contains a reading list of 13 books that concern the death of a grandparent, parent, son or daughter, plus 3 others that explore attitudes about death.

Psychological aspects of cancer. National Library of Medicine, Literature Search No. 77-17, April 1973 through December 1977. (Available without cost from Literature Search Program, National Library of Medicine, 8600 Rockville Pike, Bethesda, MD 20014.) This computer-generated bibliography prepared by Geraldine D. Nowak updates *Attitude towards death* (q.v.). It contains 269 citations in English listed alphabetically, each with major and minor topical headings for computer indexing.

Reed, J. *From private vice to public virtue: The birth control movement and American society since 1830.* New York: Basic Books, 1978. Pages 439-447 contain a bibliographical essay in cultural history following the part-division of the book's text.

Rheingold, J. C. *The mother, anxiety, and death: The catastrophic death complex.* Boston: Little, Brown, 1967. Pages 229-254 list 430 numbered references following the order of citation in the text.

Romero, C. E. Children, death and literature. *Language Arts*, 1976, *53*(6), 674-678. On page 678 is a bibliography of 21 books for primary and intermediate reading, plus 3 designed for adult/child reading.

Romero, C. E. *The treatment of death in contemporary children's literature.* (ERIC Document Reproduction Service No. ED 101 664) Computer Microfilm International, P.O. Box 190, Arlington, VA 22210. This master's thesis, submitted to Long Island University in 1974, analyzes 22 books of juvenile fiction and 3 instructional books designed for adult/child reading. It also contains an unannotated bibliography of 47 items.

Ross, E. S. Children's books relating to death: A discussion. In E. A. Grollman (Ed.), *Explaining death to children.* Boston: Beacon, 1967. The bibliography (pp. 288-296) lists 115 items.

Russell, O. R. *Freedom to die: Moral and legal aspects of euthanasia.* New York: Human Sciences Press, 1975; Dell, 1976. Pages 282-316 list sources, divided into references (367 entries previously mentioned or quoted in the text), bibliography (223 additional entries arranged alphabetically by subject headings), cases (53 court cases, opinions, or cases not taken to court), and bills and resolutions (a variety of legislative proposals and resolutions in the United States and England).

Sadker, D., Sadker, M., & Crockett, C. Death: A fact of life in children's literature. *Instructor*, March 1976, *85*(7), 73–84. This article discusses 10 recent books on death for children.

Sarvis, B., & Rodman, H. *The abortion controversy.* New York: Columbia University Press, 1973. Pages 201–217 list 335 items.

Schrank, J. Death: Guide to books and audiovisual aids. *Media and Methods*, 1971, *7*(6), pp. 32–35; 64. Pages 35 and 64 of this article include a brief teacher-student bibliography of various books, organizations, current music, feature films, and short films.

Schulz, R. *The psychology of death, dying, and bereavement.* Reading, MA: Addison-Wesley, 1978. Pages 172–187 list 303 items.

Schwartz, S. Death education: Suggested readings and audiovisuals. *The Journal of School Health*, December 1977, *47*, 607–609. This is a list of 89 books and 17 audiovisual items for elementary and high school students, and for lay or professional audiences.

Science for society: A bibliography. (Available from the Office of Science Education, American Association for the Advancement of Science, 1776 Massachusetts Avenue, N.W., Washington, DC 20036.) This is one in a series of annual bibliographies focusing on "ideas having to do with the interrelationships of humankind, the environment, science, and technology." The sixth edition (1976), a 114-page brochure prepared by Joseph M. Dasbach, provides annotated references to books and articles in 11 areas of science-society issues: aging and death; conflict; energy; environmental manipulation; ethics, values, responsibility, and science; health care; natural resources; pollution; population; technology and humankind; and transportation. Each area has its own structure of topical headings and subheadings. References in the sixth edition are to selected books published from 1972–1975, and to articles appearing from July 1974 through July 1975. This includes approximately 350 books and 100 articles carried over from the fifth edition.

Sell, I. *Dying and death: An annotated bibliography.* New York: Tiresias Press, 1977. This bibliography provides paragraph-length annotations, with author and subject indices, of 382 articles, 71 books, and 53 audiovisual items. It is intended primarily for nursing practitioners, educators, and students, but can be used by many others.

Shaffer, T. L. *Death, property, and lawyers: A behavioral approach.* New York: Dunellen, 1970. Pages 273–284 contain a "table of references" which lists 99 books, 7 anthologies, and 141 articles and papers.

Shibles, W. A. *Death: An interdisciplinary analysis.* Whitewater, WI: The Language Press, 1974. Without comment or annotation, 1305 entries are listed on pages 525–558.

Shneidman, E. S. *Deaths of man.* New York: Quadrangle, 1973; Baltimore: Penguin, 1974. Pages 225–232 list 140 entries.

Shusterman, L. R. Death and dying: A critical review of the literature. *Nursing Outlook*, 1973, *21*, 465–471. This article offers a narrative review of sociological, psychological, and medical literature concerning research on the experience of dying in a modern general hospital, together with 45 references.

Siggins, L. Mourning: A critical survey of the literature. *International Journal of Psycho-analysis*, 1966, *47*, 14–25. The author reviews and classifies the literature and provides 92 references.

Simpson, M. A. *Dying, death, and grief: A critically annotated bibliography and source book of thanatology and terminal care.* New York and London: Plenum Press, 1979. This is the first published bibliography by the author, although it was preceded by earlier editions in 1970–1973 (in Britain), 1973–1974 (in Canada), and again in 1975. The contents of this edition are as follows: an annotated list of 492 numbered books listed alphabetically with critical comments and a five-star rating system; a supplementary list of 216 other books that were recently received or that are not recommended for reading or reference—many are not annotated; a 41-category subject index to the preceding lists, with entries identified by number and arranged in order of rating stars under each heading; an author index; an annotated list of 16 journals; an annotated list of 212 numbered films listed alphabetically; an alphabetical list of film distributors and libraries; an annotated list of 57 audiovisual materials (audiotapes and audiocassettes, one record, videotapes, and videocassettes); an annotated list of 42 teaching materials and kits—mostly filmstrips; unannotated lists of French, Scandinavian, German, and Dutch literature (137 items in all); an unannotated list of 622 journal references arranged in 21 topical categories; a list of 56 films and audiovisual media available in Great Britain, together with addresses for distributors; and 55 partly-annotated "stop press additions." Simpson set out to be a very critical evaluator; his comments have variously pleased, delighted, disturbed, and outraged.

Smith, A. J. K., & Penry, J. K. *Brain death: A bibliography with key-word and author indexes.* (DHEW Publication No. (NIH) 73–347). Washington, DC: United States Department of Health, Education, and Welfare; Public Health Service; National Institutes of Health; National Institute of Neurological Diseases and Stroke; Applied Neurological Research Branch, June 1972. This 36-page brochure offers a 9-page list of 340 references presented in alphabetical order under 8 major topical headings and various subheadings. Articles published in a foreign language are indexed under the English translation of their titles. There is also a 17-page, double-column key-word subject index, and a 2-page triple-column author index.

Sollitto, S., & Veatch, R. M. *Bibliography of society, ethics and the life sciences, 1974.* Hastings-on-Hudson, NY: Institute of

Society, Ethics and the Life Sciences, 1974. This well-known bibliography includes a section on death and dying with annotations for some entries. See also subsequent issues or supplements for 1975, 1976-77, 1977-78, and 1979-80.

Somerville, R. M. Death education as part of family life education: Using imaginative literature for insights into family crises. *The Family Coordinator*, 1971, *20*, 209-224. The last two pages of this article include an unannotated bibliography of 24 items of selected fiction dealing with death and bereavement, as well as a list of 51 references.

Spiegel, Y. *Bibliography on 1) grief, 2) depression, stress and crisis, 3) death and dying, 4) related literature.* Germany: Anthropologisches Institut, University of Mainz, 1972. Mimeographed.

Stanford, G. Methods and materials for death education. *The School Counselor*, 1977, *24*, 350-360. In the course of its discussion, this article covers a variety of resources for elementary and secondary teaching, including 3 teaching units, 10 general books, 7 books for elementary students, 14 books for junior high and high school students, 19 films, and 5 other audiovisual items.

Steinzor, B. Death and the construction of reality: A revisit to the literature from 1960. *Omega*, 1978-1979, *9*, 97-124. According to the author, "this presentation will largely restrict itself to the studies, both clinical and experimental, on children and adolescents in their ordinary experience of death." It is a review article with 85 numbered references.

Stoddard, S. *The hospice movement: A better way of caring for the dying.* Briarcliff Manor, NY: Stein & Day, 1978. Pages 247-258 list 233 items.

Strugnell, C. *Adjustment to widowhood and some related problems: A selective and annotated bibliography.* New York: Health Sciences, 1974. This bibliography is a project of Harvard's Widow-to-Widow Program, whose interests define its scope and principles of selection. It lists a total of 660 entries under the following primary and secondary topical headings: concerning bereavement—bereavement in general (104), widowhood in general (79), elderly widowed (35), widowhood—cross-cultural (27), and childhood bereavement (104); problems related to widowhood—loneliness (33), and role of women (107); helping relationships—what is helping? (38), nonprofessionals (75), and mutual help groups (38); related bibliographies (20). Entries are generally restricted to Anglo-American publications appearing before 1972. Many are annotated, usually briefly but sometimes quite lengthily. Annotations are omitted if access could not be obtained to the reference, or if it was thought to be well enough known or its title sufficiently explicit to obviate the need for comment.

Sudden cardiac death. National Library of Medicine, Literature Search No. 76-18, January 1974 through March 1976. (Available without cost from Literature Search Program, National Library of Medicine, 8600 Rockville Pike, Bethesda, MD 20014.) This computer-generated bibliography was prepared by Charlotte Kenton and contains 277 citations in English listed alphabetically, each with major and minor topical headings for computer indexing.

Sudden Infant Death Syndrome, selected annotated bibliography 1960-1971. (United States Department of Health, Education, and Welfare; Public Health Service; National Institutes of Health; DHEW Publication No. (NIH) 74-237). Washington, DC: U. S. Government Printing Office, 1974. This brochure lists 239 annotated references.

Sudden Infant Death Syndrome, selected annotated bibliography 1972-1974. (United States Department of Health, Education, and Welfare; Public Health Service; National Institutes of Health; DHEW Publication No. (NIH) 76-237). Washington, DC: U. S. Government Printing Office, 1976. Dr. Marie Valdes-Dapena prepared this 52-page brochure, which lists 205 annotated references.

Sudden unexpected death in infants. National Library of Medicine, Literature Search No. 76-17, January 1974 through March 1976. (Available without cost from Literature Search Program, National Library of Medicine, 8600 Rockville Pike, Bethesda, MD 20014.) This computer-generated bibliography, prepared by Patti Burmeister, contains 159 citations in English listed alphabetically, each with major and minor topical headings for computer indexing.

The thanatology librarian or **The thanatology library.** See *R. Halporn.*

Trautmann, J., & Pollard, C. *Literature and medicine: Topics, titles & notes.* Philadelphia: Society for Health and Human Values, 1975. This is an extensive listing (151 pages), arranged chronologically and with paragraph-length annotations, of poems, plays, and fictional literature dealing with medical themes. The 39 subject indices include such topics as death, dying, euthanasia, grief, and suicide.

Triche, C. W., II, & Triche, D. S. *The euthanasia controversy, 1812-1974: A bibliography with select annotations.* Troy, NY: Whitston, 1975. According to the editors, this is a "near complete selectively annotated bibliography." It contains an alphabetical listing of 150 books and essays, and 1213 entries for periodical literature arranged under 19 primary subject headings and some subheadings. There is an author index.

Ulin, R. O. *Death and dying education.* Washington, DC: National Education Association, 1977. Pages 63-72 contain an unannotated bibliography of 48 general items, 24 examples of literary materials, 15 examples of audiovisual resources, and 6 instances of other media items.

Valdes-Dapena, M. A. Sudden and unexpected death in infancy: A review of the world literature, 1954-1966. *Pediatrics,* 1967, *39,* 123-138. This review article gives 105 references.

Veatch, R. M. *Case studies in medical ethics.* Cambridge, MA: Harvard University Press, 1977. Pages 368–401 list 630 items organized according to chapter divisions and subtopics. The section in the bibliography (pp. 396–401) corresponding to Chapter 13 lists 100 items under the general heading of death and dying, with several subheadings.

Veatch, R. M. *Death, dying, and the biological revolution: Our last quest for responsibility.* New Haven: Yale University Press, 1976. Pages 307–318 list 193 items arranged topically according to the main themes of the text.

Vernick, J. J. *Selected bibliography on death and dying.* Washington, DC: U. S. Department of Health, Education, and Welfare; Public Health Service; National Institutes of Health, 1970. This 61-page brochure contains a 29-page numbered list in alphabetical order of 1494 entries. There is also an author/subject index and an abbreviation listing of journals indexed. The entries include medical, psychological, psychiatric, religious, and literary items from the past 100 years or so. The bibliography is based on an interest in dying children, and is intended to serve physicians, educators, parents, and relatives or patients with terminal illnesses.

Walters, L. (Ed.), et al. *Bibliography of bioethics* (5 vols.). Detroit: Gale Research Co., 1975–1979. These volumes represent an attempt at a bioethics thesaurus or index language for cataloging purposes, as well as a comprehensive listing of English-language materials in the field. The subject index in each volume lists items alphabetically (with data and appropriate thematic descriptors) under topical headings. There are 800 documents in Volume I (1973 publications); 1218 in Volume II (1973–1974 publications); 1512 in Volume III (1973–1976 publications); 2000 in Volume IV (1973–1977 publications); and 1601 in Volume V (1973–1978 publications). Each volume also contains a list of journals cited, as well as title and author indices.

Wass, H., & Shaak, J. Helping children understand death through literature. *Childhood Education,* November/December 1976, *53*(2), 80–85. An argument for open discussion of death at home and the value of children's literature as a resource in that endeavor, this article includes a selective, annotated bibliography of 29 items organized by age groups.

Weisman, A. D. *The realization of death: A guide for the psychological autopsy.* New York: Jason Aronson, 1974. Pages 195–201 list 81 items organized according to the 5 chapter divisions of the text.

Zimmerman, M. K. *Passage through abortion: The personal and social reality of women's experiences.* New York: Praeger, 1977. Pages 213–220 list 126 items.

Periodicals

Our aim in this section is to provide information and guidance concerning journals and other periodical resources that are of importance for death education. In order to achieve this goal and to define the scope of the present section, we must first note that there are numerous journals and periodicals that occasionally publish an article relating to our field. Even a brief glance at the major bibliographies cited in the previous section shows that their references are drawn from a very broad spectrum of sources. For example, Poteet's 1976 bibliography alone, which is essentially restricted to literature on the psychology of death, searched over 500 journals for its entries. Our own list of articles dealing directly with the pedagogy of death education (in the first section of this book) is also taken from quite a diverse group of sources.

We have not attempted to list here all of the journals and other periodicals that have published or might publish articles on some aspect of death, dying, or bereavement. No individual could keep up with such a wide range of continuing publications. Even if that were possible, the results would hardly be proportionate to the investment of time and energy required. The overall number of such sources is too large, many are quite specialized, and others offer only an occasional piece that meets our needs. Those who desire access to such sources might do better not to concentrate on specific journals as a whole, but to proceed by identifying particular topics or references of interest to them. Individual citations can be obtained directly from the many fine bibliographies that now serve our field. Other references can be discovered indirectly through the topical indexes of general reader's guides to periodical literature, or from the very helpful abstracting services that focus on the concerns of individual disciplines and professions. *Psychological Abstracts*, *Sociological Abstracts*, *Nursing Abstracts*, and the *Index Medicus*—to name only a few of the best known—all provide ongoing guides to periodical literature in their respective fields, with detailed topical indexes and full bibliographical citations.

In the following list we have concentrated on a relatively small number of journals and newsletters that are primarily or exclusively concerned with topics of death, dying, and bereavement. This far more manageable group contains journals that appeal to the broadest audiences in our field, journals that are most likely to reward the reader's attention and to merit an individual or institutional subscription. Similar criteria have led us to include some newsletters in this section. We recognize that newsletters are a distinct form of periodical literature and that they are often made available only to those who are members of a particular group or organization. However, many newsletters publish short articles, editorials, and book or film reviews. Newsletters are an invaluable resource for keeping up with recent developments, forthcoming meetings, and potential speakers. In many cases, the conscientious death educator will find it worthwhile to join an organization in this field simply to learn about its activities and to receive its newsletter. In this section, we provide information about newsletters that seem to have the broadest appeal and value, but the reader should note that several other newsletters are also listed in Part III in our survey of organizations as resources.

Entries in this section are arranged in alphabetical order. In each case we give the full title of the journal or newsletter and the relevant publication data (format, frequency, cost, and names and addresses of editors and publishers). Beyond that, we offer a brief description of the scope and character of each journal or newsletter, and of the services it provides. These descriptions combine statements from editors or publishers and our own comments. Where no address is given for an editor, communications should be sent in care of the publisher.

Aged Care Services Review. Begun at the outset of 1978, this review is edited by Ruth Bennett and Barry Gurland, and published by

The Haworth Press, 149 Fifth Avenue, New York, NY 10010. The review provides summaries and abstracts of recent journal articles concerning aged care services. Each issue contains a topical index— one of whose entries is "death and dying"—to current abstracts; every sixth issue of this bimonthly publication will include a cumulative subject/author index to the volume as a whole. Individual issues also provide a review article dealing with critical issues and problems concerning services, programs, and intervention for the elderly. Annual subscription rates are $20.00 per volume for individuals, and $30.00 for institutions. Canadian orders, add $2.00; other foreign orders, add $5.00.

The Archives of the Foundation of Thanatology. This is a quarterly periodical published by the Foundation of Thanatology, 630 West 168th Street, New York, NY 10032 (see Part III for a further description of the Foundation and its activities). Begun in 1971, this journal "is designed to acquaint professional personnel with details of the ongoing programs and activities of the Foundation; to serve as a constantly updated reference source of the Foundation's Professional Advisory Board; to serve as an outlet for prompt publication of original brief reports of a research, philosophical, observational, or editorial nature in these areas; to advise new readers about meetings and programs of interest; and to notify readers of new Foundation of Thanatology publications (books, monographs, reprints, etc.)." Subscriptions are $30.00 per year or $8.00 per issue.

The Bioethics Digest. This is a monthly publication edited by Madeline M. Nevins, P.O. Box 6318, 5632 Connecticut Avenue, N.W., Washington, DC 20015, and published by Information Planning Associates, Inc., 2 Research Court, Rockville, MD 20850. Started in 1976, the digest provides approximately 150 abstracts per issue taken from books, conference proceedings, and scientific material, as well as articles screened from 175 journals in philosophy, medicine, and the social sciences, and 200 law journals. Abstracts are grouped topically under the following headings: general works, mental health, death and dying, human experimentation, professional/ patient relationships, genetics, population control, medical technology, and health care. The digest also offers author and subject indexes, plus a journal source list. Subscriptions are $60.00 per year.

Bioethics Quarterly. A new periodical sponsored by the Northwest Institute of Ethics and the Life Sciences, edited by Jane A. Boyajian Raible, and published by Human Sciences Press, 72 Fifth Avenue, New York, NY 10011. The journal intends to publish articles on the full range of bioethical issues, including themes in death, dying, and bereavement. Subscriptions are $20.00 per year for individuals, and $40.00 for institutions.

Bulletin of the Continental Association of Funeral and Memorial Societies, Inc. The association's address is Suite 1100, 1828 L Street, N.W., Washington, DC 20036 (a further description of its activities appears in Part III). This bulletin is a newsletter distributed to members of the association and its regional and local affiliates. Begun in 1959, the bulletin now appears four times per year. In general, it reports activities of the association and its affiliates, as well as legislative, regulatory, and other items of interest to its membership.

The Compassionate Friends National Newsletter. This is published by the national office of The Compassionate Friends, a support group for bereaved parents, whose address is P.O. Box 1347, Oak Brook, IL 60521. The subscription rate for the newsletter, which began publication in the winter of 1978 and appears quarterly, is $5.00 per year. It offers news, reports of activities in the national office and at local chapters, book reviews, and other items of interest to those who have experienced the death of a child.

Concern for Dying. This newsletter (formerly entitled *Euthanasia News*) is sponsored by Concern for Dying, an Educational Council (formerly Euthanasia Educational Council), 250 West 57th Street, New York, NY 10019. Begun in 1975, this newsletter is distributed to members of the organization and to many others without cost (although donations and membership will be solicited). It provides announcements and reports of meetings, editorials and personal statements, notice of books and other educational resources, and reports of events in the news—all of which are concerned with euthanasia, the right to die and/or to refuse treatment, and the care of the dying. See Part III for a further description of the parent organization and its activities.

Death Education: Pedagogy, Counseling, Care—An International Quarterly. This journal is edited by Hannelore Wass, College of Education, University of Florida, Gainesville, FL 32611, and published by Hemisphere Publishing Corporation, 1025 Vermont Avenue, N.W., Washington, DC 20005. It is a quarterly journal of approximately 400 pages per year that began publication in 1977. In the words of its statement of information for authors, *Death Education* "publishes papers in the areas of death and dying education, counseling, and care." It also offers brief communications, letters to the editor, and news and notes. In addition, the Media Exchange section in each issue provides reviews of books and audiovisual materials and an annotated bibliography that includes both print and nonprint items. Subscription rates are: for libraries and institutions $40.00 in the United States and Canada and $42.00 elsewhere, and for individuals $20.00 in the United States and Canada and $22.00 elsewhere. To many, it appears that *Death Education* is rapidly becoming the broadest journal in the field, serving an international readership of educators, counselors, and caregivers.

Eclipse: The Shanti Project Newsletter. The Shanti Project is a volunteer counseling service in the San Francisco area for patients and families facing life-threatening illness. Its address is 1137 Colusa Avenue, Berkeley, CA 94707. (See Part III for a further description of the Project and its activities.) Started in 1977, *Eclipse* is a 12-page quarterly newsletter that is sent to volunteers, contributors, and others who are interested in the work of the Shanti Project. It reports on the activities of the project and provides brief articles, book reviews, bibliographic references, and announcements of meetings.

Educational Gerontology: An International Quarterly. Edited by D. Barry Lumsden, College of Education, North Texas State University, Denton, TX 76203, this journal is published by Hemisphere Publishing Corporation, 1025 Vermont Avenue, N.W., Washington, DC 20005. Begun in 1976, *Educational Gerontology* is a quarterly journal of approximately 400 pages per year. It "publishes original papers in the field of gerontology, adult education, and the social and behavioral sciences," as well as some announcements, letters to the editor, and reviews of books and other learning resources. Subscription rates are: for libraries and institutions $39.60 in the United States and Canada and $42.00 elsewhere, for individuals $19.50 in the United States and Canada and $21.50 elsewhere. There are other journals in the field of gerontology, such as *The Gerontologist* and the *Journal of Gerontology* (both of which are bimonthly publications of the Gerontological Society, 1835 K Street, N.W., Washington, DC 20006), but *Educational Gerontology* is the one that seems to be closest to our interests.

Essence: Issues in the Study of Aging, Dying and Death. This is the major Canadian periodical in the field. Edited by Stephen Fleming (Department of Psychology, Atkinson College, York University, Downsview, Ontario, Canada) and Richard Lonetto (Department of Psychology, University of Guelph, Guelph, Ontario, Canada), *Essence* is published by Atkinson College Press, 4700 Keele Street, Downsview, Ontario, Canada. It is a quarterly journal of approximately 240 pages per year. The subscription rate is $12.00 per year. In the introductory editorial statement to Volume I (1976), the editors say that *Essence* "will try to encourage articles from individuals in any discipline. We want to offer opportunities to authors and readers who feel the traditional journal channels leave a good deal to be desired." In addition to articles (which tend, perhaps, to emphasize the perspectives of caregivers and the social sciences), *Essence* publishes some news items, announcements, and an occasional book review.

Forum for Death Education and Counseling: Newsletter. The Forum for Death Education and Counseling, P.O. Box 1226, Arlington, VA 22210, is a young organization that is striving to become the primary national group bringing together and representing all who are interested in death education and counseling. (See Part III for a further description of the Forum and its activities.) Its newsletter is sent to all members of the forum 10 times per year (with only one publication during the summer months). Edited by Joan McNeil, 2020 Hunting, Manhattan, KS 66502, and begun in 1977, the newsletter offers news and announcements, editorials, interviews, book reviews, reports of meetings, and other items of interest.

The Hastings Center Report. This journal is edited by Margaret O'Brien Steinfels and published by the Institute of Society, Ethics and the Life Sciences, 360 Broadway, Hastings-on-Hudson, NY 10706. It is a bimonthly publication of approximately 300 pages per year, begun in 1971. Annual dues ($19.00 for individuals and libraries, $15.00 for students, and $30.00 for institutions) entitle associate members of the institute to receive the report, as well as a partially annotated and selective annual *Bibliography of Society, Ethics and the Life Sciences* (see "Bibliographies") and other materials. The report, "which is devoted entirely to discussions of bioethics, contains brief, timely observations on new developments, longer essays, scholarly articles, a regular guide to the most recent literature, specific case studies, a calendar of events across the country, and reactions from the Associate Members." Like the parent institute, the report takes death and dying as one of its primary fields, along with population control, genetic counseling and engineering, behavior control, health policy, and the foundations of ethics. See Part III for a further discussion of the institute and its activities.

International Journal for Medicine and Law. This is a new journal published by the World Association for Medical Law, International Center, P.O. Box 6451, Haifa, Israel. The journal began quarterly publication in 1979. It deals with all aspects of medicine and law including medical, legal, philosophical, and sociological dimensions of euthanasia, abortion, human experimentation, artificial insemination, and organ transplantation. It encompasses articles, analyses of court decisions, discussions of new legislation, book reviews, and news items.

The International Journal of Aging and Human Development. This journal is edited by Robert J. Kastenbaum, Department of Psychology, College 1, University of Massachusetts, Columbia Point Campus, Dorchester, MA 02125, and published by Baywood Publishing Co., Inc., 120 Marine Street, Farmingdale, NY 11735. It is a quarterly whose title from 1970-1972 was *Aging and Human Development.* The journal now fills approximately 400 pages per volume and costs $45.00 per year. It proclaims that its "emphasis is upon psychological and social studies of aging and the aged. However, the journal also publishes research that introduces observations from other fields that illuminate the 'human' side of gerontology, or utilizes gerontological observations to illuminate problems in other fields."

Journal of Thanatology. See *New Advances in Thanatology.*

Make Today Count. This is the newsletter of an organization by the same name founded in 1974 by Orville E. Kelly to encourage mutual help and self-help for individuals with a life-threatening illness. See Part III for a further description of the parent organization and its activities. The newsletter is edited by Robert Hansen and published by Make Today Count, P.O. Box 303, Burlington, IA 52601. It is a tabloid-size newspaper of eight pages per issue that appears approximately six to eight times per year. Subscription costs are $10.00 per year. The newsletter contains editorials, personal statements, and news reports from the national office, local chapters, and interested individuals.

New Advances in Thanatology. This is a quarterly journal begun in 1977 as a successor to the *Journal of Thanatology*. It is a project of the Foundation of Thanatology, 630 West 168th Street, New York, NY 10032 (see Part III for a further description of the foundation and its activities), and is published by MSS Information Corporation which, in turn, is distributed by Arno Press, P.O. Box 978, Edison, NJ 08817. In the words of an advertisement, *New Advances in Thanatology* "publishes full-length manuscripts derived from investigations throughout the country as well as those reporting on the Foundation's own research and investigations." The subscription rate is $15.00 per year.

Newsletter of the National Hospice Organization. NHO is a young organization that attempts to represent and guide the development of the hospice movement in the United States. The organization now has two offices, at 765 Prospect Street, New Haven, CT 06511, and 301 Maple Ave. West, Vienna, VA 22180. (See Part III for a further description of this organization and its activities.) The newsletter, which began publication in 1978 and which seems to appear on an irregular basis, is circulated to all members of the organization. It provides news items and information about developments of interest to those concerned with the hospice movement, and care of dying or bereaved persons.

Omega: Journal of Death and Dying. This journal sprang from a quarterly newsletter begun by Richard Kalish and Robert Kastenbaum in 1966. It has appeared as a journal since 1970, originally bearing the subtitle "An International Journal for the Psychological Study of Dying, Death, Bereavement, Suicide and Other Lethal Behaviors." At present, *Omega* is edited by Robert Kastenbaum, Department of Psychology, College 1, University of Massachusetts, Columbia Point Campus, Dorchester, MA 02125, and published by Baywood Publishing Company, Inc., 120 Marine Street, Farmingdale, NY 11735. The subscription rate is $45.00 per year for four issues totaling about 400 pages. In its first issue, the editor's statement said that "our primary focus will be upon behavioral and psychiatric sciences and upon social and health services," although its pages were to remain "open to any kind of article from any individual." For the most part, this description is still accurate. *Omega* publishes articles, some announcements or news items, and an occasional book review. It is fairly regarded as one of the leading journals in the field. Recently, the Forum for Death Education and Counseling announced that it will assume sponsorship of this journal.

St. Francis Burial and Counseling Society Newsletter. Published
at least quarterly, this is the principal ongong publication of the St.
Francis Burial and Counseling Society, 1768 Church Street, N.W.,
Washington, DC 20036. The society is well known for its advocacy
of spiritual versus material values at the time of death, and for its
services in supplying simple wooden coffins and ash boxes at a
modest price. (See Part III for a further description of the society
and its activities.) The newsletter was originally published as the *St.
Francis Burial and Counseling Society Quarterly* from 1975–1977. It
provides "a forum for sharing 'how to' information concerning the
legal, medical, religious and practical aspects of funeral pre-planning,
as well as a way to learn froïn experts in the field of death and
dying." Issues typically include news and notes, letters to the editor,
an information exchange, brief articles, book reviews, and bibliographical references. Individual subscriptions are $10.00 per year;
group subscriptions for 10 copies are $20.00 per year.

Suicide and Life-Threatening Behavior. This journal is the official
publication of The American Association of Suicidology, an organization whose interests and activities are further described in Part III.
The journal was originally published from 1971–1974 (Vols. 1–4)
under the title *Life-Threatening Behavior*. In 1975 (Vol. 5) that
name was changed to *Suicide*, and in 1976 it took on its present title.
The journal is edited by Edwin S. Shneidman, Neuropsychiatric Institute, University of California at Los Angeles, 760 Westwood Plaza,
Los Angeles, CA 90024, and published by Human Sciences Press, 72
Fifth Avenue, New York, NY 10011. It offers the following description of its scope and interests: "*Suicide and Life-Threatening Behavior* is devoted to emergent approaches in theory and practice relating
to self-destructive, other-destructive, and life-threatening behaviors.
It is multidisciplinary and concerned with a variety of topics: suicide,
suicide prevention, death, accidents, sub-intentioned destruction,
partial death-threats to life's length and breadth from within and
without." Annual subscription costs for this quarterly of approximately 250 pages per volume are $35.00 for institutions and $15.00
for individuals.

Thanatology Abstracts. Begun in 1978 *Thanatology Abstracts* is
published annually by MSS Information Corporation, c/o Arno Press,
P.O. Box 978, Edison, NJ 08817. A project of the Foundation of
Thanatology, 630 West 168th Street, New York, NY 10032, it is
described as "a compilation of abstracts of the current periodical
literature of thanatology. This new multi-volume series will serve as a
review of current research activities in all disciplines concerned with
thanatology." Subscriptions cost $15.00 per year. See Part III for a
further description of the foundation and its activities.

The Thanatology Librarian. This four-page newsletter is published by Roberta Halporn, a book seller who owns and operates
Highly Specialized Promotions, 228 Clinton St., Brooklyn, NY
11201. Started in 1976, *The Thanatology Librarian* is an ongoing

supplement to *The Thanatology Library*, a 32-page pamphlet that Halporn published in June 1976. Both the newsletter and the original pamphlet provide capsule descriptions of books, audiovisuals, and other materials pertaining to death, bereavement, loss, and grief. *The Thanatology Librarian* describes new titles and older items, categorizes them by subject, and adds information about free or inexpensive pamphlets available from various sources. This newsletter is obviously intended to advertise the services provided by Halporn's company, but it is also a useful source of bibliographic and mediagraphic information, and a convenient basis for purchasing materials from the only specialized book dealer serving our field. The original *Thanatology Library* sold for $1.00; subscriptions to *The Thanatology Librarian* are $3.50.

Thanatology News. This is a bimonthly publication (begun in 1975) published by the Foundation of Thanatology, 630 West 168th Street, New York, NY 10032. Available only to associate members of the foundation, "this periodical is intended to assure for the first time the prompt, inter-disciplinary dissemination of information relative to all the allied health sciences and to other study areas in the field of thanatology." See Part III for a further description of the foundation and its activities.

Thanatology Today Newsletter. A new newsletter for professionals in the fields of dying, death, grief, and bereavement, this periodical is edited by Jean De Sapio and published by Atcom, Inc., Atcom Building, 2315 Broadway, New York, NY 10024. This monthly newsletter offers such services as a calendar of events, reports on current developments, interviews, reviews of books and journals, and a reader exchange. The subscription rate is $45.00 per year with reductions for multiyear periods.

Thanatos: A Realistic Journal Concerning Dying, Death and Bereavement. This quarterly journal is edited by Noranel Neely and published by the Florida Consumer Information Bureau, Inc., P.O. Drawer 7698, St. Petersburg, FL 33734. Although this fact is not mentioned in the journal or in much of its advertising literature, readers might wish to know that it is a wholly owned subsidiary of the Florida Funeral Directors Association. Perhaps because of this background, *Thanatos* appears rather more like a trade magazine than a professional journal. Its dramatic covers are strikingly attractive and its text is lavishly illustrated with photographs and colorful art work. The text consists of brief articles and an occasional editorial on various subjects related to death, dying, and bereavement. Subscription costs are $12.00 per year, for four issues of 22 pages each. Publication began in December of 1975.

Theta: A Journal for Research on the Question of Survival After Death. Begun in 1973, this is a quarterly journal edited by W. G. Roll and published by the Psychical Research Foundation, Inc., Duke Station, Durham, NC 22706. Subscription costs are $8.00 for one year or $12.00 for two years, for approximately 80 pages per year. The journal offers the following description of its own scope: "*Theta* is concerned with the most profound mystery of man's universe: Does consciousness continue beyond physical death? *Theta* presents the full spectrum of survival research, including studies of near-death experiences, mediumistic communications, reincarnation memories, and investigations of poltergeists and hauntings. Studies are also reported of such altered states of consciousness as out-of-body experiences and field consciousness, which may involve survivable aspects of the self." *Theta* also provides reports on activities of the foundation, announcements of meetings, news briefs, correspondence from readers, abstracts of articles, and book reviews. See Part III for a further description of the foundation and its activities.

WPS Insights. This four-page newsletter is published quarterly by the Widowed Persons Service of the National Retired Teachers Association and the American Association of Retired Persons, 1909 K Street, N.W., Washington, DC 20049. See Part III for a description of this organization and its activities. *WPS Insights* reports on activities of its parent associations and provides information about news items, legislative action, meetings, and publications that are of concern to widowed persons. This newsletter is made available without charge to interested parties.

Research
and
Assessment
of Death
Attitudes

When a new movement develops, more attention is given to immediate needs than to long-range implications. The death education movement is no exception. Energies have been poured primarily into developing a sound rationale for programs, and into curriculum development. As a consequence, research on and evaluation of death attitudes have been neglected. This clearly is reflected in the paucity of systematic studies reported. However, a change for the better is indicated by the recent appearance of two excellent works that focus on methodological problems and point to the relative lack of validated instruments for assessing death attitudes. The first is Richard Schulz's book, *The Psychology of Death, Dying, and Bereavement* (see p. 86). Schulz discusses death anxiety research and compares various instruments. The second is the review article by R. T. Kurlychek (see the bibliography of this section), which examines death attitude scales and reviews research using the scales. There is an obvious need for investigators to undertake the arduous task of effectively assessing death attitudes and attitude changes presumably caused by death education.

This section presents a short bibliography of known assessment instruments and techniques. A wide variety of methods, both direct and indirect, have been employed in attempting to measure various aspects of death-related attitudes. Direct techniques include interviews, questionnaires, checklists, and assorted rating scales. Indirect methods include projective techniques such as the Thematic Apperception Test (TAT) and physiologic measurements such as the galvanic skin response (GSR) in a word association test. By far the most widely used methods are direct.

When selecting an instrument for research purposes it is important to consider several factors. One major factor is test validity, i.e., does the device measure what it is intended to measure? Reliability should also be examined. Test-retest reliability, probably the most often used, refers to the stability of the instrument over time, i.e., to permanent characteristics of the individual. Sample characteristics should be considered (e.g., the age of the subjects). Is the instrument accessible to the researcher? What is the administration time and what limitations are placed upon the investigator, as well as the respondent? These are but a few of the concerns of the researcher.

The instruments and studies presented in the bibliography represent the groundwork of thanatological investigations. The broad selection offered is representative of the approaches used in the study of attitudes about death and dying.

Alexander, I. E., & Alderstein, A. M. Affective responses to the concept of death in a population of children and early adolescents. *Journal of Genetic Psychology*, 1958, *93*, 167–177. The authors measured affective responses to death words in a population of males aged 5–16. For a word association list response times, galvanic skin responses and response words were recorded. Three age subgroups were defined and discussed in the study.

Bakshis, Robert; Correll, Michael; Duffy, Myra; Grupp, Stanley E.; Hilliker, James; Howe, Thomas; Kawales, Gail; & Schmitt, Raymond L. "Meanings" toward death: ATST strategy. *Omega*, 1974, *5*(2), 161–181. This paper describes a new method for operationalizing attitudes toward death using the Twenty Statements Test format. Respondents are asked to structure 20 statements in answer to the question, "What is death?" The protocols were subjected to control analysis and 17 categories were generated. The reliability of the categorization of the responses was studied, and all protocols were coded twice by independent coders. The function of the test is to develop a new strategy for the determination of the "meanings" that individuals have toward death.

Boyar, J. I. The construction and partial validation of a scale for the measurement of fear of death (Doctoral dissertation, University of Rochester, 1964). *Dissertation Abstracts*, 1964, *25*, 2041. (University Microfilms No. 64-9228). An 18-item scale of an inventory was designed to measure intensity of fear of death. Split-half reliability was .83 but reliability based upon item-statistics was only .21. Test-retest reliability was .79 after a 10-day interval. Validity has been studied using two groups of students and embedding the FDDS items in other subject-related items. This instrument is easy to administer.

Bromberg, W., & Schilder, P. Death and dying: A comparative study of the attitudes and mental reactions toward death and dying. *Psychoanalytic Review*, 1933, *20*, 133–185. A 32-item questionnaire concerning death (included in the article) was presented to 10 psychiatric patients and 70 normal individuals. A comparison of the groups showed that the normal view of death is based on early experience and the personality integrity structure of the individual. The psychiatric patients revealed an intensification of death fears which were repressed more often than in the normals.

Bromberg, W., & Schilder, P. The attitudes of psychoneurotics toward death. *Psychoanalytic Review*, 1936, *23*, 1–28. Case histories are presented describing a variety of neurotic patients who manifested death fears. The authors discuss, after each case, the death components and the meaning death has for each patient.

Callas, M. A. The effect of an experience of death education on death attitudes and concepts and on self-perception. (Doctoral dissertation, The Catholic University of America, 1976). (University Microfilms). This study attempts to evaluate the effects of a 10-hour workshop on the psychology of death in changing death attitudes and concepts. The study involved 50 adults in the experimental group and 52 in a nonparticipating control group, and employed a pre- and posttest (plus a 2-month follow-up) design using the Templer Death Anxiety Scale, the Dickstein-Blatt Consciousness of Death Scale, and various measures of self-regard. The author concludes that the workshop did lower measured death anxiety, decrease negative images, heighten conscious ability to consider death as important in establishing life values, and increase self-acceptance and self-regard.

Christ, Adolph. Attitudes toward death among a group of acute geriatric psychiatric patients. *Journal of Gerontology*, 1961, *16*, 56–59. Using a word association test with death words embedded in the list, the author interviewed 100 patients aged 60 or older. Death-related words produced more bizarre responses and involved more blocking than other words. The author interpreted this as an indication of higher anxiety about death.

Cohen, R., & Parker, C. Fear of failure and death. *Psychological Reports*, 1974, *34*, 54. A group of 47 male undergraduate students wrote stories to four modified TAT pictures and completed the Collett-Lester Fear of Death scale. It was predicted that those having a high fear of failure would also have a high fear of death. No positive correlation was found.

Collett, L., & Lester, D. Fear of death and fear of dying. *Journal of Psychology*, 1969, *72*, 179–181. Scales were developed to assess fear of death, fear of dying of one's self, fear of death of others, and fear of dying of others. There was a test and retest of 25 female undergraduates. A 38-statement format was used with each item on a 6-point scale. The low correlations between scores on these scales indicated potential usefulness of differentiating between these four fears.

Degner, L. The relationship between some beliefs held by physicians and their life-prolonging decisions. *Omega: Journal of Death and Dying*, 1974, *5*, 223. A sociological scale was developed by the author to determine if significant differences occur in physicians' life-prolonging decisions on the basis of their beliefs concerning God, afterlife, and death. Degner discusses results of the study and describes the Life-Prolonging Scale used.

Deveries, A. G. A potential suicide personality inventory. *Psychological Reports*, 1966, *18*, 731-738. The author discusses the origination and construction of a 55-item Potential Suicide Personality Inventory (PSPI). The PSPI was administered to a group of suicidal males and a nonsuicidal group. Chi square analysis showed that the inventory clearly differentiated between the two groups at the .05 level.

Dickstein, L. Death concern: Measurement and correlates. *Psychological Reports*, 1972, *30*, 563-571. The author describes the conceptualization, construction, and scoring procedure of the Death Concern Scale, a 30-item scale each containing four response alternatives. Relationships between the Death Concern Scale and other anxiety scales as well as measures of selected personality variables are presented.

Dickstein, L. Self report and fantasy correlates of death concern. *Psychological Reports*, 1975, *37*, 147-158. Comparison of scores on the Death Concern Scale with scores on other scales were made, providing support for the construct validity of the Death Concern Scale.

Dickstein, L. Attitudes toward death, anxiety and social desirability. *Omega*, 1977-1978, *8*(4), 369-378. The Death Concern Scale is compared with three other death scales and other measures of anxiety and social desirability. The four death scales show a moderate commonality and are correlated with the other measures. The author suggests that relationships between death attitudes and other dimensions of personality need to be explored.

Dickstein, L. S., & Blatt, S. J. Death concern, futurity and anticipation. *Journal of Consulting Psychology*, 1966, *30*, 11-17. Male undergraduates at Yale were selected from the upper and lower quartiles of a death-concern questionnaire. They were then given the WAIS, Picture Arrangement, which measures future time perspective, to show a relationship between death concern and future time perspective. Those with low death concern showed greater extension into the future and scored higher on the Picture Arrangement subtest than did those with high death concern.

Diggory, J. C., & Rothman, D. Z. Values destroyed by death. *Journal of Abnormal and Social Psychology*, 1961, *63*, 205–210. A heterogeneous sample (in terms of age, community role, and socio-economic factors) of 563 respondents was given a questionnaire concerning the "consequences of one's own death." The overall conclusion was that which consequences are feared most depends on the role the individual has or expects to have, therefore on the goals to which he or she is most committed.

Durlak, J. Measurement of the fear of death: An examination of some existing scales. *Journal of Clinical Psychology*, 1972, *28*, 545–547. This study investigated the validity of four scales. The subjects were 94 psychology students. The data were analyzed for males and females separately, and results and discussions were presented.

Epting, F. R., Rainey, L. C., & Weiss, M. J. Constructions of death and levels of death fear. *Death Education*, 1979, *3*(1), 21–30. Students were administered the Threat Index (an instrument derived from personal construct theory) and Feifel's measures of the conscious, the fantasy, and the nonconscious level of fear of death in order to study the relationship of the Threat Index to Feifel's various levels of death fear and to assess the interrelationship among Feifel's levels. Results are reported and discussed.

Feifel, H. Attitudes of mentally ill patients toward death. *Journal of Nervous and Mental Disease*, 1955, *122*, 375–380. Hospitalized mentally ill patients were asked to indicate when they thought "people in general" were most afraid of death. They were then asked to rank their answers from childhood through old age. Patients were also asked to answer other death-related questions. The results indicate that old age is the time when there is greater perceived fear of death.

Feifel, Herman. Religious conviction and fear of death among the healthy and the terminally ill. In R. Fulton (Ed.), *Death and Identity* (Rev. ed.). Bowie, MD: The Charles Press, 1976. The group studied consisted of 95 healthy individuals and 92 terminally ill patients. Conscious fear of death responses were obtained by asking, "Are you afraid of your own death? Why?" and then classifying answers into a five category grouping. Death imagery was obtained by asking, "What ideas or pictures come to your mind when you think of your own death?" Below-the-level-of-awareness ideas were measured by a word association test. Results indicate no significant differences between religious and nonreligious respondents.

Feifel, H., & Branscomb, A. Who's afraid of death? *Journal of Abnormal Psychology*, 1973, *81*, 282–288. Attempting to select the major demographic variables related to fear of personal death, the study analyzed 371 physically ill, emotionally disturbed, or healthy individuals. The subjects' responses were measured on a conscious level, a fantasy level, and below the level of awareness. Fear of death was dealt with as distinct from fear of dying.

Feldman, M. J., & Hersen, M. Attitudes toward death in nightmare subjects. *Journal of Abnormal Psychology*, 1967, *72*, 421–425. On a 10-item death scale included in article, 168 college students were questioned as to their conscious death concerns. They were also asked to reveal the frequency of frightening dreams. Those with more frequent nightmares indicated a history of more deaths of relatives and close friends especially before the age of 10.

Fulton, R. Discussion of a symposium on attitudes toward death in older persons. *Journal of Gerontology*, 1961, *16*, 44–66. Included were death concerns in normal aged individuals, attitudes toward death in an aged population and attitudes toward death among a group of acute geriatric psychiatric patients. The author relates the methods used and comments on all reports.

Haley, H. B., Jr., Juan, I. R., & Gagan, J. F. Research in medical education. Factor-analytic approach to attitude scale construction. *Journal of Medical Education*, 1968, *43*, 331–336. The article discusses the construction of the Cancer Attitude Survey, a 52-item instrument which is being administered to medical students in a longitudinal study of the development of physicians' attitudes. Factor analytic techniques were used in the construction of the scales.

Hall, G. S. A study of fears. *American Journal of Psychology*, 1896, *8*, 147–249. This paper discusses the chief fears (the 19th of which was the fear of death) of 1701 people, mostly under 23 years of age. The methods of compiling this information lacked uniformity.

Handal, P. J. The relationship between subjective life expectancy, death anxiety, and general anxiety. *Journal of Clinical Psychology*, 1969, *25*, 39–42. A questionnaire was administered to 66 male and 50 female graduate students regarding their estimate of life expectancy (SLE) for their own sex. These data were then ranked from highest to lowest. Also administered were Zuckerman's Affective Adjective Checklist of Anxiety as well as a modified version of the Livingston and Zimet Death Anxiety Scale. A signficant negative relationship was found between SLE and death anxiety for females but not males. Evidence indicated that males are relatively more defensive about death than females.

Handal, P. J., & Rychlak, J. F. Curvilinearity between dream content and death anxiety and the relationship of death anxiety of repression-sensitization. *Journal of Abnormal Psychology*, 1971, *77*, 11–16. A prediction was made that both high and low scorers on the Death Anxiety Scale (DAS) will report more unpleasant and death dreams than will the subjects in the middle range. Besides the DAS, the Repression-Sensitization Scale was used. The subjects were two groups of college students with 1 year between test and retest. Both reported curvilinearity between DAS and dream content. The R-S scale did not coincide with the DAS, and the article discusses some possible reasons for this difference.

Hardt, D. Development of an investigatory instrument to measure attitudes toward death. *The Journal of School Health*, 1975, *45*, 1975, 96–99. A 20-item checklist designed to measure attitudes toward the concept of death was administered to 692 subjects aged 13–26 with mean age of 17.2 years. Reliability was studied using the split-half method, which yielded a coefficient of .87. The author suggests that this scale could be used to identify those with either extremely unfavorable or extremely favorable attitudes toward death.

Jeffers, F., Nichols, C., & Eisdorfer, C. Attitudes of older persons toward death: A preliminary study. *Journal of Gerontology*, 1961, *16*, 53–56. This 2-day multidisciplinary examination involved 269 community volunteers aged 60 or older. Two questions were asked: "Are you afraid to die?" (90 percent answered no); and "Do you believe in life after death?" (77 percent said yes). The authors felt that direct questioning might be an inappropriate way to tap death attitudes because of denial mechanism.

Kalish, R. A. An approach to the study of death attitudes. *American Behavioral Scientist*, 1963, *6*, 68–70. The author reports the findings of a pretest of a questionnaire concerning death attitudes. The 75 Likert-type attitude items were drawn from essays on "How I Feel about Death." These items are directed at death, dying, types of destruction of life, and religious beliefs. The pretest sample consisted of 280 students and 427 residents of Los Angeles.

Kalish, R. A. Some variables in death attitudes. *Journal of Social Psychology*, 1963, *59*, 137–145. This study is an exploratory investigation of attitudes toward different methods of destroying life, and the relationship of these attitudes to religious beliefs. Sixteen items were embedded in a 32-item questionnaire (items are included in the article). Results were factor analyzed with three factors emerging, 1) social liberalism, 2) destruction accepting factor, and 3) a religious justice factor.

Kalish, Richard, & Reynolds, David K. *Death and ethnicity: A psychocultural study.* Los Angeles: The University of California Press, 1976. This is a review of one of the broadest research efforts concerning death attitudes to date, an investigation into some cross-cultural views as well as opinions held by specialists in death-related areas, e.g., physicians, ministers, morticians, coroners. The 178-item questionnaire (containing demographic as well as attitude items) is included in the Appendix. This work presents results from a study that examined relationships among aspects of personality, culture, and orientations toward death of four major ethnic groups in the Los Angeles area.

Klug, L., & Boss, M. Factorial structure of the death concern scale. *Psychological Reports*, 1976, *38*, 107–112. A factor analysis of the Death Concern Scale yielded two distinct factors that are in agreement with Dickstein's (the author of the scale) two-part definition of "death concern." The present authors suggest using separate scales for each of the two factors.

Krieger, S., Epting, F., & Leitner, L. M. Personal constructs, threat, and attitudes toward death. *Omega*, 1974, *5*, 299. The authors discuss the use of the Threat Index, created for this study, and compare it and Lester's Fear of Death Scale as well as Templer's Death Anxiety Scale. The Threat Index is assessed by means of a structured interview and the use of 10 element cards that are presented to the respondent in groups of three. The article explains the procedure, outlines scoring, presents correlations among the measures, and discusses the validity of the Threat Index.

Kurlychek, R. T. Assessment of attitudes toward death and dying: A critical review of some available methods. *Omega*, 1978–1979, *9*, 37–47. Here is an excellent review article that discusses and compares various death attitude scales. Validation procedures, when attempted, are examined.

Lester, D. Experimental and correlational studies of the fear of death. *Psychological Bulletin*, 1967, *67*, 27–36. A review of the techniques used to measure the fear of death is provided. The effects of demographic variables and personal characteristics are discussed, and attention is drawn to the lack of consistency and the validity of the instruments used.

Lester, D. Inconsistency in the fear of death of individuals. *Psychological Reports*, 1967, *20*, 1084. The author reports on a study that showed inconsistency in attitudes toward death appears to be accompanied by a greater fear of death and that this finding is not due to an acquiescence response.

Lester, D. Studies in death attitudes. *Psychological Reports*, 1972, *30*, 440. This article briefly reports the result of three studies on death attitudes: inconsistency in the fear of death of individuals; sex differences in death anxiety and utility of semantic differential ratings of the concept of death as a measure of death attitudes.

Lester, D., & Lester, G. Fear of death, fear of dying, and threshold differences for death words and neutral words. *Omega*, 1970, *1*, 175–179. In this investigation of the difference between recognition thresholds for neutral and for death-oriented words, 25 subjects were used. The Collett-Lester (1969) fear of death scale was administered to each subject.

Lucas, Richard A. A comparison study of measures of general anxiety and death anxiety among three medical groups including patient and wife. *Omega*, 1974, *5*(3), 233–243. This paper presents a comparative study among three different groups of physically ill males and their wives. A 40-item Death Questionnaire (DQ) was devised by the author to be used as a comparison instrument. Reliability and validity have not been determined.

Lynch, J. H. The contexts of death imagery: An investigation of suggested categorical distinction among 25 death associated images (Doctoral dissertation, University of Oregon, 1976). (University Microfilms No. 76-27, 661). From the Context of Death Imagery (CDI), the Death Imagery Potency Scale (DIPS) was developed. It utilizes forced-choice pairings between image statements of five subscales: religious, social, somatic, medical, and existential. The 4-statement subscales produced 160 pairs which were divided into

Forms A and B (80 items each). Internal consistency has been studied. The results support the religious, social, and somatic subscales but reject the postulated association within the existential subscale. The medical subscale was tenuous.

Martin, D., & Wrightsman, L. S. Religion and fears about death: A critical review of research. *Religious Education*, 1964, *59*, 174-176. The authors state that past research has been lacking in methodological approaches. They feel that the relationship between religion and fear of death can now be studied and investigated with more discrete answers.

Maurer, A. Adolescent attitudes toward death. *Journal of Genetic Psychology*, 1964, *105*, 75-90. Two essay-type questions were asked of 172 senior high school female students. Judges rated the essays for maturity of content and further sorted them into content categories. Fear appeared more often than any other category. Mature responses were associated with academic achievement, while poor achievement was associated with greater fear, separation anxiety, belief in ghosts, disease, and violence. The authors feel that immature adolescents may need more help in making decisions aiming toward successful mastery of the human dilemma.

Meissner, W. W. Affective responses to psychoanalytic death symbols. *Journal of Abnormal and Social Psychology*, 1958, *56*, 295-299. Death symbol words were embedded in a randomly selected word list and presented to 40 Roman Catholic seminarians, aged 23-45. GSR recorded emotional responses. Significant differences were obtained between death and nondeath words.

Neimeyer, R. A. Death anxiety and the threat index: An addendum. *Death Education*, 1978; *1*(4), 464-467. The article reports on two reanalyses of previously collected data, one comparing high and low death threat groups on the Threat Index after they were confronted with anxiety-arousing situations involving death, another focusing on the possibility of modifying the Threat Index to tap death anxiety directly.

Nogas, Catherine, Schweitzer, Kathy, & Grumet, Judy. An investigation of death anxiety, sense of competence, and need for achievement. *Omega*, 1974, *5*(3), 245-255. The authors describe a death anxiety scale that was composed from an earlier scale by Farley as well as Collett and Lester. It includes 18 items scored on a 6-point scale ranging from strong agreement to strong disagreement. The participants were 80 female undergraduates enrolled in a psychology course. Reliability and validity were not studied.

Paris, J., & Goodstein, L. N. Responses to death and sex stimulus materials as a function of repression-sensitization. *Psychological Reports*, 1966, *19*, 1283-1291. Subjects were given equal numbers of male-female sensitizers chosen on the basis of their scores on the Repression-Sensitization (RS) scale. One third were given highly erotic materials, one third materials dealing with death, and one third neutral control words. There was no significant difference in ratings of anxiety either as a function of RS or of the materials. Thus the hypothesis that sensitizers would express more anxiety to literary material dealing with both sex and death than would repressers, was not proven.

Rainey, L. C., & Epting, F. R. Death threat constructions in the student and the prudent. *Omega*, 1977, *8*(1), 19-28. Two experiments were carried out to test the validity of the provided-construct Threat Index, a death orientation instrument based on cognitive construct theory. The mean death threat scores of thanatology students were found to be lower than those of a control group. However, there was no pre-post test decline among thanatology students in two death education courses.

Ray, J. J., & Najman, J. Death anxiety and death acceptance: A preliminary approach. *Omega*, 1974, *5*(4), 311-315. The construction of a new scale in Likert format designed to tap death-acceptance attitudes is reported. Consisting of seven items, this scale was embedded in several other inventories including Templer's Death Anxiety scale, and was administered to 206 sociology students. There was a low negative correlation between death acceptance and death anxiety.

Rhudick, P. J., & Dibner, A. S. Age, personality and health correlates of death concern in normal-aged individuals. *Journal of Gerontology*, 1961, *16*, 44-49. The MMPI and Cornell Medical Index were administered to 58 individuals ranging in age from 60-86. The Thematic Apperception Test (TAT) was presented to get at personal death concerns. High death concern was associated with elevations on the MMPI of Hypochondriasis, Hysteria, Dependency, and Impulsivity. The writers interpreted this as showing concern over death involving neurotic preoccupation particularly in relation to bodily symptoms.

Rigdon, M. A., Epting, F. R., Neimeyer, R. A., & Krieger, S. R. The threat index: A research report. *Death Education*, 1979, *3*(2), 245-270. This paper describes the Threat Index (TI) in its theoretical basis on George Kelly's Personal Construct Theory. Scoring procedures and modifications after 12 studies using the TI. Reliability and validity information is given. The research using the TI is summarized and evaluated. Most helpful to the researcher interested in using the TI in their study of death orientation.

Rotter, J. B. Generalized expectancies for internal vs. external control of reinforcement. *Psychological Monographs*, 1966, *80*(1) (No. 609). A 29-item, forced-choice test including 6 filler items purports to measure internal versus external control of reinforcement. Internal consistency, test-retest reliability and correlations with other tests are discussed. It is useful in determining the degree of control individuals perceive themselves as having in a given situation or period of time.

Sanders, C. M., Mauger, P. A., & Strong, P. N., Jr. *A manual for the grief experience inventory.* (Available in mimeograph form from

C. M. Sanders, Aging Studies Program, University of South Florida, Tampa, FL 33620). This 135 true-false self-report inventory is designed to assess feelings, attitudes, and experiences of bereavement. The inventory is comprised of 11 scales.

Sarnoff, I. Castration anxiety and the fear of death. *Journal of Personality*, 1959, *27*, 374-385. The author reports on an experiment designed to test the hypothesis that persons who have a high degree of castration anxiety would show a greater increase in fear of death after the arousal of their sexual feelings than would persons who have a low degree of castration anxiety. The subjects were 55 male undergraduates of Yale College. They filled out booklets containing a scale designed to measure the fear of death, a questionnaire concerning moral standards of sexual behavior, and a measure of castration anxiety under conditions of low and high levels of sexual arousal.

Schilder, P. The attitudes of murderers toward death. *Journal of Abnormal and Social Psychology*, 1936, *31*, 348-363. A 35-item questionnaire concerning death (included in the article) was administered to 31 defendants awaiting trial for murder. Case studies were presented along with their responses to the questionnaire. Three groups were identified: the young slayer who does not think about his death; the holdup man who indicated deep-seated psychotic tendencies; and the killer after an insignificant quarrel who displayed a preoccupation with death. To them, murder or death was a punishment. The author discusses the individual differences noted.

Schulz, R., Alderman, D., & Manko, G. Attitudes toward death: The effects of different methods of questionnaire administration. Paper presented at the annual meeting of the Eastern Psychological Association, New York, April, 1976. These writers report significantly lower death anxiety among college students when they were tested individually rather than in groups. The writers suggest that there might be a private component to death anxiety and that private attitudes are less likely to be expressed when the respondent signs his or her name.

Shneidman, E. S. Death questionnaire. *Psychology Today*, 1970, *4*, 67-72. This is a 75-item (18 of which are demographic questions) inventory dealing with death attitudes. A response of 30,000 added weight to the results of the study that was published in the same journal in June 1971 (see below). The questionnaire has been used in part, totally, or in adapted form, in a number of studies but to date no published data on validity or reliability is available.

Shneidman, E. S. You and death. *Psychology Today*. 1971, June, 67-72. In this article the author summarizes the results of the death attitudes survey in the preceding item.

Shrut, S. D. Attitudes towards old age and death. *Mental Hygiene*, 1958, *42*, 259-266. Attitude toward death was assessed using a psychological test battery on 2 groups of 30 ambulatory aged, female persons in 2 types of institutional residency. The group living in independent apartments showed less fear of death than did those living in the traditional institution. Further, the first group manifested better mental health, social alertness, and productivity.

Simpson, M. A. Studying death: Problems of methodology. *Death Education* (in press). The article reviews the methods and problems of research in the psychology of death, including ethical difficulties.

Swenson, Wendell M. Attitudes toward death among the aged. *Journal of Gerontology*, 1961, *16*, 49–52. The respondents, 34 persons over 50 years old, were asked to write a brief essay concerning thoughts on death. The material was screened for descriptive statements, which were used to measure death attitudes in larger groups. A death attitude checklist was then presented to 200 respondents over 60 years of age. Three groups emerged on basis of responses: those looking forward to death (45%); those avoiding any thought of death (44%); and those fearing the death experience (10%). Swenson feels that the fear of death is relatively nonexistent in the conscious thoughts of the aged.

Templer, D. The construction and validation of a death anxiety scale. *Journal of General Psychology*, 1970, *82*, 167. A 15-item true-false format was used to measure concurrent death anxiety. Internal consistency and test-retest reliability have been examined. Construct validity was established using both psychiatric patients and college students. This instrument has been used in a variety of studies.

Templer, D. I., & Lester, D. An MMPI Scale for assessing death anxiety. *Psychological Reports*, 1974, *34*, 238–240. An attempt to construct an MMPI scale for measuring death anxiety was made. The Death Anxiety scale and MMPI were administered to both college students and psychiatric patients. The reliability of the scale seems to be limited by the small number of items (there were only nine). The authors concluded that it was not feasible to derive a useful MMPI measure of death anxiety.

Templer, D. I., & Ruff, C. F. Death anxiety scale means, standard deviations and embedding. *Psychological Reports*, 1971, *29*, 173–174. A table of means and standard deviations on the Death Anxiety Scale for 23 categories of subjects is presented. A test of college students attempted to determine if the embedding of the items has an effect upon DAS scores. The embedding apparently had little or no effect upon scores.

Thompson, T. G., Crown, B., & O'Donovan, D. Attitudes toward death. *Psychological Reports*, 1967, *20*, 1181–1182. A group of 45 males rated 17 statements concerning attitudes toward death. Edwards' Social Desirability technique was used. Statements differed on 2 dimensions: Healthy vs. unhealthy, and hysterical vs. obssessive. The attitude toward death items are included in article. Results showed that healthy sensitivity was most socially desirable, and that unhealthy sensitivity was least socially desirable.

Tolor, A., & Reznikoff, M. Relationship between insight, repression-sensitization, internal-external control, and death anxiety. *Jour-*

nal of Abnormal Psychology, 1967, *72*, 426–430. The interrelation-ships among four scales that tap various elements in an individual's defense system were explored. The measures used were the Byrne (1960) Repression-Sensitization scale, the Rotter IE scale (1966), the Tolor-Reznikoff Insight test (1960), and a death anxiety scale. The subjects were 79 male college students who were seen in two weekly sessions. Results and discussion of these results are included in the paper.

Williams, R. L., & Cole, S. Religiosity, generalized anxiety, and apprehension concerning death. *Journal of Social Psychology*, 1968, *75*, 111–117. A sample of 161 college students was divided into three groups of high, intermediate, and low religiosity. Death-related words were presented tachistoscopically and GSR was measured. Those with high religiosity manifested the least anxiety, and those with low religiosity revealed the greatest generalized insecurity.

PART II

Audiovisual Resources

Introduction

Presented here is the largest and most complete annotated list of educational audiovisual materials available in the field of death and dying.

Items are listed alphabetically by title. Initials immediately preceding the annotation suggest audiences for which the items would be appropriate:

GS — Grade School
MS — Middle School
HS — High School
A — Adult: general audiences, undergraduates and professionals
      in training
P — Professionals with specialized interests

Following the discussions of the content of the items are the names of one or more distributors and other factual information: kind of medium (film, videotape, filmstrip, audiocassette), running time, and release or publication date, if known.

SOURCES OF MEDIA

Current addresses of distributors are provided in a separate listing at the end of this section. Distributor identification and addresses given here have been checked and rechecked against all current directories and catalogues, but users of audiovisuals must be alert to unexpected changes. Distributors move, change their names, go out of business, sell their holdings to or merge with other companies; films, like books, go "out of print" or are simply removed from the market, or from one or another distributor, by their producers or sponsors. In other words, the audiovisual industry, unlike the more controlled world of books and libraries, can occasionally be frustrating to deal with. For this reason we have tried to present the most up-to-date information possible. In addition, we offer specific hints for "keeping up" with the changing and growing audiovisual market.

It is important to realize, too, that in most cases the distributor or distributors listed for each item in this book are not the only ones handling the item; they are simply the ones we have used or have seen advertised nationally. Teachers should be alert to distributors or other sources of media in their own areas or communities, and should remember that media libraries—in medical schools, colleges and universities, clinics, hospitals, public libraries, schools, churches, or funeral homes—often make materials available for substantially lower cost than do commercial distributors. In addition, the following organizations (described in depth in Part III) also maintain large audiovisual collections, especially in topics of interest, and should be consulted, as should other such regional or local resources, before resorting to rental companies:

American Cancer Society
American Citizens Concerned for Life
American Lung Association
Concern for Dying
International Order of the Golden Rule
Leukemia Society of America
National Association for Mental Health
National Council of Senior Citizens
National Council on the Aging
National Funeral Directors Association
National Right to Life Committee
Planned Parenthood Federation of America

Write for catalogues of available films and ask to be put on mailing lists for information about new releases.

COSTS

We have decided not to include the rental and/or purchase prices and terms of audiovisual materials, mainly because such information changes rapidly. If one is operating on a limited budget one must double-check with the distributor in any event, and must be sure to search out alternative sources of supply, perhaps with the aid of librarians or media specialists. We wish to point out emphatically, however, that teachers *can* save money on audiovisuals by combining careful consideration of alternative media on a given topic with a judicious search for and selection of distributors. One of the authors recently taught a 4-week course using 23 films and videotapes, all critically acclaimed, available from four local sources. The only expense involved was return postage for eight of the items.

SELECTING EDUCATIONAL AUDIOVISUALS
FOR THE CLASSROOM

The most useful feature of this mediagraphy, aside from its descriptions of perhaps 95 percent or more of available audiovisual materials in the field as of late 1979, is the accompanying subject index. Topics and subtopics in the field of death and dying are suggested and annotated, then the numbers of relevant audiovisual items are listed under each heading. Many audiovisuals, of course, appear in several categories. Teachers searching for appropriate materials for their courses should find the Topical Index for this section, page 289, a helpful tool in making their choices.

USING FEATURE FILMS
IN DEATH AND DYING COURSES

Of the thousands of full-length feature films created in this century, many provide insights into a whole range of thanatological topics. But until there is a thorough history and critical analysis of death and dying in film, a teacher has to depend largely on his or her own knowledge and experience when selecting feature films for instructional purposes.

Difficulties occur in using feature films, too. They are often more costly to rent than shorter "educational" films, and have running times of well over 1½ hours. Besides, feature films, like novels, usually deal with a multiplicity of topics and some may include themes not closely related to death and dying. An instructor must prepare his or her students to be analytical and selective as they view a feature film, and at the same time must facilitate student awareness of the interrelationships of themes, characters and plots, especially in the better crafted film stories.

Indeed, if feature films are to be well used, a teacher must employ an understanding of the nature and techniques of film art for the benefit of the student. Like novelists, filmmakers—including the best producers of "educational" films—call upon a variety of resources and techniques to create complex aesthetic, intellectual, and emotional responses in their audiences. Lighting, color, camera angle, composition, sound effects, and music are but a few of the elements of film that must be appreciated for their contribution to the human action that is the heart of the film message. In a word, the task of studying death and dying in feature films is a complex one, though the rewards, in terms of a richly satisfying learning experience, more than repay the effort.

Finally, if a teacher does not wish to make the time or money commitment to specially schedule a feature film, he or she can still make the most of films that happen to come to campus, to local theaters, or to television. Speaking of television, note that many "films" these days are made especially for TV. "The Gathering," for example, a 2-hour "special" appearing on ABC-TV during the last two Christmas seasons, is bidding fair to become a holiday TV staple. It is a fine story of a man trying to atone for his past and to bring his family together again now that he is facing his death. Television series like "Roots" or "Holocaust" also offer frequent insights into a variety of death and dying topics.

Plans are now going forward to televise in January 1980 a 3-hour special, "Joan Robinson: One Woman's Story," a study of Mrs. Robinson's 2-year struggle with terminal cancer, the involvement of family members, and the role of various medical professionals— together with an analysis of ethical issues raised in her case: medical culpability, pain management, her "right to die." The National Cancer Institute; various state humanities organizations; the Public Broadcasting Service; Concern for Dying; Hospice, New Haven; and perhaps Courses By Newspaper are involved in this production, and it is expected that a good deal of advertising, related publications, suggestions for viewing and for teaching, etc., will "spin off" from this television program.

With a little ingenuity, and by simply being aware of forthcoming and current media events, a teacher, through ad hoc use of popular cultural resources, can effectively supplement classroom instruction.

To suggest something of the scope of the feature film as a potential resource for death education, we present here for the sake of example a selected, briefly annotated list of 50 films incorporating various thanatological themes.

Abandon Ship Who should survive, why, and who says so—in a lifeboat.

All the Way Home The great Agee novel, *A Death in the Family.*

The Andromeda Strain Biological warfare.

The Autobiography of Miss Jane Pittman A survivor of slavery, who has a long and noble life.

Bang the Drum Slowly A ballplayer's terminal illness changes the lives of his teammates.

Bonnie and Clyde Our national passion for violence, our predisposition to glorify criminal behavior.

Brian's Song A dying football player in his last season, and a noble friendship.

Bye Bye Braverman Four of a man's friends attend his funeral.

Coma Will there soon be a black market in body parts? A medical chiller.

Cries and Whispers Two women and their dying sister—a Bergman classic.

Death Be not Proud John Gunther's account of his son's dying.

Death in Venice The Thomas Mann short story as a fine Visconti film: passion and plague.

Death of a Salesman The Arthur Miller play of a broken family, broken career, and suicide.

Dr. Strangelove A satirical treatment of nuclear holocaust.

The Duelists Private hate in the midst of a battle, as obsessive and as baseless as the larger war.

Elvira Madigan Romantic insanity and suicide.

The End Believe it or not, a comic approach to dying of cancer.

Fail Safe Nuclear holocaust viewed seriously.

A Farewell to Arms Anything and everything by Hemingway is rich in implication: What is life? What is a man? How should death be faced?

Forbidden Games War through children's eyes—a classic antiwar film.

The Godfather Life and death in the Mafia, or at least the popular conception of it.

The Grapes of Wrath A poor family struggling to survive in an oppressive society, sharing a number of death experiences.

Hamlet Suicide, madness, violence, murder. What is life? What is a man?

Harold and Maude Satire on, among other things, suicide and funerals.

Hearts and Minds The war in Vietnam and its effects on victims, soldiers, and our society.

I Heard the Owl Call My Name A missionary learning of life and death from the Eskimos he serves.

I Never Sang for My Father Detailed study of a death in the family and the clash between the generations.

Ikiru Classic Kurosawa film. Told of his terminal illness, a man learns what life is all about.

In Cold Blood Insights into the criminal mind and the issue of capital punishment.

The Last Laugh On aging.

Little Big Man Annihilation of the American Indian.

Lord of the Flies Given the chance, kids are as much killers as adults: life and death reduced to their cruel elements.

Love Story A perfect young marriage, then sadness and tears as terminal illness ends it.

The Loved One A hilarious satire on funeral and memorial customs in the U.S.

The Omega Man Biological warfare.

The Ox-Bow Incident Lynch law in action.

The Prisoner of Shark Island Plague, yellow fever.

Romeo and Juliet Life among the adolescents: violent passions, murder, suicide—all for love.

Rush to Judgment The assassination of John F. Kennedy.

The Seven Samurai Kurosawa's masterpiece, an epic of violence and action.

The Seventh Seal Death as universal destroyer, no respecter of persons. Bergman's award-winning film.

The Shootist Violence-filled western with a gunman dying of cancer.

Slaughterhouse Five A film of the Vonnegut novel about the cruel meaninglessness of the firebombing of Dresden.

Something for Joey A family loses a child.

Soylent Green The demography of death in an overpopulated future.

Umberto D On aging.

West Side Story Musical, with modern Romeo and Juliet figures.

The Wild Bunch Violence graphically portrayed.

Wild Strawberries On aging.

Wrong Box Comic treatment of wills and greedy beneficiaries.

KEEPING UP

This book presents thorough coverage of virtually all audiovisual materials in the field of death and dying produced before 1979. Individual teachers now need only to stay current.

For those of us blessed with excellent library facilities and staff, keeping up will simply be a matter of putting one's people to the task. Another source of ready information and advice if one is in a hurry, or has particular questions or problems, is the Educational Film Library Association, 43 W. 61st St., New York, NY 10023 (telephone 212-246-4533). The rest of us can easily stay abreast of the steady outpouring of audiovisuals by occasionally checking any of a number of periodicals and library reference tools.

Periodicals

Audiovisual Instruction. Published by the Association for Educational Communications and Technology, 1126 16th St., N.W., Washington, DC 20036. Appearing 10 times a year, September–June, this journal was founded in 1956. Subscription rate is $18.00. A regular feature is an index to audiovisual reviews in other publications. The emphasis is on instruction in grade schools and high schools.

Biomedical Communications. Published by United Business Publications, Inc., 750 Third Ave., New York, NY 10017. Established in 1973, it appears bimonthly with a subscription rate of $5.00 a year. This journal publishes articles discussing "concepts or applications of media in medical education, continuing education, in-service education, patient-public education, and health care delivery." The May issue annually presents a lengthy but unannotated list of available audiovisual materials on over 40 medical subjects, using the MeSH headings of the National Library of Medicine.

EFLA Evaluations. Published by the Educational Film Library Association, 43 W. 61st St., New York, NY 10023. Begun in 1946, this is published 10 times a year in looseleaf sheet format and is available only to members of the association. It covers over 400 16mm educational films per year, describing the items, suggesting uses, and providing availability and cost information—all in capsule form.

Film Library Quarterly. Published by the Film Library Information Council, Box 348, Radio City Station, New York, NY 10019. Subscriptions are $10.00 a year to nonmembers. Founded in 1967, *F.L.Q.* supplies information on 16mm films useful for public, academic, and school libraries, and regularly reviews new films.

Landers Film Reviews. Published by Landers Associates, Box 69760, Los Angeles, CA 90069. Five issues per year are produced, with a subscription rate of $45.00. The sole task of this periodical, which was founded in 1956, is the presentation of detailed evaluative reviews of new nontheatrical films on all subjects for all audience levels. A revised directory of producers and distributors is offered annually.

Media and Methods. Published by North American Publishing Co. 401 N. Broad St., Philadelphia, PA 19108. The subscription rate is $10.00 a year for 10 issues, September–May. Established in 1965, this is the best available periodical in the audiovisual field for middle and secondary schools. It regularly prints articles on effective and creative use of AV in the classroom, reports on new and forthcoming materials, including TV programs, and reviews feature films, educational films, audiocassettes, LPs, and other media.

Media Mix. Published by Claretian Publications, 221 W. Madison St., Chicago, IL 60606. Subscriptions are $9.00 a year for eight issues. Established in 1969, *Media Mix* is a basic resource for reports on and reviews of new films, filmstrips, TV programs, tapes, LPs, kits, teacher aids, etc. The focus is on materials appropriate for secondary schools, but college level media are reviewed on occasion.

Previews: Audiovisual Software Reviews. Published by the R. R. Bowker Co., 1180 Avenue of the Americas, New York, NY 10036. Subscription rate for 10 monthly issues, September–June, is $15.00. Founded in 1972, the journal contains detailed evaluative commentary by audiovisual specialists, teachers, and librarians on new media of all types for all audience levels, preschool through adult.

Sightlines. Published by the Educational Film Library Association, 43 W. 61st St., New York, NY 10023. This appears quarterly and subscriptions are $15.00 a year. Founded in 1967, *Sightlines* is a basic source of information about and reviews of new 8mm and 16mm films for schools and libraries. Also included are summaries of reviews from other sources.

Library Reference Tools

AVMP 1979: Audiovisual Marketplace: A Multimedia Guide. New York; R. R. Bowker, 1979. This book lists addresses of producers and distributors; public radio and TV program libraries that lend, sell, or rent programs they have produced; audiovisual cataloging services; reference books and directories (annotated and cross-indexed); and over 140 periodicals, newsletters, and trade journals that regularly review and report on media.

Educational Film Locator: Of the Consortium of University Film Centers and R. R. Bowker Company. New York: R. R. Bowker, 1978. An annotated and cross-indexed union list, this includes over 37,000 rental films in the collections of 50 university libraries across the country.

Feature Films on 8MM, 16MM and Videotape (6th ed), by Jim Limbacher. New York: R. R. Bowker, 1979. Presented here are titles and full descriptive and availability information on no fewer than 20,350 items.

The Health Sciences Video Directory, edited by Lawrence Eidelberg. New York: Esselte Video, Inc., 1977. Here are annotated listings of over 4400 video programs and series, each cross-indexed at least three times in accordance with the MeSH system of the National Library of Medicine. Names and addresses of producers, distributors and video subscription services are also listed. Supplements are being published quarterly.

Humanities Index: Moving Picture Reviews. For feature films.

Index to Educational Audio Tapes; Index to Educational Videotapes; Index to 16MM Educational Films; Index to 35MM Educational Filmstrips. Los Angeles: National Information Center for Educational Media (NICEM), University of Southern California, 1977. This set of indexes—which includes a separate directory of producers and distributors as well as separate listings of records, slides, overhead transparencies, and 8MM motion cartridges—is one of the most massive available. It is, perhaps, *the* basic source. Listed both alphabetically and under detailed subject headings, each item is annotated for content, audience level, and availability. It is projected that new editions will appear biennially; the next is scheduled for publication in December 1979. Supplements, titled *Up-date of Non-book Media*, are issued quarterly in intervening years.

Medical and Health Information Directory, edited by Anthony T. Kruzas. Detroit: Gale Research Company, 1977. Among other things, this reference book offers annotated entries for audiovisual producers and services, computerized information systems and services, Medline Network centers, libraries and information centers, and medical research centers and institutes.

Medical Media Directory. This is the separately available May issue of *Biomedical Communications* (see above).

National Library of Medicine Audiovisuals Catalogue. Bethesda, MD: U.S. Department of Health, Education and Welfare, National

Library of Medicine, 1977—. Each yearly volume from 1977 on will collect citations appearing in the year's quarterly N.L.M. catalogues. Earlier citations appear in the 1975/1976 issue of the N.L.M. *Avline* catalogue. Items of more specialized professional interest under headings "Attitude to Death," "Death," and "Terminal Care."

National Medical Audiovisual Center Catalogue: Audiovisuals for the Health Scientist. Atlanta, GA. U.S. Department of Health, Education and Welfare, National Medical Audiovisual Center, 1977. Lists items of more specialized professional interest, under these topic headings: "Attitudes to Death," "Death," and "Terminal Care." Annual supplements are being published.

New York Times Film Reviews, 1913–1968. Biennial supplements are being issued. For reviews of feature films.

New York Times Index. Motion Pictures—Reviews. For reviews of feature films.

Reader's Guide to Periodical Literature. Motion picture reviews.

A Reference List of Audiovisual Materials Produced by the United States Government. Washington, DC: General Services Administration, National Archives and Records Service, National Audiovisual Center; 1978.

Note. See the section, *Periodicals*, for other excellent sources of information and reviews of new audiovisuals in the field.

Listings

1. **Abandon Ship.** (HS, A) A feature film. See *The Right to Live: Who Decides?*

2. **Abyss.** (HS, A) This personal experience film may be useful in triggering discussion of sudden death, the will to survive, and beating the odds. A mountain climber falls to what his companions think is his certain death. Days later he manages to come back down the mountain and is reunited with his grieving friends. Phoenix Films, color, 17 minutes.

3. **Accident.** (HS, A) In this personal experience film the central figure is the filmmaker. He returns to the scene of his near-fatal accident and explores his emotional state as he faced death and, having escaped, as he adjusts to a new and heightened outlook on life. *Accident* would be useful in triggering discussion of sudden death and near-death and their effects. Doubleday Multimedia, or University of California, Berkeley, 17 minutes, 1975.

4. **The Admiral.** (HS, A) Facing certain defeat in a sea battle, the old admiral decides to commit suicide. The sea and the shattered

ships of his fleet are depicted pouring out of the wound in his head. This vividly impressionistic film would make a fine trigger for discussion. University of Nebraska, color, 6 minutes, 1971.

5. **Adolescent Suicide.** See *American Association of Suicidology: Proceedings of the Conference, 1978.*

6. **Adolescent Suicide: A Documentary.** (A) Dr. Herman Farberow and other staff members at the Suicide Prevention Center in Los Angeles discuss factors in the alarmingly high rate of adolescent suicide, the effects on survivors, and possible methods of prevention and intervention. Included are interviews with youths who have attempted suicide. The Charles Press, 54 minutes, 1973.

7. **After Our Baby Died: Sudden Infant Death Syndrome.** (A) This well-made, impressive film, winner of a blue ribbon in mental health at the 1976 American Film Festival, was created to help professionals and others who come into contact with SIDS parents to better understand the syndrome. Parents are interviewed, and offer telling lessons and insights for caregivers. Free loan from Modern Talking Picture Service, or National SIDS Foundation, or Bureau of Community Health Services (HEW), color, 20 minutes, 1976.

8. **The Aged.** (HS, A) The film depicts the variety of services offered by the "geriatrics project," a helping group for the aged. Carousel Films, color, 17 minutes, 1973.

9. **Aging.** (A) While playing cards two elderly men discuss their past lives and present loneliness. This film can help sensitize audiences to the problems of the aged and to their potentially useful and valuable roles within their families. Indiana University, 30 minutes, 1967.

10. **Aging.** (A) General concepts on the aging process—psychological and biological—are presented, then the film offers commentary on the roles of the aged in contemporary society. The emphasis throughout is on the positive. By exploring a variety of attitudes and life-styles of older people, the film helps break down stereotypes. Communication Research Machines, color, 22 minutes, 1973.

11. **Aging and Dying: A Positive View.** (A) This is a set of five audiocassettes that include extensive interviews. New Dimension Foundation, 30 minutes each.

12. **Agua Salada.** (A) This look at a brutal side of life may start discussion on the meaning of life and death. Excellently photographed amid scenic splendor, the film shows an old fisherman casting his nets as he has done for years and bringing from the water the body of his son. Viewfinders, Inc., black and white, 12 minutes.

13. **Aldermaston Pottery.** (A) Here are telling juxtapositions of images of pottery-making near Aldermaston, England, site of an atomic energy plant; and medical photographs of victims of the Hiroshima atomic bomb attack. Viewfinders, Inc., color, 18 minutes.

14. **All the Way Home.** (HS, A) The novel on which this fine film is based, *A Death in the Family,* is one of the most profoundly moving, most searching, and best written analyses of family reactions

to the death of a member in all literature. Particularly important are the many cameo portraits of grief: the dead man's wife, his two very young children, and various other relatives. Religious belief—or lack of it—as a conditioning factor in responding to death is studied in minute detail. The novel is essential reading for everyone trying to understand death, and the film also makes a major contribution. Films, Inc., black and white, 103 minutes, 1963.

15. **American Association of Suicidology: Proceedings of the Conference, 1978.** (P) Various conference papers are available on audiocassette: "The Psychological Autopsy as a Model for Managing Staff Reactions"; "Suicide Rates and Macrosociology"; "Suicide Prevention in the Hospital"; and "Dichotomous Thinking and Suicide Complexes." Highly Specialized Promotions, 4 audiocassettes.

16. **American Association of Suicidology: Proceedings of the Conference, 1978: A Set of Presentations on Adolescent Suicide.** (P) Titles include "Suicide and Children," "Suicide Methods and Potential in Ages 4–12," "Intent and Death Attitudes of Adolescents," and "Mobilizing Help in Adolescent Suicide." Highly Specialized Promotions, 4 audiocassettes.

17. **American Attitudes toward Death and Dying.** (A) See *Perspectives on Dying*.

18. **American Attitudes toward Death and Funerals.** (A) Two marketing professors at Ohio State University discuss the results of their poll on the subject. Allied Memorial Council, color film or videotape, 30 minutes.

19. **American Cancer Society: National Conference on Cancer Nursing—Precepts, Principles, Practices: Meeting Highlights.** (A, P) American Cancer Society, 2 audiocassettes.

20. **American Cancer Society: National Conference on Childhood Cancer: Meeting Highlights.** (A, P) American Cancer Society, film, 2 hours, 1974.

21. **American Cancer Society: Second National Conference on Human Values and Cancer, Chicago, 1977: Meeting Highlights.** (A, P) American Cancer Society, two audiocassettes, album.

22. **The American Funeral.** (A) This taped conversation with a mortician, a minister, and a sociologist explores the real function of the funeral, analyzes high funeral costs, and traces the historical development of contemporary funeral customs and the funeral industry. Center for Cassette Studies, 28 minutes.

23. **And I Want Time.** (HS, A) This item is a separately available 28-minute segment of the feature film *Love Story* (1970). Marketed by Paramount Pictures together with a study guide, the clip is said to be suitable for use in death and dying courses. *Love Story*, of course, is well known as a rather romanticized presentation of a simply perfect young marriage suddenly and sadly ended by terminal illness and death. Paramount Communications, color, 28 minutes, 1978.

24. **Anna and Poppy.** (A) Faced with the death of her grand-

father, Poppy, young Anna comes to learn that memories of shared love and happy times together can overcome the effects of sadness. This film can foster discussion and sensitize audiences to death in the family, and the nature and function of the bonds of love. Association Films, or Media Guild, color, 15 minutes, 1977.

25. **Annie and the Old One.** (GS, HS) Annie, a Navajo girl, loves her grandmother the Old One, very much. When the grandmother tells Annie she expects to "return to the earth" when a new rug she is weaving is taken from the loom, Annie tries to delay its completion. Based on a book by Miska Miles, the film is a beautiful portrayal of death and the meaning of the generations from a child's point of view. Indiana University, or University of Illinois, color, 16 minutes, 1976.

26. **The Art of Age.** (HS, A) The film presents four elderly people, happily retired and satisfied with their varied and active lives. Their point is that the later years of life, like the early and middle ones, are best if lived constructively. ACI Films, color, 27 minutes, 1972.

27. **Arthur and Lillie.** (A) This film is a kind of brief history of the motion picture and of a man at the center of that history, Arthur Mayer, aged 89, and his wife Lillie, aged 86. The film records their success-filled life and well-handled old age. In telling about their useful and creative careers, Arthur and Lillie show us what "old" can be. Viewfinders, Inc., or Pyramid Films, color, 30 minutes.

28. **At 99.** (A) Louise Tandy Murch lives alone in the family house, practices yoga, sings and plays the piano, and has a remarkable philosophy at age 99—age is a function of how you act. She says she might worry about death when she gets to be 100. Viewfinders, Inc., or University of California, Berkeley, color film, 24 minutes, 1975.

29. **Attempted Suicide: What Constitutes Appropriate Medical Care?** (P) This is a taped panel discussion at a conference on clinical ethics. The approach and suggested answers to the title question are interdisciplinary. University of California, Los Angeles, Medical Center, videotape, 60 minutes, 1974.

30. **Attitudes towards Death and Dying.** (A, P) Thomas Hunter, M.D., Professor of Society and Science Concerns and former Dean of the University of Virginia Medical School, is interviewed on a variety of sociomedical issues. In clear, well-organized commentary, Dr. Hunter surveys medical professionals' attitudes toward death and dying, cost factors in extended illness, the death with dignity concept, the living will, informed consent, the definition of death, and individual versus social rights in continuation or withdrawal of extraordinary care. University of Virginia, color videotape, 30 minutes, 1973.

31. **Autopsy.** (P) Autopsy techniques are demonstrated on this videotape. The program could be useful to sensitize properly prepared caregivers. University of Texas Health Sciences Center, color, 35 minutes, 1969.

32. **The Autopsy.** (A) This short experimental film could be used to trigger discussion and to sensitize audiences. The film rather daringly cuts back and forth from various life scenes to an ongoing autopsy. Serious Business Company, color, 4½ minutes.

33. **The Ballad of Alma Gerlayne.** (A) An allegorical story with a moral about what is important in life. Finally achieving material success, a young singer tries to find true happiness with a man whose own negative philosophy of life only demoralizes her and drives her to suicide. The film may help start discussion. Paulist Productions, or Association Instructional Materials, color, 27 minutes.

34. **Ballad without End.** (HS, A) A young Civil War soldier kills an off-guard, unarmed enemy, then rejects war and killing after examining the dead man's personal effects. Viewfinders, Inc., or Phoenix Films, color, 12 minutes.

35. **Bang the Drum Slowly—A Series.** (HS, A) The story of a team of baseball players who change and grow—for the first time, it seems, they come to understand something important about the nature of life, human relationships, and death—when one of their teammates becomes terminally ill. Films, Inc., 2 Storystrips (about 350 frames), 1976.

36. **Barabbas.** (HS, A) A 15-minute segment of this Columbia Pictures feature film is available, concentrating on the issue of violence for the pleasure of it. The selection—and indeed the film itself—can serve to foster discussion of this and other death-related issues. Learning Corporation of America, color, 1972.

37. **Battle of San Pietro.** (HS, A) This film about what war is really like, particularly as it affects innocent civilians, was banned by the U.S. government as potentially demoralizing when John Huston made it in 1944. It is still a powerful indictment of war, making audiences understand that it is human beings who fight wars and die in them. The film can thus sensitize viewers to key issues of life and death. Viewfinders, Inc., black and white, 30 minutes.

38. **Beneficent Euthanasia.** (A) This televised dialogue from a humanist perspective is part of the series, "Moral Values in Contemporary Society." It is also available on audiocassette, and is accompanied by a discussion guide. The Humanist Alternative, videotape, 30 minutes.

39. **Bereavement.** (A) Dr. C. Murray Parkes discusses grief and bereavement particularly as they affect the widowed. The nature and symptomology of the normal and the abnormal grief processes are introduced, and suggestions for treatment and counseling are offered. Royal College of General Practitioners, reel-to-reel tape recording with 5 slides, 26 minutes, 1967.

40. **Bereavement and the Process of Mourning.** (A) Professor Paul Irion discusses loss as a disruption of social relationships and argues that the funeral and other social rituals facilitate the expression of grief and thereby lead to a healthy social restructuring. The Charles Press, audiocassette, 54 minutes, 1972.

41. **Between the Cup and the Lip.** (A) Symbolic in style and theme, this animated film presents life as a series of figures moving in a never-ending procession interspersed occasionally with the snuffing out of a candle to represent the passing of one of its members. The available discussion guide may help audiences with potential problems of interpretation. Mass Media Associates, color, 11 minutes, 1971.

42. **Beyond Shelter: Ideas on Housing for the Elderly.** (A) This item depicts the lack of options facing the aged today. Mixed housing, sheltered housing, and special housing for the handicapped are shown as alternatives to current institutions. Educational Film Library Association, black and white, 25 minutes.

43. **The Big Shave.** (HS, A) Some critics, at least, have said this would make a good trigger film. A nice young man starts his usual morning shave. He lathers, he strokes, then loses control and "shaves himself to death." University of California, Berkeley, color, 6 minutes, 1968.

44. **Biography of a Cancer.** (A) In this CBS-TV presentation, the famous Dr. Tom Dooley is interviewed as he is diagnosed and treated for his cancer. Especially valuable are his reactions to the news and his determination to maintain a positive attitude: the personal, human responses are timeless. The level of medical insight is, of course, dated, but comparison with current knowledge and treatment methodology may be informative. Association-Sterling Films, 2 reels, 54 minutes, 1960.

45. **Bless the Beasts and the Children.** (HS, A) A 15-minute segment of this Columbia Pictures feature film is available, concentrating on the love of killing for its own sake. The selection as well as the film can trigger discussion. Learning Corporation of America, color, 1972.

46. **Breath Death.** (HS, A) Filmmaker Stan Vanderbeck has become famous for this surrealistic antiwar film, an experimental piece that incorporates fifteenth-century woodcuts of the "Dance of Death." Indiana University, black and white, 15 minutes, 1964.

47. **The Bridge.** (A) The bridge in question is the Golden Gate, site of many suicides and suicide attempts. The film discusses causal factors and describes suicide prevention techniques. Montage Educational Films, color, 26 minutes, 1976.

48. **But Jack Was a Good Driver.** (HS, A) His schoolmates begin to suspect that Jack's death in an auto accident may have been a suicide. Subsequent discussion shows the students considering their own attitudes toward suicide, dispels some myths, presents the warning signs to look for, and offers suggestions relating to and working with suicidal persons. University of California, Berkeley or McGraw-Hill Films, color, 15 minutes, 1974.

49. **A Call for Help.** (A) This is a training film for police officers, rescue workers, and emergency room personnel, although a general range of caregivers will find it valuable. Specific lessons are offered for dealing with cases of Sudden Infant Death Syndrome. A study guide is available. Free loan from the Bureau of Community Health

Services, or National Sudden Infant Death Syndrome Foundation, color, 20 minutes, 1976.

50. **Cancer Pain: A Report on the Pain Clinic Experience.** (P) This audiocassette records a presentation by Dr. Ruben Tenicela during a symposium on pain at the University of Pittsburgh. University of Pittsburgh School of Medicine, 30 minutes.

51. **Cancer Patient, Supportive Care: Fear, Hope and Fulfillment in the Care of the Cancer Patient.** (P) This is a videotape of an extended panel discussion about a leukemia patient with a particularly complex set of medical and emotional problems, and is of value for raising issues of broader concern. M. D. Anderson Hospital and Tumor Institute, color, 60 minutes, 1974.

52. **Cancer Series I: The Nature of Cancer and Its Diagnosis.** (P) This set of five filmstrips and accompanying audiocassettes provides an understanding of the nature of cancer as an alteration in a normal cell, the development of neoplasms and their effects on the host, and diagnostic procedures. While not dealing directly with death and dying, this series provides the informational background for the two other series described below. Student nurses are the primary audience.

53. **Cancer Series II: Focusing on Feelings.** (P) Two of the four filmstrips in this series are designed to sensitize nurses and other caregivers to their possible emotional responses to patients with various cancer-related problems. The other filmstrips present case studies of typical patient concerns, and how the caregiver can best address them. General adult audiences would find this series informative and valuable, too.

54. **Cancer Series III: Treatment Modalities with Implications for Nursing Care.** (P) Modern cancer treatment, complex and sophisticated as it is, requires of the nurse a high degree of knowledge and technical skill as well as sensitivity to the patient's needs. This set of seven filmstrips and audiocassettes introduces the current treatment modalities (surgery, radiotherapy, and chemotherapy), and analyzes the physical and psychological effects which may result from their use.

Each Series filmstrip set includes an instructor's manual containing script narrations, presentation guidelines, previewing questions, study questions, and bibliographies. Individual filmstrip-cassette programs may be purchased separately. The three Series are high quality, carefully crafted productions. The topics are presented in depth, the narrations are clearly written and skillfully delivered, and the visual support has high impact. Concept Media.

55. **Cancer—The Wayward Cell.** (HS, A) The nature of cancer, methods of treatment, and prospects for control of the disease in the future are surveyed in this film, which includes commentary of a young cancer victim. Document Associates, Inc., color film, 26 minutes, 1976.

56. **Care for the Dying and Bereaved: How Can We Help?** (A, P) Guidance Associates, three color filmstrips and audiocassettes or

records, 55 minutes, and accompanying printed materials. These are selected items from *Death and Dying: Closing the Circle* (see below).

57. **The Care of the Bereaved.** (P) In this lecture the Rev. Dr. Michael Wilson of the University of Birmingham offers to a medical-professional audience a variety of introductory information on grief and bereavement, and on the responsibilities of doctor and nurse to the recently bereaved. Royal College of General Practitioners, reel-to-reel audiotape, 35 minutes, 1971.

58. **Care of the Dying Patient.** (P) These programs serve to increase nurses' awareness of the psychological and physical needs of their dying patients. Signs of approaching death are presented, and instruction is given in after-death procedures. Train-Aid Educational Systems, two filmstrips with record or audiocassette, 9 and 15 minutes, 1970.

59. **Care of the Patient Who Is Dying.** (P) This filmstrip introduces the physical and emotional needs of the near-death patient, and the related problems of family and staff. Indications of approaching death and procedures for caring for the body are then covered. Trainex Corporation, color filmstrip and audiocassette or record, 20 minutes, 1975.

60. **Care of the Patient with Terminal Cancer.** (P) Many aspects of physical care and psychological support necessary for patients with terminal cancer are presented here. Trainex Corporation, color filmstrip with audiocassette or record, instructor's guide.

61. **Care of the Terminally Ill.** (P) Addressing itself to an audience of nurses, this program introduces the "five stages of dying," and reminds the learner to be aware of family and staff needs as well as the needs of the dying patient. Career Aids, filmstrip with audiocassette or record.

62. **A Case of Suicide.** (A) The suicide is that of Kate, a 17-year-old British wife and mother. The girl's estranged husband, mother, and friends are asked if they had any suspicion of Kate's intentions. Analysis reveals that warning signs had been present, but were not acted upon. Kate's survivors all demonstrate the guilt frequently seen in similar cases after the fact. This fascinating and moving case study will trigger further discussion for general and professional audiences. Time-Life Films or University of California, Berkeley, black and white, 30 minutes, 1968.

63. **The Cemetery.** (HS, A) A representative of the American Cemetery Association discusses history and growth of cemeteries and their operating procedures. Allied Memorial Council, color videotape.

64. **Chickamauga.** (HS, A) Based on the Ambrose Bierce short story, the film graphically portrays the terror and the folly of war from the perspective of a 6-year-old deaf-mute. Viewfinders, Inc., or University of California, Berkeley, black and white, 33 minutes.

65. **Childhood Cancer: Emotional Effects.** (P) This videotape is available for medical professionals. M. D. Anderson Hospital and Tumor Institute, color, 58 minutes, 1975.

66. **Children and Death.** (A) Included in this program are discussions about childrens' experiences with death, their perceptions and questions about it, and a series of related suggestions for adults. J. A. B. Press, three audiocassettes.

67. **Children and Death.** (A) Dr. Simon Yudkin gives an overview of essential aspects of this topic: the importance of death education for children, the significance of religious training, and the need to allow children to participate in death rituals and mourning. Royal College of General Practitioners, reel-to-reel audiotape, 40 minutes, 1967.

68. **Children and Death: A Guide for Parents and Teachers.** (A) This program provides general answers to a number of questions: How does one tell a child about death? What should one say and not say? What form should death education take, and when? Should children be allowed to attend funerals? Allied Memorial Council, or Educational Perspectives Associates, audiocassette, teacher's guide. (See also *Understanding Death Series*.)

69. **Children and Dying Conference, University of Chicago, 1977: Proceedings.** (A, P) Seven audiocassettes are available on these topics: "Care for the Caregivers," "The Child and Sudden Death," "What Shall We Tell the Children?" "The Dying Child at Home," "The Dying Child in the Hospital," and "Parental Loss and Childhood Bereavement." Highly Specialized Promotions, available as a set or individually.

70. **Children Die Too.** (P) See *Physician's Role with the Dying Patient.*

71. **Children in Crisis: Death.** (A) The titles of the five filmstrips in this series accurately suggest the content: "Death as a Reality of Life," "Expressing Grief," "Ages of Understanding," "Explaining Death to Children," and "The Importance of Funerals." Reviewers (for example, *Death Education*, 1977, *1*(3), 351–353) suggest the program may have value for general audiences or beginning death educators, but lacks depth. Parent's Magazine Films, 5 color filmstrips and audiocassettes or record, scripts and discussion guide.

72. **Children's Conceptions of Death.** (A, P) This critically acclaimed program is well organized and informative. Children at various ages—under 5, between 6 and 9, and 10 and older—have different and developing attitudes to death, and differing needs in the face of it. Teachers, caregivers and parents will find these lessons most helpful. University of Wisconsin-Milwaukee, School of Nursing, color videotape, 40 minutes, teacher's guide, 1974.

73. **A Child's Eyes: November 22, 1963.** (A) This short film provides valuable insights into the minds of children and into basic human questions of life and death. A number of 5- and 6-year-olds react to the assassination of President Kennedy through crayon drawings and their own narrative. Julian Morris Agency, color, 9 minutes.

74. **Chipper.** (HS, A) The story is best described as a parable about the angel of death and one man's confrontation with it.

Chipper passes through the stages of dying to a kind of acceptance, instructed by a friend not to fear either death or God, but to see death as defining life and as marking the beginning of a new order of life. The film is stimulating, well made, and well acted. The Media Guild, or Paulist Productions, or Association Films, color, 27 minutes, 1975.

75. **Christian Medical Ethics.** (A) Father Charles Curran, a distinguished Roman Catholic moral theologian, discusses ethical issues as diverse as sterilization, transplant, experimentation, genetics, abortion, death and dying, and allocation of scarce medical resources—all from a Catholic point of view, in a relaxed, informal style appealing to professional and lay audiences. The Thomas More Association, 6 audiocassettes, approximately 6 hours.

76. **Cipher in the Snow.** (A, HS) This excellent film tells a moving story of a school boy's sudden and unexplained death, and how he had been written off as a zero (or so he felt) by his parents, classmates, and teachers, none of whom, as they realize after the fact, really knew the boy. Is it possible to die physically as well as emotionally from lack of love? Saying "yes" in a convincing but not maudlin way, the film could trigger discussion of the essential relationship between love and life. Brigham Young University, or University of Iowa, or University of Utah, color, 25 minutes, 1974.

77. **The Clergy in Cancer Management.** (P) The film explores the broadening role of the clergy as part of the rehabilitation team. Clergymen of many faiths are depicted interacting with a variety of patients and their families. Many questions are raised and some solutions offered, all in an effort to stimulate further discussion between the clergy and medical professionals. American Cancer Society, color film or videotape, 27 minutes, 1976.

78. **Clinical Oncology Grand Rounds: Contributions of Pharmacology to Clinical Cancer Chemotherapy.** (P) This videotape is available to medical professionals. M. D. Anderson Hospital and Tumor Institute, color, 59 minutes, 1975.

79. **Come and Take My Hand.** (A) Center stage in this film is a Dominican nun at the Holy Family Home in Cleveland. She is a warm and caring health professional who relates successfully with dying patients and their families. Her work could serve as a model for others, though according to critics the film is not particularly well made. NBC Educational Enterprises, or Films, Incorporated, color, 25 minutes, 1972.

80. **Concepts of Grieving.** (P) This is one of many available videotaped presentations with Dr. Elisabeth Kübler-Ross discussing the stages of dying and the nature of proper and beneficial professional relationships with dying patients. As usual, Dr. Kübler-Ross supports her arguments with a wealth of case studies. Milwaukee Regional Medical Instructional Television System, Inc., color, 55 minutes, 1971.

81. **A Conference on the Dying Child.** (P) A pediatric head nurse, a nursing supervisor, and a nursing instructor share their experiences and opinions about working with dying children. Emotions are a major issue, for nurse and family alike. Also discussed are children's concepts of death and their origins, how nurses should respond in given situations, and how, when and whether the truth should be told. American Journal of Nursing Company, film or videotape, black and white, 44 minutes, 1967.

82. **Conflicts between Patient's Religion and Medical Opinion.** (A, P) Legal, moral, and medical aspects of cases involving religious objection to medical treatment are surveyed in this videotaped panel discussion. A hypothetical case study is analyzed from varying perspectives to suggest the range of problems raised by such cases. University of Virginia, black and white, 60 minutes, 1973.

83. **Confrontations of Death.** (A) The film records a series of sensitivity sessions during which participants were led to confront their personal feelings about death. They listened to music and poetry, role-played, built a death machine, wrote their own eulogies, viewed slides, and then held discussions. Viewing the program may help educators planning similar activities for their students. University of Oregon, or University of Iowa, color, 35 minutes, 1972.

84. **Confronting Death.** (HS, A) This round-table discussion including Dr. Elizabeth Kübler-Ross and Rev. Carl Nighswonger would be useful in introducing audiences to basic concepts about death and dying. Thomas More Association, audiocassette.

85. **The Confused Person: Approaches to Reality Orientation.** (A) See *Perspectives on Aging.*

86. **Conscious Dying.** (A) Ram Dass shares his experiences and insights from his work with the dying in this videotaped interview. Interface, 30 minutes.

87. **A Conversation with a Widow.** (A, P) The widow interviewed in this videotape program lost her husband four weeks before. Her grief and other emotional reactions to the death are revealed. She is better able to handle the experience because of help she received from hospital staff during her husband's last days. University of Arizona, color, 30 minutes, 1977.

88. **Conversation with Lynn Caine, Widow.** (A) Ms. Caine, author of the best-selling book, *Widow,* relates some of her experiences adjusting to the death of her husband and to her life. The book and, more briefly, this audiocassette offer some of the most insightful and well-expressed personal commentary on the subject available. The Charles Press, 27 minutes.

89. **Conversations with a Dying Friend.** (A) Reporter Connie Goldman interviews a cancer patient whose disease has progressed hopelessly despite a mastectomy. The patient tells the effects her dying has had on her personal relationships, then describes her dying

as an "identity crisis" which her inner resources helped her confront. Specific suggestions for caregivers are offered. The Charles Press, audiocassette, 1972.

90. **Coping.** (A) This film documents a series of interviews between a doctor, a young boy terminally ill with leukemia, and his parents. What is remarkable about the boy and his family is the level of acceptance of the disease and of death that they have reached together; they understand the prognosis, and discuss it openly and honestly. The film demonstrates the great value of healthy familial relationships when someone is dying. Children's Memorial Hospital, or University of California, Berkeley, color, 22 minutes, 1974.

91. **Coping with Death and Dying: Emotional Needs of the Dying Patient and the Family.** (A) Here perhaps is the "essential Kübler-Ross," at least in audiocassette format. This 180-minute tape series is certainly the longest and most detailed presentation of her views outside of her writing, and follows the format of argument and explanation familiar to readers of *On Death and Dying*. On tape one, "The Fear of Death: Verbal and Nonverbal Symbolical Language," Dr. Kübler-Ross reports how her research began and the early distrust and hostility of her medical colleagues. Then she explains that many patients see death as an impersonal, catastrophic force, and that caregivers should be able to pick up on verbal and nonverbal expressions of these attitudes and feelings. Clinical examples are used to illustrate. Tapes two and three present the now-familiar "stages of dying" in considerable detail and with a wealth of illustrative case studies. "Children and Death" is the topic of tape four. Again citing case studies, Dr. Kübler-Ross treats the basic concerns of truthtelling, problems caused by denying parents, helping parents cope, children's conceptions of death and how those conceptions develop during the process of dying. On tape five sudden death is discussed from the viewpoint of emergency room personnel. How does one tell the waiting survivors, or others injured in the same accident? How does one give such information on the telephone? Should emotional outpouring be encouraged? Do survivors need to see the body? What of the emotional needs of medical professionals, after their efforts have failed? Psychology Today Cassettes, or Highly Specialized Promotions, or Ross Medical Associates, 5 audiocassettes, 30 minutes each, 1973.

92. **Coping with Fatal Illness.** (A) See *Dimensions of Death Series.*

93. **Crib Death: Or Sudden Infant Death Syndrome.** (P) This is a videotaped lecture by a physician, Dr. Barbara Bruner. Georgia Regional Medical Television Network, black and white, 47 minutes, 1972.

94. **Crib Death: Sudden Infant Death Syndrome.** (A) In this round-table discussion, Dr. John Coe reviews current research and statistics on SIDS. Nurse Carolyn Szybist and parents who have lost children to SIDS discuss their bad experiences—the fears, the guilt,

th ignorance of outsiders—as well as great benefits offered by the SIDS Foundation and its self-help activities. Additional suggestions for caregivers are offered. The Charles Press, audiocassette, 59 minutes, 1972.

95. **The Crisis of Loss.** (P) This is a lecture for student nurses on the subject of crisis intervention: supporting patients as they deal with loss and the mourning process. Crisis theory is emphasized, while examples illustrate the importance of the patient maintaining a sense of control and responsibility. American Journal of Nursing, color film or videotape, 30 minutes, 1975.

96. **Crisis: The Hospitalized Child.** (A) A chaplain, a 16-year-old cystic fibrosis patient, and her family discuss the disease, treatment methods, and the inevitable outcome. Communications in Learning, audiocassette, 37 minutes.

97. **Crisis: The Terminally Ill Patient.** (A) This discussion highlights the role of the chaplain in working with dying patients, and through several case studies offers suggestions to chaplains and other caregivers for improving their work. Communications in Learning, audiocassette, 45 minutes.

98. **Cross-Cultural Aspects of Death.** (A) See *Dimensions of Death Series.*

99. **Crunch Crunch.** (A) This is a simple animated film that could trigger discussion of elemental issues of life and death. A little bug is "crunched" by a bigger one, and that one by another bigger still. Enter man to destroy the biggest nonhuman creature, then turn on fellow humans: not for food but for possessions and power. In man's death little bugs complete the cycle, but the film ends ironically: the memory of humanity lingers on in the form of a monument depicting him as hero slaying a dragon. Viewfinders, Inc., color, 9 minutes.

100. **A Cry for the Children.** (A) This short film studies the effects upon fire fighters witnessing children die in fires. Film Communicators, color, 11 minutes, 1977.

101. **The Cry for Help.** (A) The "cry" in the title comes from the potential suicide. This film primarily addresses police officers and other emergency personnel, but the case studies presented—dramatizing a variety of reasons why people consider suicide—and the techniques of response and understanding advocated have the broadest relevance. Kansas Department of Health and Environment, or National Naval Medical Center, color film or videocassette, 15 minutes, 1963.

102. **Cryonic Suspension of Two Patients.** (HS, A) The procedures used to prepare a body for indefinite cryonic storage are explained and illustrated in this program, consisting of 65 color slides and an 11-page printed text. Trans Time, Inc.

103. **The Day Grandpa Died.** (HS, A) David comes home from school one afternoon to be told that his beloved grandfather has died. "I don't want Grandpa dead," he cries. Then his mind gradually

fills with happy memories of shared experiences. David's father is particularly helpful and understanding: "You've lost your grandpa and your friend, but I've lost my father," beautifully making an essential point about "generations." The graveside ceremony helps David come to terms with the fact of the death so he can resume living, rich in his memories. BFA Educational Media, or University of California, Berkeley, or University of Michigan, color film, 12 minutes, 1970.

104. **A Day in the Death of Donnie B.** (A) Donnie B. is a young inner city drug addict, and his death at the end of a short, miserable life is a foregone conclusion. Voice-over commentary on the drug problem by mothers, doctors, police officers, ex-addicts and members of the clergy adds chilling irony to the reality of Donnie's dying. National Institute of Mental Health, black and white film, 18 minutes.

105. **The Day Manolete Was Killed.** (HS, A) Spain's greatest bullfighter, pressured from retirement by a would-be rival, dies in the bullring. Graphic stills from that last fight force the audience to ask why. Viewfinders, Inc., or University of California, Berkeley, black and white film, 20 minutes.

106. **Day of the Dead.** (A) The title of the film comes from the October festival day in Mexico celebrating the oneness the people feel with their dead. Skulls, skeletons, coffins, and altars for the dead are everywhere. Flowers and food are brought to the cemeteries, ostensibly as memorial gifts to the dead, but the living eat the food in an atmosphere of joy and merry dancing. Studying the death attitudes and rituals of other cultures can be enlightening. Pyramid Films, or University of Washington, Audio-visual Services, or University of Southern California, color, 15 minutes, 1957.

107. **The Dead Bird.** (GS, HS, A) Cartoon pictures and voice-over narration tell the Margaret Wise Brown story of a group of children who discover, bury, and mourn a dead bird. There are insights here into children's attitudes toward death. Indiana University, or University of Wisconsin, Madison, color film, 13 minutes, 1972.

108. **Dead Birds.** (A) The primitive Dani tribe of New Guinea do not fight wars the way the great civilizations do. When a conflict starts they fight until one member of the enemy tribe dies, then hostilities cease. The film ends portraying the funeral rites for a dead child, the first and only casualty in the most recent war. Included are filmed segments of mourning customs and rituals. Viewfinders, Inc., or Phoenix Films, or McGraw-Hill Films, or University of California, Berkeley, color, 83 minutes, 1962.

109. **Dead Man.** (A) The camera moves slowly around the naked body of an old man in a morgue. While some critics have been affronted by this stark and shocking film, most have been awestruck and stimulated. In coldly realistic yet reverent terms, the film declares that this was life, this *is* death. Highly recommended for sensitizing audiences and stimulating discussion, this film should be pre-

viewed by teachers before showing to their classes. Foundation of Thanatology, or Highly Specialized Promotions, black and white, 4 minutes, 1972.

110. **Dealing with Loss and Grief.** (A, P) See *Death and Dying: Closing the Circle.*

111. **Dealing with the Critically Ill Patient.** (A, P) See *Death and Dying: Closing the Circle.*

112. **Dealing with the Terminally Ill Patient.** (P) In this videotape presentation Dr. Elisabeth Kübler-Ross discusses her concept of the five stages of dying and the responses of caregivers and survivors. Network for Continuing Medical Education, black and white, 16 minutes.

113. **Dear Little Lightbird.** (A) The subject, an incurably ill "blue baby," is the 3-year-old son of the filmmaker. Viewfinders, Inc., color film, 19 minutes.

114. **Death.** (HS, A) Buddhist views of death, its relationship to life, and the concept of reincarnation are presented in this film. Comparisons are drawn between Eastern and Western beliefs and customs. Indiana University, black and white, 29 minutes.

115. **Death (Arthur Barron).** (A) This award-winning film documents conditions and treatment for terminal cancer patients at Calvary Catholic Hospital in the Bronx in 1968. Of course since that time the medical professions have come a long way in the quality of care offered the dying. But as this film studies the dying of Albro Pearsall, we watch him receiving less than optimum care, listen to his unresolved doubts about the quality of his life and fears about his pain, and see the family struggle unassisted with their own grief and in their misguided counseling efforts. We are reminded of how much more we have to learn. As a model of care, Calvary Hospital and the dying of Albro Pearsall can be meaningfully contrasted with, for example, the St. Christopher's Hospice program as analyzed in several audiovisual media noted in this section of this book. Filmmakers Library, or University of Michigan, or University of Iowa, or University of California, Berkeley, black and white, 43 minutes, 1969.

116. **Death (CBS Sandpile Series).** (HS) Designed for older youth, the film may be used to stimulate discussion about life, death, and humanity's relationship to God. Several role-playing situations—death of a parent, resistance to war and the draft, drug and alcohol abuse—are presented, then a discussion is led by Professor of Theology Dr. William Hamilton. Association-Sterling Films, black and while, 26 minutes.

117. **Death—A Natural Part of Living.** (GS) In addition to making the key point referred to in the title, this program surveys a variety of contemporary death-related issues, and examines attitudes toward death in other lands and at other times. Marsh Film Enterprises, filmstrip (65 frames) and audiocassette or record, 1977.

118. **Death: A Time to Remember.** (HS, A) This film presents a historical survey of funeral and burial practices from many cultures, reaching back to the dawn of recorded history. Mass Media Ministries, color, 28 minutes, 1977.

119. **Death and Dying (NNMC).** (P) Designed for nurses' training programs, this videotaped discussion treats the problems, feelings, and rights of terminal patients, and explores the roles of the institution and the caregiving staff. National Naval Medical Center, black and white, 58 minutes.

120. **Death and Dying (PRI)** (A, P) For information on the items in this series of videotapes see entries for the separate programs: *Death and the Doctor, The Dying Patient, The Family,* and *Living with Dying.*

121. **Death and Dying (Proceedings of the American Health Congress).** (A, P) These are taped highlights of Congress sessions on caring for dying patients, extraordinary care, the rights of dying patients, and the nature and function of hope in the dying trajectory. Teach 'em, Inc., two audiocassettes.

122. **Death and Dying: A Conversation between Dr. Lee Beach and Dr. Elisabeth Kübler-Ross.** (A) One positive characteristic of this videotaped dialogue is that Dr. Kübler-Ross's views, by now familiar to most people, are presented from a fresh perspective in conversational give and take. In addition to discussing the stages of dying, Drs. Kübler-Ross and Beach touch on cultural differences in dying, caregivers' roles and attitudes, and the helpfulness (or lack of it) of clergy during the dying process. University of Washington Health Sciences Television Center, black and white, 30 minutes, 1971.

123. **Death and Dying: A Conversation with Elisabeth Kübler-Ross, M.D.** (A) In this videotaped interview, in addition to presenting her views on the stages of the dying process and the proper attitudes of caregivers and family members, Dr. Kübler-Ross discusses her emerging beliefs in life after death. Public Television Library, color, 29 minutes, 1974.

124. **Death and Dying: Closing the Circle.** (A, P) This extensive introductory program on death and dying consists of five color filmstrips, with accompanying audiocassettes or records, and a discussion guide and study outline. Consultants are Robert Jay Lifton, M.D., and Professor Austin H. Kutscher. In part 1, "The Meaning of Death," Dr. Lifton surveys death in our society. Part 2, "A Time to Mourn, A Time to Choose," examines death, burial and memorial rites and society's underlying beliefs, assumptions and attitudes about them. In part 3, "Walk in the World for Me," Doris Lund retells her son Eric's 5-year struggle with leukemia. Part 4, "Dealing with the Critically Ill Patient," features an interview with a man with cardiovascular disease. He relates his reaction to his disease, while suggestions are offered for caregivers working with high-risk patients. Part 5, "Dealing with Loss and Grief," consists of interviews with survivors of a young cancer victim, and provides commentary and analy-

sis of the nature of grief. This set of programs is one of the better introductory surveys in the field. Guidance Associates.

125. **Death and Grief.** (A) In this videotaped conversation on a Baltimore television talk show Dr. Edgar Jackson, an authority on grief and bereavement, discusses such matters as the varieties of grief in individuals and cultures, stages of grief, abnormal grief, and the functions of funerals. University of Maryland, black and white, 16 minutes, 1971.

126. **Death and Life.** (HS, A) This audiocassette can best be described as an anthology of views on life and death. A variety of people are interviewed on their conceptions of death, their fears about it, and how death affects their philosophy of life. Center for Cassette Studies, or Canadian Broadcasting Corporation, 60 minutes.

127. **Death and the Child.** (A) Dr. Edgar Jackson tells parents, health professionals, and teachers to be honest, truthful, and realistic in teaching children about death, in answering their questions, and in helping them through death crises. Anything less can cause emotional problems. Specific approaches, resources and skills are suggested. The Charles Press, audiocassette, 45 minutes, 1972.

128. **Death and the Creative Imagination.** (A) See *Dimensions of Death Series.*

129. **Death and the Doctor.** (P) Six physicians share their experiences with dying patients and explore their own attitudes toward life, death, and the effectiveness of their relationships with patients. Professional audiences will find this conversation stimulating. Professional Research, Inc., videotape or film, 20 minutes, 1975.

130. **Death and the Family: From the Caring Professions' Point of View.** (A, P) Professor Delphie Fredlund lectures on effective treatment of dying children and on the preparation and responsibilities of caregivers of the dying. The Charles Press, audiocassette, 30 minutes, 1972.

131. **Death and the Self.** (A) Death attitudes are learned at an early age, Dr. John Brantner explains, and develop and change as we grow. Imperfect attitudes can cause problems in adult living; attitudes should be reexamined occasionally to help enrich life experiences. The Charles Press, audiocassette, 28 minutes, 1970.

132. **Death as a Part of Living.** (A) This is a fine film to trigger discussion. Close to death, a nursing home patient is deliberately isolated from his friends and fellow patients. As a result, they wonder more fearfully what it will be like when they will be in his place. National Audiovisual Center, color, 3 minutes, 1976.

133. **Death as a Practical Matter.** (A) See *Dimensions of Death Series.*

134. **Death Be Not Proud.** (HS, A) This is a film version of John Gunther's famous 1949 memoir of the dying and death of his 17-year-old son, victim of a brain tumor. Learning Corporation of America, color, 99 minutes, 1976.

135. **Death by Request.** (A) After a lifetime of suffering with multiple sclerosis, Meg Murray feels entitled to speak out: laws should be changed to allow persons to help others commit suicide when their lives have lost the quality they wish. A dynamic speaker, she makes a compelling case. Concern for Dying, color film, 25 minutes.

136. **Death: Coping with Loss.** (A) People from various walks of life, and from a variety of perspectives, discuss their attitudes toward life and death, their conceptions of death and their fears. Grief, bereavement, and funeral customs are treated, too—by parents who have lost a child, by a clergyman, funeral director, and physician. Coronet Instructional Films, color, 19 minutes.

137. **Death, Drugs and Walter.** (HS, A) The protagonist of this story is a 12-year-old heroin addict. His short and unhappy career is followed to the end, to the toilet in a Harlem tenement where, wearing a Snoopy T-shirt, he finally overdosed. Interviews with Walter's grieving aunt and his friends raise many points for discussion about the dangers of drugs, the unmet needs of children, and the kind of society in which this sort of thing can happen. Viewfinders, Inc., or Pyramid Films, color, 13 minutes.

138. **Death Education.** (HS) George Daugherty, author of a variety of death education materials for school use, talks about different courses already implemented in grade and high schools. Excerpts from various visual presentations used in those courses are shown. Allied Memorial Council, color videotape or film, 30 minutes.

139. **Death: Family of Man Series.** (HS, A) Produced by BBC-TV, this film is a detailed and insightful cross-cultural study of death attitudes and customs. Cremation ritual in England, for example, is constrasted with cremation in India. A witch doctor conducting funeral rites in Botswana is presented, then a sorcerer in New Guinea. Part of a series studying the life-cycle of man, this program has been favorably reviewed and is enthusiastically recommended for courses wanting cross-cultural insights into death and dying. Time-Life Films, color, 45 minutes, 1971.

140. **Death, Grief and Mourning.** (A) See *Dimensions of Death Series.*

141. **Death: How Can You Live with It?** (GS, HS) This 19-minute clip from the Walt Disney film, "Napoleon and Samantha," focuses on the reaction of a young boy to the dying of his grandfather. The producers believe the film would be effective in triggering discussion, a guide for which is included. Walt Disney Educational Media Company, color, 19 minutes, 1977.

142. **Death in America.** (A) Dr. George LaMore, head of the Department of Religion and Philosophy at Iowa Wesleyan College, addresses a group of clergymen. A most dynamic speaker, LaMore surveys basic issues in the field of death and dying. Washington State Funeral Directors Association, audiocassette, 90 minutes.

143. **Death in Literature.** (HS, A) This program presents a great variety of literature, from Psalm 104 and Ecclesiastes through Shake-

speare to John Gunther, Tom Stoppard, and Simone de Beauvoir. Commentary introduces each piece of literature and its historical and cultural context. In addition, certain themes like the loss of friends and suicide are developed in the literary selections. Guidance Associates, two color filmstrips and audiocassettes or records, teacher's guide.

144. **Death in the Family.** (A) Eda LeShan, author of *Learning To Say Goodbye*, discusses the pain and the grief of survivors. Children, too, experience great suffering. Ms. LeShan analyzes their emotions and suggests ways of helping them cope. Psychology Today Cassettes, audiocassette.

145. **Death: Its Psychology.** (A) A terminally ill woman talks with her husband about her feelings and her acceptance. The presentation refers to Dr. Kübler-Ross's five stages of dying. Center for Cassette Studies, or Canadian Broadcasting Corporation, audiocassette, 60 minutes.

146. **Death Notification.** (P) Police officers who must often notify survivors about deaths are the audience for this presentation of what to do, what to say, and why. Harper and Row Media films, color, 23 minutes, 1977.

147. **Death of a Gandy Dancer.** (HS, A) This brilliant little film story explores how the dying of Grandfather Ben affects other members of the Matthews family. Ben's daughter and son-in-law are concerned and loving, but both want to hide the truth. Grandson Josh is the focal point of Ben's last days and, as it turns out, the best hope that the grandfather's principles and ideals will live on in his progeny. Casting and acting are superb, and the story rich in insight for students of death education. Family dynamics in the dying trajectory, the importance of memory and progeny, truth-telling, and the advantages of choosing one's manner of dying are just a few topics which discussion can explore. Learning Corporation of America, color, 26 minutes, 1977.

148. **Death of a Newborn.** (A, P) Presented in this videotape program is an interview with a young couple who lost their firstborn infant at age 3 weeks. Valuable insights are offered into parental grief and mourning and into intervention techniques that do and do not work. Case Western Reserve University, color, 32 minutes, brochure, 1976.

149. **Death of a Peasant.** (HS, A) A Yugoslavian peasant escapes from a Nazi firing squad, is chased, then manages to find a death of his own choosing. The film is superbly made, well acted, and builds to a tense and exciting conclusion. It can stimulate discussion of basic philosophical and ethical questions about the nature and purpose of life, and the extent of individual control of that life. Mass Media Associates, or University of California, Berkeley, color, 10 minutes, 1972.

150. **Death of a Sibling.** (A) Beginning with an actual case of a child's accidental death in a house fire, the film portrays and inter-

views the parents as they struggle to tell the surviving sibling and work through their fears, guilt, and other emotions. Then two physicians review these events and generalize about anticipated emotional and other problems in such cases, questions for caregivers to expect, and what methods of helping would be most appropriate. Network for Continuing Medical Education, color videotape, 19 minutes, 1972.

151. **The Death of Socrates.** (A) Based on the death as reported in Plato's *Crito* and *Phaedon*, this dramatization can foster discussion on the nature and value of suicide, the individual's right to determine the manner of dying, and the relationship between the quality of a death and the quality of the life. McGraw-Hill Films, or Time-Life Films, black and white film or videotape, 45 minutes, 1969.

152. **Death of the Wished-for Child.** (A) Glen W. Davidson, Professor of Thanatology at Southern Illinois University School of Medicine, interviews a mother who lost a wished-for child at birth and who developed emotional problems because of errors in intervention made by her caregivers. Dr. Davidson makes quite clear what should be done and said in such situations. O.G.R. Service Corporation, or Professor Davidson (P.O. Box 3926, Springfield, IL 62708), color flim, 28 minutes.

153. **Death, the Enemy.** (A) Noted thanatologist Edwin S. Shneidman discusses suicide, intentioned and subintentioned deaths, and the impact of grief upon survivors. Psychology Today Cassettes, audiocassette.

154. **Death Themes in Literature.** (HS) See *Perspectives on Death: A Thematic Teaching Unit.*

155. **Death Themes in Music.** (HS) See *Perspectives on Death: A Thematic Teaching Unit.*

156. **Death through the Eyes of the Artist.** (HS) Presented on this 87-frame color filmstrip are photographs of masterpieces of world art treating death in various ways. Audiocassette commentary analyzes the themes of death illustrated in each work, and generalizes about the universality of death and its portrayal in art. Educational Perspectives Associates; see also *Perspectives on Death: A Thematic Teaching Unit.*

157. **Deathstyles.** (HS, A) Clips of Richard Nixon speaking about death, together with scenes from newsfilm on the Kennedy assassination in Dallas and the Kent State shootings are just a few of the ingredients of this admittedly experimental film about "a nightmare automobile journey to death and dehumanization through a monstrous landscape." The film encourages discussion. Time-Life Films, color, 50 minutes, 1972.

158. **Decisions: Life or Death.** (A) Father Charles Curran and Dr. Michael DeBakey discuss the ethical implications of heart transplants and other medical innovations. Association Films, or Macmillan Films, black and white film, 30 minutes.

159. **Depression/Suicide: You Can Turn Bad Feelings into Good Ones.** (HS, A) The subject of this film is teenage suicide. Young people who have attempted suicide are interviewed and explain what motivated them. They now successfully control remaining suicidal urges, and are putting their lives back in order. University of California, Berkeley, color, 28 minutes, 1976.

160. **Desert.** (HS, A) The scene is a former battlefield. As a boy and his dog play with a rusting cannon, pitted helmets, and other relics, dead soldiers come to life and aim the cannon at the boy. The topic, of course, is youth and war: the film can spur discussion of this and other basic issues of life and death. Viewfinders, Inc., black and white, 16 minutes.

161. **The Detour.** (A) From the perspective of an elderly woman unable to move or speak as she dies in the hospital, we witness the thoughtlessness, the coldness of a number of caregivers including a doctor, a minister, and hospital staff. She would rather do without them, she thinks; but they come back in force when the machines say her body needs the resuscitation she does not want. This well-made, ironically humorous film can generate discussion of institutional treatment of the very ill and the aged. Viewfinders, Inc., or Phoenix Films, color, 13 minutes, 1977.

162. **Developmental Concepts of Death.** (A) See *Dimensions of Death Series.*

163. **Dialogue on Death.** (A) In a fine conversation, three prominent thanatologists—Dr. John Brantner, Professor Robert Slater, and Dr. Robert Fulton—survey a host of major issues of interest and relevance to all beginning students of death education: U.S. attitudes toward death, contemporary funeral customs, isolation of the seriously ill and the dying, and various weaknesses in professional care and treatment modes. The Charles Press, audiocassette, 59 minutes, 1970.

164. **The Dignity of Death.** (HS, A) ABC News visited St. Christopher's Hospice in London and interviewed its founder, Dr. Cicely Saunders, patients, and others. In this excellent filmed report, the principles of hospice philosophy and modes of spiritual and emotional, as well as physical and medical, treatment are introduced. This is a significant film with much to offer all audiences from high school through adult to medical professionals in training. ABC News, color, 30 minutes, 1973.

165. **Dimensions of Death Series.** (A) This collection of 10 separate filmstrip-audiocassette programs is the only available audiovisual resource of such ambitious scope addressed to general and college audiences rather than to the schools, and is thus of more than passing interest to the death educator attempting to meet the needs of college students and adults. To illustrate the wide range of topics covered, here are the titles of the ten units and the subject matter or discipline of each:

1. "Death and the Creative Imagination": painting, sculpture, music, poetry, and prose fiction.
2. "Cross-cultural Aspects of Death": history and anthropology.
3. "Religious Viewpoints on Death": Judaism, Catholicism, and Protestantism.
4. "Death as a Moral and Ethical Issue": philosophy, particularly ethics.
5. "Man's Attitudes to Death": sociology, psychology.
6. "Developmental Concepts of Death": psychology.
7. "Death, Grief and Mourning": the psychology of grief.
8. "Coping with Fatal Illness": psychosocial counseling.
9. "The Funeral in American Culture": U.S. history.
10. "Death as a Practical Matter": consumer education.

The best organized and most detailed programs are 5, 6 and 7, those dealing with death and dying from sociological and psychological perspectives. While 1 and 4 are comparatively weak, the others may be useful for general audiences. Educational Perspectives Associates, 10 color filmstrips or slides and audiocassettes, available as a set or individually.

166. **The Discovery of Faith.** (HS, A) A terminally ill patient produced this videotape about his own dying and his deep religious faith. His story is intensely moving, and may be of value to both believers and nonbelievers in demonstrating the impact religious faith can have in the dying process. Creative Christian Communications, color, 45 minutes, 1974.

167. **Do Funerals Help the Mourners?** (A, P) Edgar Jackson answers in the affirmative, and offers reasons. Jeffrey Norton Publishers, Audiocassette, 28 minutes, 1963.

168. **Do I Really Want to Die?** (A) Ordinary people under great stress—a widow, a student, a druggist's assistant, an office worker out of a job—discuss their suicide attempts and continuing suicidal feelings. The point made strongly is that suicidal thoughts and behavior are not so much cowardly as they are cries for help. This is a fine film to trigger discussion. Polymorph Films, color, 31 minutes, 1977.

169. **Do Persons Have the Moral Right to Commit Suicide?** (A) A psychiatric nurse practitioner lectures on moral issues pertaining to suicide and suicide prevention. PSF Productions Corporation, audiocassette, 60 minutes.

170. **Dr. Cicely Saunders: A Medical Pilgrim.** (A) The founder of St. Christopher's Hospice in London and pioneer in the field discusses hospice philosophy and treatment methods. This is perhaps the best audiocassette introduction to the hospice concept. The Charles Press, 40 minutes, 1975.

171. **Drama of Death: Counseling the Dying and Their Families.** (A) This instructional program on the topic includes two audiocassettes (or phonograph record) and study guide. Creative Resources, 2 hours, 22 minutes.

172. **Dying.** (A) Director Michael Roemer presents the last days of four individuals and their families through actual conversations, interviews, and filmed day-to-day experiences and activities. The artistic beauty of the film results from the brilliant camera work and thoughtful editing. Its human significance is found in the individuals who are facing the stark reality of death. Three family groups respond heroically, with great dignity and poise, yet in uniquely individual ways. In the fourth, as a result of the long, slow dying of a husband and father of two sons, relationships crumble. The wife, Harriet, fearful at the prospect of her widowed life, inadequate to the task of raising her sons alone, and angry at her husband and his dying for laying such a burden upon her, cannot come to terms with reality. Bill's last days and Harriet's troubled reactions as a result are not as uplifting or as inspiring as the other stories in the film, but they are no less human or instructive. This is an important film for all audiences, even the most experienced professionals. WGBH/Distribution, color videotape or film, 97 minutes, 1976.

173. **Dying and Death in Contemporary America.** (A) Dr. Herman Feifel, one of the leading thanatologists in the U.S., presents a brilliant lecture in which he surveys modern attitudes to death and makes a strong plea for the healthy, realistic acceptance of death as a part of life. Dr. Feifel's concluding remarks suggest very well the theme of his talk: "To die is the human condition, to live well and to die appropriately, this is man's privilege." Psychology Today Cassettes, audiocassette.

174. **Dying Child.** (A) Dr. Elisabeth Kübler-Ross addresses herself in this videotaped lecture to the problems and needs of dying children, their parents and caregivers. She offers several specific suggestions on ways of getting children to express their feelings about their deaths: poetry, play therapy, and art activities, for example. Medical College of South Carolina, color, 42 minutes, 1975.

175. **Dying Is a Problem for Young and Old.** (A) The topic of this videotaped discussion is kidney disease and the particular problems associated with it. University of Arizona, color, 42 minutes, 1974.

176. **The Dying Patient.** (P) This videotape is aimed at health care professionals, attempting to make them aware of the feelings and needs of dying patients, and to suggest modes of care and understanding. Professional Research, Inc., color videotape or film, 19 minutes, 1975.

177. **The Dying Patient.** (P) In the first part of this professional training film a woman dying of cancer is interviewed. In the second half two doctors discuss the dynamics of the interview, general interviewing techniques, and the attitudes and fears of dying patients most likely to be revealed by structured interview. Indiana University School of Medicine, or University of California (Irvine), black and white, 68 minutes, 1971.

178. **The Dying Patient and His Family.** (A) Presentations by four experts at a critical care medicine symposium were recorded:

Dr. P. G. Gaffney, "The Dying Child"; Dr. Ned Cassem, "The Dying Adult"; Ms. Margaret Wynn, "The Social Worker's Role"; and Rev. G. E. Jackson, "The Clergyman's Role." University of Pittsburgh, 4 audiocassettes, 1974.

179. **Early American Cemeteries: Clues to a Nation's Heritage.** (HS, A) As its title suggests, this filmstrip-cassette program investigates U.S. historical and cultural heritage as revealed by stones in old graveyards. Changing attitudes toward life and death are traced, symbols on stones are analyzed, and, in general, the graveyard as an outdoor museum of art and history is discussed. Educational Perspectives Associates, or Allied Memorial Council, 26 minutes.

180. **Echoes.** (HS, A) Visiting the ancestral farmhouse, an 11-year-old girl walks through the cemetery with her grandfather and finds the grave of an 11-year-old relative who died in 1883. In the house she finds the girl's picture and doll. Again she visits the grave and leaves the doll and a fresh flower, sensing the nature of the generations and the bonds that cement them. Guidance Associates, color film, 11 minutes, 1974.

181. **Emily: The Story of a Mouse.** (GS) A simple story designed to introduce the concept of death at the elementary level, the film tells the life of a field mouse growing from a "child" to an adult, raising her children, then dying. Even in her death life goes on, for her body provides warmth and nourishment for new life. Viewfinders, Inc., 5 minutes, 1975.

182. **Emotional Reactions to Cancer in Clinical Practice.** (A, P) This film presents conversations between patients and their physicians about the disease, possible treatment methods, and complications. Then physicians discuss among themselves successful modes of counseling their seriously or terminally ill patients. These conversations can spark audience discussion about emotional reactions to cancer and proper professional intervention. American Cancer Society, color, 26 minutes, 1973.

183. **Emotional Support for Dying Patients.** (A) Dr. Jimmie Holland lectures on common attitudes toward and conceptions of death, and provides helpful suggestions for dealing with dying children and their families. Communications in Learning, audiocassette and slides, 38 minutes.

184. **Emotions and Cancer.** (A) Lawrence LeShan, psychotherapist and author of *You Can Fight for Your Life*, discusses emotions as possible causative factors in cancer, and psychotherapeutic techniques effective in handling emotional aspects the disease. Psychology Today Cassettes, audiocassette.

185. **The End of One.** (HS, A) This short film might be well used to initiate discussion on death attitudes and societal reactions to death. A seagull falls to earth from a soaring flock and dies unnoticed by his fellows. Learning Corporation of America, color, 7 minutes.

186. **Epitaph: The Lingering Heart.** (HS, A) A young father is diagnosed as having leukemia, approaches his death and dies within

15 months. At the same time the film studies his wife and daughters and records their grief, bereavement, then readjustment to a new life. WKYC-TV, color, 25 minutes, 1975.

187. **An Equal Knock on Every Door.** (HS, A) This public service program gives factual, practical information about funeral customs and ritual, and available options. The role of the funeral director in helping a family work through their grief is also explained. WKYC-TV, color videotape, 30 minutes.

188. **Espolio.** (HS, A) This film can trigger discussion of guilt versus duty, of the extent of responsibility, and of the validity of the common excuse, "I was just following orders." How culpable is the carpenter who made the cross for the crucifixion, or the soldier who kills in war, or anyone who hurts another, even for "good reason"? Viewfinders, Inc., color, 7 minutes.

189. **The Ethical Challenge: Four Biomedical Case Studies.** (A) This program illustrates the dilemmas faced by patients, doctors, and society as a result of medical advances. Examined in some detail are cases involving allocation of scarce medical resources, behavior control, genetic screening, and refusal of treatment in the face of death. The Center for Humanities, two audiocassettes or records, 40 minutes, and 160 accompanying color slides, 1975.

190. **Ethical-Legal Aspects of Nursing Practice.** (P) Using several vignettes to illustrate basic points, this program deals with a number of medical-ethical topics with nurses' needs and possible options in mind: euthanasia, the living will, a patient's right to refuse care and family rights in such situations, and the proper use of human subjects in medical experiments. American Journal of Nursing Company, Educational Services Division, color film or videotape, 30 minutes, 1974.

191. **Everyday Heroics of Living and Dying.** (A) Interviewed on his deathbed, Ernest Becker, author of *The Denial of Death*, discusses his theory that the fear of death gives rise to human creativity and heroism. Psychology Today Cassettes, audiocassette.

192. **The Excuse.** (A) Poet Ruth Stone talks about being a widow, about her husband's suicide, and how those life experiences have affected her philosophy of life and the nature of her poetry. University of California, Berkeley, color film, 16 minutes, 1975.

193. **Experience in Dying.** (A) This videotaped presentation is meant to be a general introduction to the process of dying and related issues for medical caregivers and family members. McMaster University, color, 30 minutes, 1976.

194. **Experience in Grieving.** (A) Relatives report on their need for support and contact with medical caregivers for some time after the death of their loved one in the hospital. McMaster University, color videotape, 30 minutes, 1977.

195. **Explaining Death to Children.** (A) Rabbi Earl Grollman, who has written extensively on this subject, offers essential introductory concepts. Available from Allied Memorial Council, color film or videotape, 30 minutes, 1974.

196. **Extending Life.** (MS, HS) This brief survey of the moral and social implications of scientific advances in "life extension" would be useful to introduce the topic to school children. BFA Educational Media, color film, 15 minutes, 1976.

197. **The Faces of "A" Wing.** (HS, A) The scene is a nursing home, and the "faces" are those of patients, relatives, and staff. The approach in this film is largely visual: watching the faces the audience can begin to sense effectively what it is like to live, to work, to be in such a place. Pennsylvania State University, black and white, 58 minutes, 1974.

198. **Exploring the Cemetery.** See *Understanding Death Series.*

199. **Facing Death.** (P) Four physicians in a panel discussion talk about the stress experienced by physicians who must tell dying patients and family members about the terminal condition. Problems are exacerbated by patients who want to pretend or deny to protect their loved ones. Solutions are based on thoughtful rapport with the patient as an individual. National Medical Audiovisual Center, color film, 20 minutes, 1968.

200. **Facing Death: The SHANTI Project.** (A) Charles Garfield lectures on this famous organization in Berkeley, California, which offers counseling and companionship for dying patients and families, and grief counseling for survivors. See also the Project in Part III. Highly Specialized Promotions, or Psychology Today Cassettes, audiocassette, 30 minutes.

201. **Facing Death with the Patient: An On-going Contract.** (P) This lecture by Dr. Vincent Hunt is directed to physicians working with the dying. They are urged first to face their own fears about death and their own human nature: physicians are not omnipotent. Then, communicating honestly with dying patients and their families, physicians can be more effective. The Charles Press, audiocassette, 30 minutes, 1972.

202. **Facts about Funerals.** See *Understanding Death Series.*

203. **Families in Crisis: Coping with Death.** (A) Death from various causes and of various types (sudden or lingering, for example) are presented, and varying effects on family members and modes of intervention are discussed. Coronet Instructional Films, color filmstrip and audiocassette or record, 35 minutes, 1976.

204. **The Family.** (P) Aimed at a medical audience, this program discusses the variety of problems faced by the families of terminally ill patients, and how caregivers can help. Caregiving community organizations are also identified. Professional Research, Inc., videotape or film, 15 minutes, 1975.

205. **The Family Coping with Breast Cancer.** (A) Fears, emotional responses, and other problems faced by the mastectomy patient, as well as related difficulties experienced by family members (in this case the husband and daughter) are discussed in some detail in this videotaped interview with a doctor. Stanford University, color, 60 minutes, 1974.

206. **The Family of the Dying Patient.** (A, P) Nationally known nursing consultant Virginia Barckley addresses an audience of nurses, though all caregivers will find her remarks useful. She observes that the families of dying patients must be well understood, too, and handled with the same thoughtful care as the patients. Different problems arise when the dying individual is a child, a parent, or an aged spouse. Whatever the case, family members have particular needs influenced by life-styles and family customs. A number of positive suggestions are offered. American Cancer Society, audio-cassette or reel-to-reel tape, 23 minutes, discussion guide, 1972.

207. **Father.** (HS, A) Starring Burgess Meredith, this fine little film is based on a short story by Anton Chekhov. Ned Kelly, a hansom cab driver in New York's Central Park, alone in the world since the recent death of his son, tries to share his grief with passengers in his cab but is coldly rebuffed or ignored. The point is made beautifully but painfully that grief must be shared. University of California, Berkeley, or New Line Cinema, black and white, 1971.

208. **Feelings of a Father.** (A) A father discusses his grief at the loss of his child. The Compassionate Friends, audiocassette.

209. **The Final Proud Days of Elsie Wurster.** (A) This film is not only a careful look into a nursing home. It also provides a great number of insights into being old and institutionalized from the knowledgeable and thoughtful point of view of the title character, a retired public health nurse now close to death, remembering her life and coming to terms with her death. Pennsylvania State University, black and white, 30 minutes, 1975.

210. **The Following Sea.** (HS, A) At the funeral of his father, an old fisherman, Charles recalls his father's life and realizes the legacy of wisdom and insight left behind which now, like a following sea, continues to move the lives of his survivors. McGraw-Hill Films, black and white, 11 minutes.

211. **Freeze: Wait: Reanimate.** (A) The commentator describes a visit to the Cryonics Plant on Long Island and interviews the management. Science fiction writer Isaac Asimov comments on the cryonics idea. Pacifica Tape Library, audiocassette, 58 minutes.

212. **Fritzi: Living and Dying with Dignity.** (A, P) In this video-taped interview with Fritzi, one of his patients, a psychiatrist demonstrates how the terminally ill must be treated as human persons, with respect and dignity. Audio Visual Medical Marketing, Inc., color videotape, 50 minutes.

213. **The Funeral: A Vehicle for the Recognition and Resolution of Grief.** (HS, A) Twenty color slides and a printed manuscript. National Funeral Directors Association.

214. **Funeral Customs around the World.** (HS) Funeral customs and rituals of various cultures, including the United States, are explored. The conclusion is that all civilizations share common bonds in the experience of death, grief and the funeral and memorial process. Educational Perspectives Associates, or Washington State

Funeral Directors Association, color filmstrip and audiocassette, teacher's guide. See also *Perspectives on Death: A Thematic Teaching Unit.*

215. **The Funeral Director.** (HS, A) The executive director of the National Funeral Director's Association, Howard Raether, discusses the role of the funeral director in the community, funeral practices and traditions, and the nature and benefits of the funeral service—all from the industry point of view. Allied Memorial Council, color videotape or film, 30 minutes.

216. **The Funeral: From Ancient Egypt to Present Day America.** (HS, A) A printed manuscript and 12 color slides. National Funeral Directors Association.

217. **The Funeral in American Culture.** (A) See *Dimensions of Death Series.*

218. **Future Unknown.** (A, P) Presented in this film for medical caregivers is a dramatized discussion between a terminally ill patient, initially hostile to intervention, and a nurse. Skillfully the nurse builds a rapport with the patient and encourages her to give vent to her fears, emotions, complaints, and concerns, which are typical of those encountered in such situations. In her helpful, specific responses to the patient's comments, and in her mode of conversational inter- actions generally, the nurse demonstrates one model of effective care. University of Pittsburgh School of Nursing, black and white, discussion guide, 20 minutes.

219. **Gale Is Dead.** (A) A 19-year-old girl dies of a heroin over- dose, and this award-winning documentary film attempts to reveal the causes of her addiction, not simply the effects. Framed at begin- ning and end by scenes from her funeral, the film interviews teachers and acquaintances, explores her early years and formative experiences, and suggests that in many ways society and its institutions, not simply the addict's own psychological condition, are at least partly to blame; they could have done more for her. Time-Life Films, color film or videotape, 51 minutes, 1970.

220. **The Garden Party.** (HS, A) Based on the Katherine Mans- field short story, the film juxtaposes upper- and lower-class attitudes, assumptions, misinformation, and fears about death and post-death rituals, as it portrays in depth the effects of death on a young girl. This is excellent for discussion purposes. ACI Films, or University of Illinois, 24 minutes.

221. **Gift of Life/Right to Die.** (A) A panel of experts discusses four problems in medical ethics: organ transplants, triage, euthanasia, and death criteria. In brief, the complexity of the issues is well sug- gested. Indiana University, or University of California, Berkeley, black and white film, 15 minutes, 1968.

222. **Graduation Day.** (HS, A) A probation officer manages to help a suicidal teenager back to a healthy sense of reality. The point is made that a worthwhile life must be based on a sense of personal identity and inner freedom. Paulist Productions, color film, 27 min- utes, 1973.

223. **Gramp: A Man Ages and Dies.** (HS, A) Based on the best-selling book by Mark and Dan Jury, this program records the last days of their grandfather dying of generalized arteriosclerosis. His end is not pleasant to watch, but the love and care demonstrated by the family as they take Gramp through his dying are inspiring. Sunburst Communications, or Human Relations Media Center, black and white filmstrip and audiocassette, 1976.

224. **The Grandfather.** (A) A 93-year-old man is interviewed about his long life, old age, and imminent death. The film will help stimulate discussion of aging and the viewpoints of the aged. Indiana University, or University of California, Berkeley, black and white, 16 minutes, 1968.

225. **The Great American Funeral.** (HS, A) Produced by CBS, this is a hard-hitting documentary critical of the funeral industry. Ministers, morticians, cemeterians, garment makers, and limousine dealers are interviewed, as is Jessica Mitford, author of *The American Way of Death.* Mass Media Associates, color videotape, 55 minutes, 1965.

226. **The Great Plan.** (HS, A) Overhearing his grandchildren questioning the fairness of the impending death of their grandmother, grandfather answers their questions and explains the nature of death as part of the Christian view of God and human life. Association-Sterling Films, color film, 20 minutes, 1961.

227. **The Great Tree Has Fallen.** (A) The king of the Ashanti Nation in Ghana has died, and an 8-day funeral marks the passage of power to a new monarch. The effect of the death on the people and the nation as well as the cultural significance and social value of funeral ritual are presented. University of California, Berkeley, color film, 22 minutes.

228. **Grief.** (A) A number of people recall what the death of loved ones meant to them and how they experienced, then worked through, their grief. One woman speaks of "black, awful feelings," and describes her compulsion and her denial. Taken together, these comments provide a convenient introduction to a complex human emotion. Concord Films, color film, 50 minutes, 1972.

229. **Grief and the Funeral.** (A) Edgar Jackson discusses the nature of grief, the function of the funeral in the grief process, and how caring professionals and clergy can be of maximum benefit to mourners. Allied Memorial Council, color videotape, 30 minutes.

230. **Grief Therapy.** (A) Originally produced as part of the CBS-TV "60 Minutes" series, this film presents several on-camera grief therapy sessions. Dr. Donald Ramsey leads a mother to "let go," to face the facts and separate herself from her daughter, whose accidental death she has been mourning intensely for over 2½ years. Insights into the nature of grief are graphically presented. Carousel Films, or University of California, Berkeley, color, 20 minutes, 1976.

231. **Group Concepts of Human Death.** (HS, A) This film compares three cultures—the American, the Bantu of Africa, and the Kiriwina of the Trobriand Islands—in terms of life-death attitudes,

funeral and burial ritual, and conceptions of an afterlife. Dancing and original music help to underscore the points made. Indiana University, black and white, 30 minutes, 1958.

232. **Growing Old: The Prospects for Happiness.** (A) This televised dialogue from a humanist perspective is part of a series, "Moral Values in Contemporary Society." It is also available on audiocassette and a discussion guide is available. The Humanist Alternative, videotape, 30 minutes.

233. **Guidelines for Consent: The Uniform Anatomical Gift Act.** (A) Medical and legal experts discuss organ transplants with special reference to the widely recognized Uniform Anatomical Gift Act. Network for Continuing Medical Education, black and white videotape, 15 minutes.

234. **Guidelines for Interacting with the Dying Person.** (A) See *Perspectives on Dying.*

235. **Handling Holidays.** (A) The title refers to the special problem faced by parents who have lost a child, and this audiocassette offers practical advice from people who have had the experience. The Compassionate Friends.

236. **The Hangman.** (HS, A) Maurice Ogden's poem on which this animated film is based presents a whole town passive in the face of a new scaffold in the town square, and a hangman who daily increases his "take" until no one, not even the enthusiastic cooperators, is left. The film could spur discussion of individual responsibility, of the individual in society, and of "taking orders." McGraw-Hill Films, color, 12 minutes, 1963.

237. **Hazards and Challenges in Providing Care.** (A) See *Perspectives on Dying.*

238. **Help and Self-Help.** (A) In a panel discussion setting, Dr. Robert Fulton, Dr. Phyllis Silverman, and others talk about grief and the process of mourning, particularly as related to widows, and offer many positive suggestions for caregiving intervention. The Charles Press, audiocassette, 40 minutes, 1976.

239. **Help Me! The Story of a Teenage Suicide.** (HS, A) Based on the story of one young girl who becomes a suicide statistic, this film explores behavior patterns of suicide-prone individuals and offers suggestions for effective intervention. S. L. Film Productions, color, 25 minutes.

240. **Help When It Is Needed.** (HS, A) Arguing that one should understand the funeral process before it is needed, this program follows a typical family as they get information about and make plans for a funeral, cemetery plot, funeral flowers and memorialization, and contact a minister and a lawyer. Allied Memorial Council, color filmstrip with audiocassette, 14 minutes.

241. **Hiroshima—Nagasaki—8/45.** (A) Using footage shot by Japanese photographers on the scene, this film documents the mass death and destruction caused by the two atomic bombs dropped on Japan by the United States in World War II. Center for Mass Communications, black and white, 16 minutes, 1970.

242. **Hodgkin's Disease.** (A) Two patients with the disease and their spouses discuss how both their individual lives and their marriages have been affected. The videotape concludes with remarks by a psychiatrist familiar with the cases. Stanford University, black and white, 38 minutes, 1972.

243. **The Hole.** (HS, A) The title refers to a construction project from which two workers emerge to eat their lunches and to discuss nuclear war, the likelihood of total destruction on all sides, and the seeming ease with which such a holocaust could begin. Their sobering analysis suggests that their hole is probably a good place to be. This nicely animated film would be effective in fostering discussion of "the last things" of our time. Viewfinders, Inc., color, 16 minutes.

244. **Home for Life.** (A) This moving presentation on old age and its problems portrays life at Chicago's Drexel Home for the Aged. Films, Inc., black and white film, 58 minutes, 1967.

245. **Hospice for the Dying: A Living Experience.** (A) Principles of hospice care for the terminally ill as developed at St. Christopher's Hospice in London is the theme of this audiocassette presentation. The Charles Press, 1975.

246. **Hospital.** (A) Another exciting documentary by Frederick Wiseman ("Titicut Follies" and "Primate"), *Hospital* spends a day in a very large and crowded urban institution. The pace is frantic, the atmosphere tense and necessarily impersonal. One wishes it were not so, and seeing the film may have positive effects on an audience, whether lay or professional, who can watch *Hospital* and perhaps see themselves. The film can effectively trigger discussion of proper attitudes to patients and effective modes of terminal care. Zipporah Films, black and white, 75 minutes, 1970.

247. **How Could I Not Be among You?** (HS, A) Like most fine poets, Ted Rosenthal has a heightened intellectual and sensuous appreciation of his experience. When he is diagnosed as having terminal leukemia, he continues to see, feel, and express as a poet, to our great benefit. This fine film is rich in Rosenthal's commentary on his condition and his life, in the insight that his dying has given him, in the wisdom he offers in the beautiful title poem, and in the suggestive color and imagery of the filmmaker, whose work won the American Film Festival Blue Ribbon in 1972. Viewfinders, Inc., or Indiana University, or Eccentric Circle Cinema Workshop, or Spectrum Motion Picture Laboratory, color, 29 minutes, 1970.

248. **How Death Came to Earth.** (MS, HS, A) For classes interested in the cross-cultural study of death this well-made little film with attractive musical accompaniment may be valuable. It retells an East Indian folk tale about a time when there were two suns and two moons and no one died. When one of each pair fell in love with each other and came to play on earth, people were afraid of the fire so a hunter was sent to kill them both. Thereupon storms, rain, and death descended upon the earth. McGraw-Hill Films, color, 14 minutes, 1971.

249. **How Do You Explain Death to Children?** (HS, A) Use of

this film is free to classroom teachers and death educators. Write for information and make booking well ahead of time. Walter J. Klein Co., Ltd., color, 28 minutes, 1976.

250. **How to Kill.** (A) This animated film, called "a cartoon for adults," might well spark discussion of basic issues such as the sanctity of life when tested by wartime pressures to kill or be killed. Viewfinders, Inc., color, 11 minutes.

251. **How Would You Like to Be Old?** (HS, A) Economic and psychological problems faced by the aged in our society are surveyed, and humane solutions are suggested. A discussion guide is included. Guidance Associates, two color filmstrips and audiocassettes or records.

252. **Human Development: Successful Aging.** (A, P) Designed for professionals of all types who work with the aging, as well as for the aging themselves, this five-film-strip/cassette series offers two programs on the topic, "successful aging" (the biological, psychological, social, and chronological components of aging, and various social-psychological theories, approaches and techniques to help achieve "success"), two programs on the widow, and one on the widower, presenting background information and helping techniques through several case histories. The set includes a manual with suggestions for teaching, discussion questions, study-review questions, bibliographies, and script narration. Concept Media, 5 color filmstrips and audio-cassettes, 1979.

253. **The Human Side of Cancer.** (A) The human, or nonmedical, side of the disease is highlighted in this informative film. Cancer patients often have difficulty communicating with family members and caregivers, must often change their life-styles may need rehabilitation or job counseling and retraining, and must adjust to marital problems and changed attitudes toward them of friends and associates. The problems are complex and solutions are not easy, but patients can overcome difficulties with the help of sympathetic, knowledgeable caregivers. The film suggests specifically how caregivers can help most effectively. American Cancer Society, color film or videotape, 13 minutes, 1978.

254. **A Humanist Funeral Service.** (HS, A) National Funeral Directors Association, color film, 15 minutes.

255. **I Heard the Owl Call My Name.** (HS, A) Based on the best-selling novel by Margaret Craven, the film tells the story of a missionary who learns noble dying from the Eskimos he is serving. Eskimo philosophy of life, death, and the purpose of things makes a strong impression on the priest at a crucial time of his life. Learning Corporation of America, or University of California, Berkeley, color, 78 minutes, 1974.

256. **I Never Sang for My Father.** (A) Here is a vivid portrayal of how death in the family highlights, changes, or disrupts long-standing family relationships. The death of his wife accentuates the difficulties of a tyrannical old man, and hurls him and his middle-aged

son, already beset with identity problems, into direct conflict. The focus of the film is on the old man, and on the problems of the elderly in a society that does not set much store by them. Macmillan Films, color, 92 minutes, 1970.

257. **I Never Saw Another Butterfly.** (A) This is a film record of a fascinating set of children's drawings, which include depictions of the happiness and joy of houses, toys and flowers, and vivid renderings of funeral scenes and death by gallows and lightning. What is special are the artists, inmates of the Nazi concentration camps in World War II. Macmillan Films, color, 15 minutes.

258. **I Want to Die.** (P) Addressing physicians, this videotape tells how to recognize and manage depression and suicidal attitudes of patients as expressed in office visits. Network for Continuing Medical Education, 19 minutes, 1974.

259. **Ikiru.** (A) A man informed of his imminent death learns how to live in the fullest sense of the term. Fighting initial apathy, he struggles to get through to uncomprehending family, friends, physicians and bureaucrats. In the face of custom and tradition he finds it difficult to act on his newfound values, but he does succeed. This masterful film is by award-winning Japanese director Akira Kurosawa. Macmillan Films, black and white, 140 minutes, 1952.

260. **The Immortalists.** (A) An introduction to the theories and techniques of cryonics. WKYC-TV, color film, 30 minutes, 1974.

261. **Immortality: A Debate.** (A) The subject is discussed from a humanist perspective in this part of the series, "Moral Values in Contemporary Society." Audiocassette format and a discussion guide are available. The Humanist Alternative, videotape, 30 minutes.

262. **Implications for Teaching.** (A) See *Perspectives on Aging.*

263. **Implications of Nursing: The Dying Patient.** (A, P) Rose Marie Chioni, on the faculty of the University of Wisconsin School of Nursing, lectures primarily to nurses on proper care of the dying patient. This care embraces family members, too, and continues consistently through all stages of the illness. It should be understood as a team effort, involving all medical staff, other caregivers (even housekeepers), and family members and friends. The presentation is clearly organized and is rich in detail and insight. Milwaukee Regional Medical Instructional Television System, color videotape, 55 minutes, 1971.

264. **In My Memory.** (GS, HS) A preteen reacts to the death and funeral of her grandmother with happy memories as well as painful questions, doubts, and feelings of guilt. These are the expected reactions of children, but the adult and caregiver responses in this film are not presented equally effectively. The film may be useful as a basis for classroom discussion of a loved one's death, but reviewers have noted the weak acting in this dramatization. Allied Memorial Council, or National Instructional Television Center, color film or videotape, 15 minutes, 1973.

265. **In Search of Life after Death.** (HS, A) Patients who have experienced "near death" or "life after life" phenomena described

by Ray Moody and others tell their stories in this film program. Pyramid Films, color, 24 minutes, 1976.

266. **The Incident.** (HS, A) A would-be suicide poises himself to jump from the top of a tall building. A crowd starts to gather below, drawn by the wailing of sirens. Police, reporters, TV crews converge, and into the crush wade venders, pickpockets—anyone with something to gain, everyone anxious for sensation and thrills. Thus human tragedy and despair become entertainment for the masses. This fine little film can provide the basis for good discussion of such topics as death and the media and death and popular culture. Phoenix Films, color, 8 minutes, 1975.

267. **The Interest in Dying and Death as it Relates to the Funeral.** (HS, A) The speaker is Howard C. Raether, Executive Director of the National Funeral Directors Association. National Funeral Directors Association, color film, 43 minutes.

268. **Interviewing and Crisis Intervention Techniques.** (P) This program series is on proper techniques of suicide prevention and intervention for medical professionals, social workers, and law enforcement and emergency personnel. See also *Suicide Prevention and Crisis Intervention: A Series of Case Histories*, the filmed basis for this audio program. Charles Press Publishers, or Jeffrey Norton Publishers, six audiocassettes with printed instructional materials, 1974.

269. **Interviews with My Lai Veterans.** (A) Five young men who participated in the total destruction of this Vietnamese village tell their stories in strangely cold and matter-of-fact language. This award-winning film demonstrates very well what war can do to normal people. Macmillan Films, color, 22 minutes, 1970.

270. **An Investment in Sight.** (HS, A) The story of a nearly blind boy whose vision has dramatically improved as a result of corneal transplant surgery, this film demonstrates the great benefits offered to the living by donations of eyes and other bodily organs after death. University of Iowa, color, 19 minutes.

271. **Is Society Ready to Face the Reality of Terminal Treatment?** (A) The emphasis here is on the legal rights of terminally ill patients, and the legal as well as medical responsibilities of their caregivers. Case histories illustrate the commentary. University of Arizona, color videotape, 56 minutes, 1974.

272. **Joe and Maxi.** (A) Joe is both Maxi's father and the subject of her film. He is dying of cancer, having lost his wife to the disease several months before, and his sons have left school and come home to run the family business. Maxi records the altered family life, Joe's gradual dying, and the newfound togetherness of the family. Maxi Cohen/Joel Gold, color, 90 minutes, 1978.

273. **John Baker's Last Race.** (HS, A) An outstanding college athlete after being told in high school he was too uncoordinated to run track, John Baker becomes a grade school and amateur track club coach. John respects each of his charges as an individual and encourages even the handicapped to "do your best despite the odds."

When he is told he has terminal cancer he first considers suicide, then decides to practice in his own life what he has been teaching his students. His last days, marked by the success of his track team and the fulfillment of his personal philosophy, are very moving, even for more sophisticated audiences. The story is true, though the script and the direction give the film a *Reader's Digest* aura. Brigham Young University, color, 34 minutes, 1976.

274. **Joseph Schultz.** (HS, A) The title character is a German soldier ordered to participate in the firing-squad execution of a group of civilians during World War II. His conscience makes him refuse to aim his weapon, so he is put up against the wall himself. This well-made little film could start a discussion of moral responsibility versus the need to "follow orders." Viewfinders, Inc., or University of California, Berkeley, or University of Michigan, color, 13 minutes.

275. **Journey to St. Christopher's: A Hospice for the Dying.** (A) Staff and patients of this world-renowned institution discuss hospice philosophy and treatment. The Charles Press, audiocassette, 29 minutes, 1975.

276. **Journey's End.** (A) Through a dramatized case study involving a father and husband who died intestate and the resulting fears and problems experienced by widow, son, and friends, the point is made that making a will and having funeral and other practical matters arranged before one's death will alleviate much stress and trouble for survivors. University of Southern California, or University of California, Berkeley, color film, 28 minutes, 1974.

277. **Joy of Love.** (HS, A) This film might prompt a discussion of the life cycle or growing old. A young couple courts, marries, raises a family, and grows old together. After his wife dies, the widower fondly remembers her when she was young. University of Michigan, color, 9 minutes.

278. **Just a Little Time.** (A) Dr. Elisabeth Kübler-Ross conducts a probing, enlightening interview with Eileen, a 49-year-old cancer patient. Revealed are some of Eileen's fears about her disease and its prognosis, her denial mechanisms, and her attitudes to life in the face of her cancer. Dr. Kübler-Ross then interviews Eileen's nurse, Mrs. Donna LeBlanc, about her long-standing relationship with Eileen and her very satisfying work with other terminally ill patients. Association-Sterling Films, color film, 21 minutes, with study guide, 1973. An audiocassette with the same title is available, presenting a "nursing conference" designed to prepare a care plan for Eileen as presented in the film. American Journal of Nursing Company, Educational Services Division, 21 minutes, 1973.

279. **A Last and Lasting Gift.** (A) Information on bequeathing one's body and/or bodily organs to medical science is presented. The specific use of different tissues and organs, as well as testing and storage techniques, are explained. The film ends with an interview of an older woman who can now see for the first time since childhood as the result of corneal transplant surgery. Inland Empire Human Re-

source Center, or San Diego Human Resource Center, color film, 26 minutes.

280. **The Last Full Measure of Devotion.** (HS, A) To help present the "positive story of funeral service," this film recounts the funerals of Presidents Lincoln, Roosevelt and Kennedy to demonstrate how this nation has cared for its dead over the last 100 years. National Funeral Directors Association, color film, 27 minutes.

281. **The Last of Life.** (A) This documentary film surveys biological knowledge of the aging process and urges professionals to treat their aged patients more sympathetically, to be aware of their strengths and their uniqueness. With minimal help many of the aged can lead active, independent lives. Filmmakers Library, color, 27 minutes.

282. **Learning to Live with Dying.** (A) During this videotaped discussion medical students, physicians, and theologians discuss the difficulties experienced by caregivers, patients, and families in trying to come in terms with dying. Network for Continuing Medical Education, color, 39 minutes.

283. **A Legacy from Paula.** (A) Paula Doherty was diagnosed as having leukemia in the third trimester of her first pregnancy. She accepted the fact better than her family and friends, and went on to deliver her daughter with no problem. It was Paula's idea to be interviewed and to express her very positive emotions and reactions to her dying as a legacy to her daughter, family, and medical caregivers. A most impressive film. Thanatology Resource Center of Massachusetts, color videotape, 50 minutes.

284. **Legend Days are Over.** (A) This award-winning film would be useful in classes studying cross-cultural attitudes toward life and death. An old woman of the Nez Percé Indian tribe recalls her past. Paulist Productions, color, 5 minutes, 1974.

285. **Lessons from the Dying Patient.** (A) Dr. Kübler-Ross presents her theories of the stages of dying, interviews patients, and underlines effective techniques for caregivers working with dying patients. Ross Medical Associates, 5 audiocassettes, 1973.

286. **Let's Rejoice.** (A) This film studies a group of nursing home residents who, despite the personal tragedies of the past, have banded together to affirm the meaning and value of their lives. They have become a new family. Viewfinders, Inc., color, 10 minutes.

287. **Leukemia Panel Discussion.** (A) Parents of leukemic children and their doctors discuss the psychological and emotional effects of the disease on the families. Stanford University, School of Medicine, color videotape, 32 minutes, 1975.

288. **Life Cycle.** (HS, A) This is symbolic portrayal of the life cycle: one red dot appears, grows in size, meets another, has a home, gives rise to other smaller dots, works, retires, then returns to the element from which it came. There is no narration, but a lively musical score accompanies the action. ACI Films, or Highly Specialized Promotions, color film, 7 minutes, teacher's guide, 1971.

289. **The Life Cycle.** (HS) Several of the individual captioned filmstrips in this series of six on growth, development, and the cycle of life would be of special interest to teachers planning death education units. The discussions are clearly presented and the visuals are helpful and attractive. Topics are: adolescence, young adulthood, marriage, separation and divorce, aging, and death. Educational Record Sales, six color captioned filmstrips.

290. **Life Cycle: The Death.** (A) In this lecture Dr. Vivian Rakoff, a psychiatrist at the University of Toronto, argues that attitudes to death are largely functions of a particular time and place, and are changed by people depending on their age and their varying attitudes to life. Canadian Broadcasting Corporation, audiocassette, 30 minutes.

291. **Life—Death.** See *Understanding Death Series.*

292. **A Life Has Been Lived.** (HS, A) Presented in this film is a contemporary, nontraditional funeral service employing guitar music, and short, personal eulogies by family members and friends. National Funeral Directors Association, color, 16 minutes.

293. **Life on Death Row.** (HS, A) This film vividly presents interviews with a number of prisoners on death row in San Quentin prison. Classes discussing capital punishment can use this film profitably, as can any group trying to understand how it feels to face death. Indiana University, black and white, 9 minutes.

294. **The Life That's Left.** (A) A number of individuals who have experienced a loss—an elderly widower, a young widow, a sibling, parents, and the mother of a stillborn baby—describe their feelings in interviews. Great Plains National Instructional Television Library, color film or videotape, 29 minutes.

295. **Lifting Shadows.** (HS, A) This brief film provides a history of U.S. funeral customs and practices based on the *History of American Funeral Directing*, a book sponsored by the funeral industry. National Funeral Directors Association, 20 minutes.

296. **The Lingering Heart.** (A) The program presents a young husband and father who is also a leukemia patient who devotes much of his time to counseling other terminally ill patients. Sunburst Communications, color videotape, 30 minutes.

297. **Living and Death.** (A) The flim features the Indian philosopher and spiritual leader Krishnamurti discussing living, love, and death as three essentially interrelated elements. The fear of death, he says, disrupts the potential fullness of living and love; by "dying every day" we rise beyond our fear of death to a more enriched life. Indiana University, black and white, 29 minutes, 1971.

298. **Living and Dying with Cancer.** (A) Lois Jaffe, dying of cancer, is interviewed. Pacifica Tape Library, audiocassette, 64 minutes, 1977.

299. **Living Together and Dying Alone.** (HS, A) Citing statistics demonstrating that the married have lower death rates than single, widowed, or divorced people for various diseases, and seem to be less

suicide- and accident-prone, this program makes a case for family life, warm human relationships generally, and traditional values. The photography makes an impact and the narration is presented clearly. Illinois Funeral Directors Association, or 20/20 Media, color film-strip and audiocassette, 21 minutes, 1978.

300. **Living with Death.** (HS) Catholic attitudes on the subject are presented in this 51-frame filmstrip. Highly Specialized Promotions.

301. **Living with Dying.** (A) Orville Kelly, founder of Make Today Count, introduces these presentations by four terminally ill individuals. Each discusses his or her disease and the steps taken to live life in spite of the prognosis. Each offers detailed comments about treatments, caregivers, attitudes, and philosophies of life that have been especially helpful. Professional Research, Inc., color video-tape or film, 18 minutes, 1975.

302. **Living with Dying.** (HS) This set of classroom materials will be a valuable resource to the teacher of death education. There is a copy of Ernest Morgan's booklet, *A Manual of Death Education and Simple Burial*, a set of 24 illustrative prints (11" × 14"), and a teacher's guide. Documentary Photo Aids.

303. **Living with Dying (Sunburst).** (HS, A) The first of the two filmstrips in this set presents death as part of the natural cycle of life and discusses various ways to achieve symbolic immortality. Fear and denial are natural but can be overcome. The second filmstrip demonstrates how our culture encourages a denial of death in children, and offers positive suggestions. The program, which won an award in 1973 from the National Council on Family Relations, ends by dramatizing the five "stages" of dying and explaining how a caregiver can be most helpful. The photography and accompanying recorded commentary are useful. Sunburst Communications, or Mass Media Associates, 2 color filmstrips and audiocassettes or records. Part 1: 72 frames, 14 minutes; part 2: 78 frames, 15 minutes. 1973.

304. **Lois Jaffe, M.S.W.** (A, P) Ms. Jaffe discusses the effects of her terminal leukemia on her family, her work, and her life, and explains the nature and particular effects of her treatment regimen. This is part of a series, "Interviews with Family Therapists." ETL Video Publishers, color videotape, 60 minutes, 1975.

305. **A Long Look at Death.** (A) Margaret Mead is interviewed on attitudes to death in a variety of cultures around the world. Pacifica Tape Library, audiocassette, 23 minutes, 1976.

306. **The Long Valley: A Study of Bereavement.** (A) As Dr. C. M. Parkes, a British psychiatrist, lectures on the nature and stages of the grief process, interviews with and commentary by other medical personnel and lay people illustrate his points. Overall, this is a most impressive and thorough introduction to the topic of grief. Time-Life Films, color film, 59 minutes, 1976.

307. **Loss and Grief.** (A) Designed to train members of all the helping professions, this extensive analysis of loss and grief treats

not just loss from death or impending death, but the loss of a spouse through divorce, of an infant given up for adoption, of a job, of children who have grown up and left home, of a son by imprisonment, of a chronic but not necessarily terminal disease, and even of moving from a familiar neighborhood. The first three filmstrips are a well-organized presentation of background information on the varieties and levels of loss and adaptive and maladaptive grief responses. The other four filmstrips present case studies which elicit feelings, stimulate discussion, and provide an opportunity to apply concepts learned in the informational section. Concept Media, seven filmstrips with audiocassettes or records, 1977.

308. **The Lost Phoebe.** (A) An elderly man cannot accept the death of his wife. He imagines she is still alive, and has nightmarish visions of her. Friends fail to reach him as his own life begins to disintegrate. The film, based on a short story by Theodore Dreiser, is well acted and well produced, and contains valuable insights. Perspective Films, color, 30 minutes, 1974.

309. **The Lottery.** (A) This film version of the famous Shirley Jackson short story of ritualized sacrifice and social terror could be used to trigger discussion on attitudes toward life and death. Encyclopaedia Britannica Educational Corporation, or University of Washington, color, 18 minutes, 1969.

310. **Love Must Not Be Wasted—When Sorrow Comes, Take It Gently by the Hand.** (A) This personal approach to bereavement reports the experiences of Isabella Taves as she shared her husband's dying and as she worked to build a new life after he died. Library of Congress, Division for the Blind and Physically Handicapped, three long-playing records, 1974.

311. **The Loved One.** (A) This hilarious film debunks some of America's most cherished funeral and burial customs, and offers a healthy contrast to the often uncritical assumptions and practices of the funeral industry. Films, Inc., color, 116 minutes, 1965.

312. **A Lover's Quarrel with the World.** (HS, A) Poet Robert Frost is featured in this film, reading from his work and commenting on his life and his happy old age. Bailey Film Associates, black and white, 40 minutes, 1966.

313. **Magic and Catholicism.** (HS, A) Funeral rites in the Bolivian highlands are a unique melding of Catholic ritual (church processions, burning votive candles before statues and pictures of saints, and so on) and ancient magical practices (ceremonies and sacrifices performed in the countryside to appease the spirits). University of California, Berkeley, color film, 34 minutes.

314. **The Magic Moth.** (HS, A) Based on the book by Virginia Lee, the film portrays the illness, death, and funeral of Maryanne, the middle child of five, and the reactions of her family and friends. The family is a model (perhaps somewhat unrealistic) of healthy relationships characterized by open discussion and honest acceptance of the reality of death. Their frankly stated Christian beliefs and point

of view may be objected to by some as simplistic. As Maryanne dies the beautiful moth of the title springs from a cocoon given to her earlier by her brother. The acting is, at times, only fair. Centron Educational Films, or Washington State Funeral Directors Association, color, 22 minutes, 1977.

315. **Magical Death.** (HS, A) The shaman of the Yanomamo Indians of Venezuela uses hallucinogenic drugs to put him in contact with the spirits of the dead who, it is believed, will help him cure. Classes studying death beliefs and rituals in other cultures will find the film useful. University of Washington, color, 29 minutes, 1972.

316. **The Magician.** (HS, A) This film is frankly antiwar, so it may help start a discussion of such basic issues as the value of life and the right to kill. The title character, attracting a crowd of children with his bag of tricks, first gets them to play with toy guns and then with real ones. Sterling Educational Films, 13 minutes, 1963.

317. **Make Today Count.** (A) Orville Kelly founded the organization Make Today Count to help terminally ill individuals like himself combat feelings of isolation and rejection by others, and to improve the quality of their remaining days. Kelly discusses his views and explains the work of his organization in this program. Alfred Shands Productions, color film, 29 minutes, 1975.

318. **A Man.** (A) The film focuses on a group of men in a consciousness-raising group after the father of one of them has died. Insights are offered into male reactions to loss, and the way they express emotions. Polymorph Films, black and white, 21 minutes, 1976.

319. **Man Blong Custom.** (HS, A) Funeral rites and related spirit customs in the New Hebrides, the Solomon Islands, and on Moro are portrayed. Time-Life Films, color film, 55 minutes, 1975.

320. **Management of Grief and Depression in Practice.** (P) Dr. Rex Pittenger gives a lecture during a course at the University of Pittsburgh. U. P. School of Medicine, audiocassette, 1974.

321. **Management of Pain in Cancer.** (A, P) Modes of pain treatment are discussed in this audiocassette, and illustrated and explained on the accompanying 13 color slides and printed handouts. Communications in Learning.

322. **Management of the Depressed Patient.** (A, P) Topics discussed by a panel of doctors include managing bereavement, prolonged depression, suicidal tendencies in the aged, theories of depression, and the uses of psychotherapy and drugs. Trainex Corporation, audiocassette, 1975.

323. **Management of the Terminally Ill: The Family.** (A, P) Dr. Kübler-Ross lectures to a medical audience on the special problems of caring for and relating with family members of a terminally ill patient. Network for Continuing Medical Education, black and white videotape, 16 minutes.

324. **Managing the Suicidal Patient.** (P) This is a videotaped lecture by Dr. Richard Lisle. Emory University, black and white, 28 minutes, 1975.

325. **Many Crises in Cancer.** (P) The American Cancer Society prepared this informational presentation for nurses, which includes a discussion guide. American Cancer Society, audiocassette or reel-to-reel tape.

326. **Marek.** (A) Marek is a 7-year-old boy who must undergo dangerous cardiac surgery to correct a birth defect. The doctors advise the parents of the risks involved and counsel the family attentively. The surgery is performed but there are complications and Marek dies. The parents are then helped through the shock of the loss. Produced by BBC-TV, the film is well made and impressive. Time-Life Films, color, 45 minutes, 1978.

327. **The Mark Waters Story.** (HS, A) The title character was a Honolulu newsman who died of lung cancer that he blamed on excessive smoking. His story, well acted by Richard Boone, is his obituary. Public Television Library, or University of California, Berkeley, color film or videotape, 29 minutes, 1969.

328. **Masque of the Red Death.** (HS, A) The theme of this famous Edgar Allen Poe story is that death is an impartial yet inevitable visitor to everyone. This animated film version would help stimulate discussion of this basic fact of life. University of Michigan, or Viewfinders, Inc., color, 10 minutes.

329. **A Matter of Indifference.** (A) This is an in-depth interview with Maggie Kuhn, founder of the Gray Panther Movement. It is an eye-opening analysis of the lack of respect and the ill treatment commonly afforded the aged in this country. Viewfinders, Inc., black and white film, 50 minutes.

330. **A Matter of Time.** (A) Photographed at the Princess Margaret Hospital in Toronto, this film presents the diagnosis and treatment of a cancer patient, then notes the effects of illness on the patient's relationships with others. Indiana University, black and white, 53 minutes, 1969.

331. **The Meaning of Death.** (A, P) See *Death and Dying: Closing the Circle.*

332. **The Meaning of Death in American Society.** (A) Dr. Herman Feifel lectures on the tendency of our society to deny death and to vulgarize it as we do, for example, in the mass media. He suggests that we need to accept death, and we should put the energies we spend suppressing death into affirming life. This is a fine presentation by a noted expert in the field. The Charles Press, audiocassette, 28 minutes, 1970.

333. **Medical and Psychological Aspects of Terminal Renal Disease.** (P) Nurses in training are the audience of this presentation by a psychiatrist and a nurse. The main topic is the team approach to terminal care, and major points are illustrated in the 40 accompanying slides and a variety of printed handouts. Communications in Learning.

334. **Medical Perspectives on the Value of Human Life.** (A, P) At a symposium at the University of Cincinnati, Dr. Michael DeBakey

discusses ethical issues raised by the increased ease and frequency of transplant surgery. He explores related changes in the definition of death. Jeffrey Norton Publishers, audiotape, 1969.

335. **Medicine, Morality and the Law: Euthanasia.** (A) Positive euthanasia, or direct action to end a life out of merciful motives, is the topic of this filmed panel discussion involving experts from various fields. After looking at case studies from legal and moral points of view, the panel concludes that "mercy killing" is clearly manslaughter or worse. University of Michigan, black and white, 30 minutes.

336. **Meeting Needs . . . Serving People.** (HS) This color slide and audiocassette program on the funeral and the service provided by the funeral director was designed especially for junior high and high schools. National Funeral Directors Association.

337. **Memorialization.** (HS, A) Two spokesmen of the memorial (monument or gravestone) industry discuss the history of and current trends in memorialization in the U.S. Allied Memorial Council, color videotape, 30 minutes.

338. **The Mercy Killers.** (A) Euthanasia is the topic of this BBC-TV production. Case histories and interviews with interested parties and medical and legal experts elicit questions about an individual's right to die, legal obligations of physicians, and the quality and relevance of motives. The presentation takes no sides, but the general level of insight may be dated as the film was made in 1967. Time-Life Films, or University of Illinois, black and white, 37 minutes.

339. **Mercy Killing.** (A) Here is a panel discussion on many aspects of the topic. Canadian Broadcasting Corporation, audiocassette, 30 minutes.

340. **Mind Over Body.** (A) The film documents the case for the mysterious ability of the human mind to control or at least materially affect bodily function. Pain control through mental effort or suggestion is one subject treated here which may be of interest to caregivers of the terminally ill. Time-Life Films, or University of Washington, or University of California, Berkeley, color film or videotape, 35 minutes, 1972.

341. **Ministering to the Terminally Ill.** (A, P) Joseph Bayly moderates a panel discussion involving Gordon Addington, B. Balfour Mount, and Merville O. Vincent. A variety of topics are presented from a Christian perspective. Highly Specialized Promotions, 3 audiocassettes, teacher's guide.

342. **Mr. Story.** (A) At age 86, self-sufficient Mr. Story is coping intelligently with the problems of growing old in our society, but his articulate condemnation of the abuses we inflict upon the aged is forceful. Viewfinders, Inc., color film, 28 minutes.

343. **Mongoloid Infant: Should We Operate?** (A, P) A panel of doctors at the University of Virginia Medical School breaks this question down into its more specific medical and ethical components, and discusses the varying types and prognoses of mongoloidism, the

"quality of life" concept, and the extent of parental rights in determining treatment. University of Virginia, black and white videotape, 60 minutes, 1973.

344. **Moral, Philosophical and Religious Considerations of the Hopeless and Dying Patient.** (A, P) This is a conference paper delivered by Dr. Stephen J. Galla. University of Pittsburgh School of Medicine, audiocassette, 1974.

345. **The Mortal Body.** (A) A Yugoslavian filmmaker creates an evocative series of photographic images (there are no words, only a musical background) that suggest basic philosophical questions on the nature and purpose of human life. The film would be useful as a discussion starter, or as a climax or summary in a death and dying program. Filmmakers Library, black and white, 12 minutes, 1976.

346. **Mountain People.** (HS, A) There remains in America at least one outpost of an older way of life in which people live to great age, still vigorously active, productive, and healthy in their communities, surrounded by children and grandchildren in three- and four-generation homes. But family life-styles are becoming "modern" even in rural Dingess, West Virginia, as these old ways, practiced now by only a few, die out. An informative, thoughtful film, a finalist at the 1978 American Film Festival. Cinema 5, color, 52 minutes, 1978.

347. **Mourning for Mangatopi.** (A) Mangatopi was leader of the Tiwis, an Australian aboriginal tribe on Melville Island. His funeral, done according to old tradition, brings together many relatives, friends, and tribesmen. This film record of the ceremonies would be useful for groups studying death and dying in other cultures. University of California, Berkeley, color, 56 minutes.

348. **My Grandson Lew.** (MS, HS, A) When, how, and what to tell children about a death in the family are questions raised by this film, based on the book by Charlotte Zolotow. Lew is thinking about his grandfather and wonders when he will visit again. Mother tells Lew that the grandfather has died and that she was afraid to tell him earlier because he was too young. They then share happy memories of grandfather. Barr Films, or University of Illinois, color, 13 minutes, 1976.

349. **My Son, Kevin.** (A) Kevin, a "thalidomide baby," has no arms or legs, but he rises above misfortune to attend a community school and be a loved and loving person. This film would interest discussion groups on policies and attitudes toward malformed fetuses, abortion, and birth defects. Viewfinders, Inc., color, 24 minutes.

350. **My Turtle Died Today.** (GS) The book on which this cartoon is based tells the story of a pet turtle getting sick, dying, then being mourned by three children until they realize that life continues. Bailey Film Associates, color film, 5 minutes.

351. **The Mystery that Heals: The Story of Karl Gustav Jung—Number 3.** (A) In this third and final segment of a documentary on his life and thought, Jung discusses his attitudes toward death, religion and the after life, when he feels the psyche may continue to

exist in some way. University of California, Berkeley, or Time-Life Films, color film or videotape, 30 minutes, 1972.

352. **Mysto the Great.** (HS, A) The dynamics of adjustment to a death in the family and the conflicts that accompany attempts of family members to go on living in their own ways are well portrayed here. When his wife dies, Mysto, an old magician, is pushed by his children to arrange for a certain kind of funeral and to settle the estate quickly. Haunted by his own memories of his wife and his long professional career, Mysto grieves in his own way. Finally done with bickering, he embarks on a new life by leaving funeral arrangements in the hands of his family and journeying to visit an old girlfriend now alone in a rest home. Perspective Films, color film or videotape, 25 minutes, 1978.

353. **Myths and Realities.** (A) See *Perspectives on Aging.*

354. **Narcotic Deaths, Parts I and II.** (P) Pathologist Dr. Milton Helpern presents basic medical and physical information about drug use, abuse and overdose. Though there is nothing here about psychological or emotional factors, caregivers of suicidal patients and in suicide intervention would find this material beneficial. National Medical Audio-visual Center, or National Audio-visual Center—GSA: part 1, color film or videotape, 38 minutes; part 2, color film or videotape, 28 minutes, 1970.

355. **National Public Radio.** (HS, A) Over the years NPR has aired dozens of broadcasts on a great variety of death and dying topics, from the problems of aging, death with dignity, grief, and the right to die, to funerals and widowhood. These programs are available on audiotape and audiocassette. Write for information and listen for new shows. National Public Radio Information, 2025 M Street, N.W., Washington, DC 20036.

356. **The Nature and Management of Terminal Pain.** (A, P) Dr. Cicely Saunders discusses concepts of treatment, and particularly of pain management, for terminally ill patients. Her ideas are more successful and certainly more humane than much current practice. For physical pain she advocates early and permissive use of any appropriate analgesic. Caregivers must understand the interrelationships of physical pain and emotional and spiritual pain, and be willing and able to address themselves to all patient needs. These and other hospice-related concepts are presented in greater depth and breadth by Dr. Saunders in more recent audiovisual programs. See the Index. Royal College of General Practitioners, reel-to-reel audiotape, 36 minutes, 1966.

357. **The Nature of Sudden Death.** (P) Three physicians discuss sudden death by heart attack. American College of Cardiology, audiocassette, 1969.

358. **The Necropsy as a Tool in Medical Progress.** (P) This talk by Dr. Edward A. Gall is delivered at the New York Academy of Medicine. Jeffrey Norton Publishers, audiotape, 24 minutes, 1968.

359. **A Need to Know: A Family Faces Death.** (A, P) Part of the videotape series "Interventions in Family Therapy," this program presents an interview between Lois Jaffe, M.S.W., a leukemia patient herself, and the family of a child with the same disease. ETL Video Publishers, color videotape, 60 minutes, 1975.

360. **Nell and Fred.** (A) The hero and heroine of this film documentary are a couple over 80 typical of so many in contemporary society, caught in the grinder of social worker, senior citizens' home and life on a pin-money budget. They talk about moving to a nicer retirement home, but doubt they can afford it. In this film, society stands accused of ignoring its responsibilities to the aged. McGraw-Hill Films, black and white, 29 minutes, 1971.

361. **Never Give Up.** (HS, A) Photographer Imogen Cunningham, as indomitable as ever at 94, is the subject of this film. She continues her art, gardens, and otherwise remains active. Aside from its value in introducing audiences to a unique human being, the film is a powerful antidote to widely held misconceptions about being old and a woman. Viewfinders, Inc., or University of California, Berkeley, color, 28 minutes, 1974.

362. **New Deal.** (HS, A) This fast-moving, impressionistic film about growing old in the U.S. was designed especially to sensitize young people and young adults. Carousel Films, black and white, 1973.

363. **Night and Fog.** (A) Produced and directed by Alan Resnais, the film vividly depicts life and death in a Nazi concentration camp by juxtaposing explicit black and white documentary film footage and photographs made by the Nazis and the liberating Allies, and color film made of the ruins of the camp. The film argues that we still live with the effects of the Holocaust, and unless we understand its implications we may be doomed to repeat it. (There are several dozen films on the Holocaust. See *Medium*, 1978, *16*, published by Jewish Media Service, Brandeis University, Lown Building, 415 South Street, Waltham, MA 02154; or write Richard A. Pacholski.) Films, Incorporated, or University of California, Berkeley, color and black and white, 31 minutes, 1955.

364. **Nine-Year-Olds Talk about Death.** (GS, HS, A) School teachers and others interested in understanding children's attitudes toward death will find this short film informative and stimulating. The format is straightforward: a group of fourth-graders are filmed as they answer questions about death posed by a teacher off-camera and comment on one another's responses. Here is yet another valuable illustration of the sometimes profound wisdom of children. International Film Bureau, black and white film, 15 minutes, 1977.

365. **November.** (HS, A) The film could trigger discussion of the cyclical nature of all life. Visual images of autumn and winter in country and city are interspersed with pictures of death, both violent and painful, and quiet and natural. Through it all, however, there are

promises of the winter cycle moving into rebirth, into spring. McGraw-Hill Films, or University of California, Berkeley, color, 10 minutes.

366. **Nursing Management of Children with Cancer.** (A, P) The purpose of this film is to illustrate the skills, commitment, and rewards involved in pediatric cancer nursing. The procedures demonstrated include infusions, mouth care, control of infections and fevers, ostomy care, and play therapy. The need for emotional support for patients and their families is explained, as is the nurse's teaching responsiblity of aiding parents to help and treat their children at home. Statistical information is provided that suggests that the prognosis of many childhood cancers is improving. American Cancer Society, color, 22 minutes, 1974.

367. **Nursing Management of the Dying Patient.** (A, P) Virginia Barckley, R.N., a nationally recognized nurse educator and consultant, urges caregivers to see each patient as an individual, even though most of them appreciate the same things: the nurse's presence, listening, caring, gifts, and even medical rituals. Caregivers occasionally need care, too—suggestions are offered. American Cancer Society, audiocassette, 21 minutes, 1972.

368. **An Occurrence at Owl Creek Bridge.** (HS, A) This gripping film version of the Ambrose Bierce Civil War short story describes a man's future passing before his eyes in slow motion while he is being hanged as a saboteur. The film is well made and the topic is provocative. Here is a nineteenth-century account of a "near-death" experience. Viewfinders, Inc., or McGraw-Hill Films, or University of Washington, or University of Southern California, black and white, 27 minutes, 1962.

369. **Of Life and Death.** (HS, A) Roman Catholic views, with special emphasis on the meanings of Catholic funeral and burial ritual and symbolism, are presented. National Funeral Directors Association, color film, 27 minutes.

370. **Old Age (The Family of Man Series).** (HS, A) Old age can be a happy, positive experience. Whether in England, Botswana, New Guinea, or a Himalayan village, old age can be enriched by continuing hard work and the presence and support of children and grandchildren. Time-Life Films, color film, 45 minutes, 1971.

371. **Old Age: Out of Sight, Out of Mind.** (HS, A) This documentary film studies hospital wards and nursing homes for their treatment of the aged and, in most respects, finds them lacking. Indiana University, black and white. 60 minutes, 1967.

372. **Old Age: The Wasted Years.** (HS, A) A case is built against society's mistreatment and abuse of the aged in these interviews with elderly people. Indiana University, black and white film, 60 minutes, 1967.

373. **Old, Black and Alive.** (HS, A) The daily lives and the personal and religious philosophies of several elderly black people from a range of backgrounds are contrasted. In a nursing home or still on

the job, these people have one thing in common: They are adjusting well to the realities of their aging and are living each day with poise. University of Michigan, color film, 28 minutes, 1974.

374. **Old People's Home: A Poetic Essay on Aging.** (A) See *Perspectives on Aging.*

375. **The Old Woman.** (HS, A) Our spirited heroine is busy with her hobbies and active around the house. So when death—a pile of bones wrapped in a sheet—knocks at the door she recognizes it right away but has so much to do it will have to wait. When death finally "dies" of impatience or boredom, she sheds a few crocodile tears for it, then sweeps it out the door. This silent animated film is a perfect delight. ACI Films, or University of Michigan, color, three minutes, 1973.

376. **On Death and Dying.** (A) This NBC-TV special interviews Dr. Kübler-Ross, who speaks about her conceptions of the five stages of dying and her philosophy of humane care of the terminally ill. Viewfinders, Inc., or Films, Incorporated, color film, 58 minutes.

377. **One Day at a Time.** (A, P) In an interview with a nurse, a 20-year-old leukemia patient shares her reactions to her illness and to the caregivers working with her. Academy of Health Sciences, U.S. Army, color videotape, 30 minutes, 1975.

378. **One in 350: Sudden Infant Death.** (A) Perhaps one of the most serious problems faced by parents who have lost a child to SIDS is the tactless ignorance of family, friends, and well-meaning caregivers. Education on the nature of the disease, and on the fact that so little is known about it, can help parents and the public alike. In this film parents share their experiences and their particular kind of grief. National Sudden Infant Death Syndrome Foundation, black and white, 30 minutes.

379. **One of the Missing.** (HS, A) In this film version of a beautifully horrifying Ambrose Bierce short story, a Civil War soldier suddenly finds himself pinned in the rubble of a blown-up building with his rifle pointed right between his eyes. This thoughtful study of fear of imminent death can provoke discussion. Macmillan Films, color, 56 minutes, 1971.

380. **One Time Around.** (HS, A) A young man takes a part-time job in a retired citizens program, and learns from the aged some basic lessons about finding the meaning of life and accepting the reality of death with poise and dignity. This is a nice study in the often irreconcilable attitudes toward life of the young and the old. University of Minnesota, or Northern Illinois University, or University of South Florida, color film, 16 minutes, 1974.

381. **The One Who Heals.** (A) Several filmed vignettes portray various situations of patient care involving both physicians and the clergy. The film suggests that the doctor should consider the patient's religious faith as a factor in treatment, and demonstrates how doctors and clergymen could work together more effectively. American Medical Association.

382. **Our Busy People.** (HS, A) Sponsored by the funeral industry, this film discusses the role of the funeral director, the cemeterian, the florist, and the memorialist. Allied Memorial Council, color, 17 minutes.

383. **The Parting.** (HS, A) A middle-aged man dies in a remote village in Montenegro. The mourning becomes a community activity, along with the laying out, the funeral ritual, and the burial. Death is very much a part of life for these people, whose approach may be healthier than ours. Viewfinders, Inc., or Wombat Productions, color film, 16 minutes, 1973.

384. **Passing Quietly Through.** (A) This award-winning film shows the relationship between a bedridden, lonely old man in a New York tenement apartment and the nurse who visits him daily. He reveals his attitudes about his life and approaching death, and she shares significant experiences in her own life. There are valuable insights here into the loneliness of old age, the inadequacy of society and its institutions to do much for the aged, and the importance of simple but sincere human relationships. Films, Incorporated, or Grove Press Film Division, black and white, 26 minutes, 1971.

385. **The Patient Is Dead.** (A, P) A panel discussion involving a funeral director, a hospital pathologist, an administrator, and a priest explains their respective roles and responsibilities upon notification of a death in the hospital. They reveal mutual misunderstandings that complicate their tasks and thus their relationships with the families of dying and dead patients. This videotape would be of interest to caregivers, institutions, and communities desirous of improving their team approach to terminal illness. Milwaukee Regional Medical Instructional Television System, color, 55 minutes, 1971.

386. **The Patient Who Is Not Going to Get Better.** (A) Practical instruction is offered to family members and other caregivers in providing for a patient on a long-term basis at home. Emphasis is placed on the team approach, with the physician, community personnel or agencies, and family members all having a role to play. Further, the patient and family have to be ready psychologically for the burdens of home care. Royal College of General Practitioners, reel-to-reel audiotape with 20 illustrative slides, 1971.

387. **The Patient with a Terminal Illness.** (A) This is a presentation for the clergy, offering suggestions for developing more effective relationships with dying patients. A number of case histories are presented. Communications in Learning, audiocassette, 60 minutes.

388. **The Patient's Right to Die.** (A) This lecture covers such important bioethical issues as the definition of extraordinary care, types of euthanasia, and other aspects of the question of maintaining life. Walter Reed Army Medical Center, black and white videotape, 60 minutes.

389. **Peacebird.** (HS, A) Deanna Edwards, a volunteer music therapist headquartered in Normal, Illinois, has written many moving

songs especially to comfort the sick and dying in clinical settings. She sings her songs accompanied by guitar and small orchestra on this record (or audiocassette, 1974) and on (A Song Is a Gentle Thing) (record or audiocassette, 1976). Her voice is warm and pleasing, and the arrangements and performances are highly professional. Teleketics.

390. **Peege.** (HS, A) A typical U.S. family visits an almost totally senile grandmother in a typical U.S. nursing home. Everyone is stiff and uncomfortable, well intentioned but patronizing, defensive and behaving stereotypically. One grandson, however, breaks the pattern, reaches out to Peege in a human way, and makes contact. The acting and the production generally are first-class, forcefully presenting essential lessons about aging and family. Viewfinders, Inc., or Phoenix Films, or University of California, Berkeley, color film, 28 minutes, 1974.

391. **People Helping People.** (HS, A) The role of the funeral director is illustrated and explained in this filmstrip (or slide) and audiocassette program. OGR Service Corporation.

392. **Perspectives on Aging.** (A) Designed for nurses and other caregivers but suitable for any interested and intelligent audience (either for self-study or as a classroom aid), this series is a well made, clearly organized, in-depth introduction to the aging process and to caring for the aged. The first program, "Myths and Realities" (25 minutes), presents information about finances, housing problems and preferences, health, transportation, and so on. "Physical Changes and Their Implications" (31 minutes), the second program, treats physiological and psychological processes as affected by aging, and the third program, "Implications for Teaching" (26 minutes), presents specific teaching and communication techniques effective with the elderly. In the fourth program, "The Confused Person: Approaches to Reality Orientation" (24 minutes), suggestions for treatment accompany information on, for example, functional as opposed to organic disorders, and reversible and irreversible brain syndromes. Finally, "Old People's Home: A Poetic Essay on Aging" (7 minutes), a photographic interpretation of W. H. Auden's poem, is a probing, emotional analysis and critique of our society's preference for putting the aged away in institutions. All the filmstrips have diagrams, charts, summary lists, and other devices to facilitate learning. The instructor's manual offers suggestions for use, topics for discussion, study questions, script narrations, and bibliography. Concept Media, five color filmstrips and audiocassettes, available as a set or separately.

393. **Perspectives on Death: A Thematic Teaching Unit.** (HS) Widely used in secondary schools, this program consists of an anthology of readings, a student activity book, teacher's resource book, and four audiovisuals. "Funeral Customs Around the World" (110-frame color filmstrip and audiocassette) is a cross-cultural survey. "Death Through the Eyes of the Artist" (87-frame color filmstrip and audiocassette) shows the work of such masters as Michelangelo, Rembrandt, Bosch, and Picasso, and explains how style, color, and

symbolism can "capture the face and mood of death." Narrators read from selected works of Shakespeare, Poe, London, Wilder, and others in "Death Themes in Literature" (audiocassette, 20 minutes), and musical selections like "Danse Macabre," Mozart's "Requiem," "Die Erl-Konig" by Schubert, "Taps" and "Deep River" are played in "Death Themes in Music" (audiocassette, 18 minutes). Components of the unit are available separately. Educational Perspectives Associates.

394. **Perspectives on Death (Sunburst).** (HS, A) The first of two filmstrip-cassette programs, "Toward an Acceptance" (12 minutes), discusses such ideas as death is annihilation, death and an afterlife are the promises of religious belief, and death can be "outlived" through work, family or a life lived well. Death is feared, of course, but accepting its inevitability and its naturalness can enhance the quality of life. The second program, "The Right to Die" (11 minutes), explores the definitions of death, active and passive euthanasia, and the concepts "right to die" and "quality of life." Both programs are well organized and attractively presented with color photography and music nicely coordinated with clear narrative. Sunburst Communications, or Human Relations Media Center, teachers guide included, 1976.

395. **Perspectives on Dying.** (A) Six filmstrips and audiocassettes, plus related instructional aids, make up this ambitious program for nursing and adult education. In "American Attitudes toward Death and Dying" (17 minutes), denial as a characteristic of our culture, as a defense mechanism, and as a complicating factor in caregiving is analyzed. "Psychological Reactions of the Dying Person" (30 minutes) investigates the dying individual's personal responses, interpersonal relationships, and complicating factors like the nature and course of the particular illness or injury. "Hazards and Challenges in Providing Care" (28 minutes) discusses both good and bad effects of the caregiver's expectations of and interaction with the dying patient. Especially valuable is a comparison of the effects of pretense and the effects of open sharing in nurse-patient relationships. Other topics discussed are the use of addicting drugs for extreme pain and the withdrawal of extraordinary treatment. "Guidelines for Interacting with the Dying Person" (22 minutes) focuses on three basic patient needs and how the caregiver can meet them: a feeling of personal dignity, a sense of security, and some element of hope. The importance of active listening is stressed. The last two programs, "Viewpoint: The Dying Patient" (31 minutes) and "Viewpoint: The Nurse" (26 minutes), present case studies of the dying and death of two patients that illustrate contrasting sets of feelings and reactions, and the modes of caregiving and related personal difficulties of the nurses involved. These programs are emotional and provocative. Included in this set are an instructor's manual, role-playing cards, personal questionnaire, and a supplementary text, *Confrontations of Death* (Oregon Center for Gerontology). Concept Media, 1973.

396. **The Philosophy of Dying.** (P) See *Physician's Role with the Dying Patient.*

397. **Physical Changes and Their Implications.** (A) See *Perspectives on Aging.*

398. **The Physician and the Dying Patient.** (P) Typical physician attitudes to dying patients, effective communication with them, and dealing with patients' fears are some of the topics explored in this program, structured on a grand-rounds basis. Hahnemann Medical College, black and white videotape, 60 minutes, 1977.

399. **Physician and the Terminally Ill Patient.** (A) Four physicians in a panel discussion make a variety of observations, none in great depth, on dying patients and their needs, physician-patient relationships, truth-telling, improving medical education, and the team approach to caring for the terminally ill. This videotape program may be useful if it is followed by further discussion. Medical Media Network, black and white, 40 minutes, 1968.

400. **Physician's Role with the Dying Patient.** (P) Three programs make up this series aimed at helping practicing physicians improve their work with dying patients. "Children Die Too" offers suggestions on treating dying children and relating effectively with family members. "Maintaining Integrity of the Profession" offers guidelines for physician-patient exchange at various stages in the dying process. "The Philosophy of Dying" discusses legal, social, and emotional factors in the dying situation. University of Arizona, three color videotapes, 50-57 minutes each, 1974.

401. **Picking up the Pieces: One Widow Speaks.** (A) Lynn Caine, author of the best-selling book *Widow*, discusses in an interview the dying and death of her husband, her bereavement, and the painful process of building a new home life and career. Public Television Library, color videotape, 29 minutes, 1975.

402. **Planting Things I Won't See Flower.** (A) Hodgkin's disease took eight years to kill Jill Bresloff. Aside from the devastating physical effects on Jill of the disease and the extensive radiation and chemotherapy, her dying also put tremendous emotional and psychological strains on her, her husband, and their already shaky marriage. This vivid documentation of Jill's dying and its impact can trigger discussion of the personal and familial dynamics of dying; it demonstrates ways by which caregivers can meaningfully intervene in similar situations. United Methodist Film Service, color film or videotape, 26 minutes, 1976.

403. **Please Let Me Die.** (A, P) With over 70 percent of his body burned in a freak accident, a 27-year-old man explains very calmly to his doctor that he wants his treatment stopped and that he simply wants to go home, even if that means he will die. Treatment, however, continues, and we see the devastation of his face and eyes, hands, arms, trunk and legs caused by the burns and subsequent plastic surgery, more of which is to be done. The young man, once active and self-sufficient, is now helpless and in great pain. Are his

rights being violated? Is he competent to decide for himself? Do the doctor and the hospital have the legal and moral right to ignore the patient's requests? This production vividly raises those issues, providing a moving case study for further discussion. University of Texas Medical Branch, color videotape, 30 minutes, 1974.

404. **The Poem as a Personal Statement—To a Very Old Woman.** (HS, A) Using Irving Layton's poem "To a Very Old Woman" as a basis, this short film praises the old woman for her years of strong and courageous survival in a life which had more than its share of hardship. Her acceptance of death as a fitting natural end is another noble characteristic of that life. Learning Corporation of America, color, 10 minutes, 1974.

405. **Poetry of Death.** (HS, A) A number of well-known poetic treatments of death, ranging from Shakespeare to contemporary song lyrics and including such chestnuts as Robert Louis Stevenson's "Requiem" and William Cullen Bryant's "Thanatopsis," are read to the accompaniment of guitar music and evocative photographs. Spectrum Educational Media, two color filmstrips and audiocassettes, with text, 1974.

406. **Point of No Return.** (A) A case of attempted suicide is presented and carefully analyzed. A panel of doctors then makes general observations on suicide prevention. The impact of suicide and suicide attempts on the survivors is also analyzed. International Film Bureau, or Kansas Department of Health and Environment, black and white film, 24 minutes, 1965.

407. **Portrait of Grandpa Doc.** (A) The filmmaker who brought us *Peege* uses the stars of that film (Bruce Davison as the sensitive young man, Barbara Rush as his mother) to create another story of the relationships between the generations. Beginning his career as an artist, Davison paints scenes from his childhood as he looks at old photographs and home movies, and remembers the grandfather he loved. Grandpa Doc's dying came without senility, so its impact on the family was very different than was the gradual deterioration of Peege. Viewfinders, Inc., color film, 28 minutes.

408. **The Potential Suicide.** (A, P) Beginning with a dramatized case history of a man who made a suicide attempt shortly after being released from a hospital, this film shows the nursing staff trying to remember the behavior and conversation of the man while he was a patient to determine if he was considering suicide all the while and should have been helped. Of course there were signs that should have been heeded. The film presents and discusses them, in an effort to teach nurses and other caregivers how to recognize and interrelate with the potential suicide. Medical Media Network, color, 20 minutes, 1970.

409. **Preparing the Doctor and the Nurse to Handle the Inevitable.** (P) This is a videotaped lecture on the topic. University of Arizona, color videotape, 56 minutes, 1974.

410. **The Price of Life** (HS, A) This short film raises basic ethical questions for discussion by presenting three situations. In the first vignette, the "rights" of civilians clash with the deeds of soldiers driven by "military necessity." The second part poses retarded human beings against their cost to society. The third segment portrays a couple considering an abortion. Paulist productions, or Association Films, color film, 12 minutes, 1973.

411. **Primitive People: Australian Aborigines: Part III, the Corroboree.** (A) Funeral beliefs, customs, and rituals of this tribe are colorfully presented. Kent State University, black and white film, 17 minutes.

412. **The Problem of Suicide in General Medical Practice.** (P) This lecture addresses the general practioner on recognizing and dealing with the suicidal patient. Communications in Learning, audiocassette, 36 minutes.

413. **Problem—To Think of Dying.** (A) Lynn Caine, author of *Widow*, and Orville Kelly, founder of the Make Today Count organization, have a wide-ranging personal conversation. They discuss their experiences with dying, death, grief, and learning to live again. Indiana University, color film; or Public Television Library, videotape, 60 minutes, 1975.

414. **The Promise of Death.** (A) Interviews with doctors, social workers, psychologists, pastoral counselors, and dying patients, both children and adults, are carefully edited into an effective introduction and survey of basic death and dying issues. The Thomas More Association, four audiocassettes, 3 hours and 50 minutes.

415. **Psychiatric Conference: The Family Practitioner and the Terminal Patient.** (P) Dr. James L. Mathis lectures on the proper relationships between the physician and dying patient, and on the physician's professional responsibilities. Medical College of South Carolina, color videotape, 55 minutes, 1974.

416. **Psychological Aspects of the Nurse-Family Relationship in Cancer.** (A, P) Nurses can often be of help to their cancer patients by relating effectively with family members under great stress as a result of the prolonged, serious illness of their loved one. Methods are suggested for active listening, clarifying the physician's instructions, and generally helping the family to improve the patient's care. American Cancer Society, black and white film, 22 minutes, 1969.

417. **Psychological Aspects of the Nurse-Patient Relationship in Cancer.** (A, P) The nurse is a key figure in the ongoing care of cancer patients. As such, he or she must be well aware of patients' emotional responses—their fear, depression, and anger—as well as related physical, social or familial, and financial problems. American Cancer Society, black and white film, 22 minutes, 1969.

418. **Psychological Reactions of the Dying Person.** (A) See *Perspectives on Dying.*

419. **Psychopharmacologic Agents in the Care of the Terminally**

Ill and Bereaved. (P) This is a set of nine audiocassettes published by the Foundation of Thanatology. Highly Specialized Promotions.

420. **A Psychosocial Aspect of Terminal Care: Anticipatory Grief.** (A) In this talk recorded at Columbia University in 1970, Dr. Robert Fulton discusses and criticizes contemporary social and medical attitudes toward, and practices in dealing with, dying patients and the chronically ill. The Charles Press, audiocassette, 32 minutes.

421. **Psychosocial Aspects of Death.** (A) The film dramatizes the dying and death of a leukemia patient, and the effects of the situation on the man's wife and a young student nurse first confronting death. Although some insights are offered into the dynamics of the deathbed, several reviewers have noted that poor acting seriously spoils any impact the film might have. Indiana University, black and white, 31 minutes, 1970.

422. **Psycho-Social Aspects of Death.** (A) Dr. Robert Fulton surveys this topic. Allied Memorial Council, color videotape, 30 minutes.

423. **Pulling the Plug—Mercy or Murder.** (HS, A) An examination of ethical and moral issues surrounding extraordinary or "heroic" life-support efforts for the terminally ill (part of a *New York Times*-sponsored series on current affairs). Educational Enrichment Materials, Inc., black and white filmstrip (70 frames), with audiocassette or record, 1977.

424. **A Question of Values.** (A) Down's syndrome is explained and moral issues related to keeping and caring for Down's syndrome and other handicapped infants are raised. Patients (three infants and three children, aged 5-21) and their families are introduced to illustrate commentary on the widely varying physical and psychological traits found in the D.S. population. This presentation tries to counter the film *Who Should Survive?* which presents the case of D.S. infant, unwanted by the parents, who was allowed to die without corrective surgery. See also *Who Speaks for the Baby?* Edward Feil Productions, color film, 28 minutes, 1972.

425. **Rabbit.** (GS, HS, A) A 9-year-old boy finds that taking care of three pet rabbits given as an Easter present is more of a chore than he thought. Finding homes for two of them, he releases the third in the woods and then is filled with sadness and guilt when he discovers it dead. His first encounter with death is complicated by the burden of responsibility. The film is a sensitive, insightful portrait of the child's responses to loss and death. Viewfinders, Inc., or Eccentric Circle Cinema Workshop, color, 15 minutes, 1974.

426. **Reactions of Children to Serious Illness, Death, and Natural Catastrophe.** (P) This is a videotaped lecture to a medical audience by Dr. Howard Hansen. University of Washington Audiovisual Services, 60 minutes.

427. **Ready or Not, Here Comes Immortality.** (A) Jerry Tucille's book, *Here Comes Immortality*, discusses current and projected life-extension techniques. He presents some of his research and his pre-

dictions for the future in this taped interview. Pacifica Tape Library, audiocassette, 36 minutes, 1973.

428. **Redesigning Man: Science and Human Values.** (A) Two programs in this 6-part series on recent and projected developments in the biomedical sciences deal with death-related issues. "Transplants and Implants" (Part III) discusses ethical, legal, and moral problems created by the increasing desire to take body parts from the "dead" in contexts in which "death" is no longer clearly or simply defined. "Search for Immortality" (Part VI) examines the problem of over-population in the face of our developing abilities to prolong life. Harper and Row Media Films, or Human Relations Media Center, six color filmstrips and audiocassettes or records.

429. **Reflections on Death.** (A) In this interview anthropologist Joan Halifax-Grof and psychiatrist Stanislav Grof discuss death attitudes and rituals in a variety of cultures, then explain their research on LSD as useful drug therapy for terminal cancer patients. Carlos Hagen, audiocassette, 58 minutes, 1974.

430. **Reflections on Death and Dying.** (P) Dr. Edwin Shneidman lectures to hospital personnel and surveys, informally, a variety of general practical issues of interest to medical professionals. Delores Ezers, audiocassette, 60 minutes, 1976.

431. **Reincarnation.** (A) The subject is studied in a variety of cultural settings and religious beliefs around the world. Modern Talking Picture Service, color film, 1973.

432. **Reinvestment-Reorganization-Recovery.** (A) The words outline a program of therapeutic action for parents who have lost a child. The Compassionate Friends, audiocassette.

433. **Religious Faith and Death: Implications in Work with the Dying Patient and Family.** (A) Dr. Carl Nighswonger, a pastor, argues that the patient, the family, and all caregivers should openly acknowledge death and express and share their fears and emotions. He feels if that is done, dying and death can be a rich personal and social experience for all concerned. The Charles Press, audiocassette, 32 minutes, 1971.

434. **Religious Viewpoints on Death.** (A) See *Dimensions of Death Series.*

435. **Remembrance and Goodbye.** (A) This very personal experimental film recalls the death of the filmmaker's mother, and explores images of death and dying in general. It may prompt discussion of personal attitudes toward death. Film-Makers Cooperative, color, 9 minutes, 1968.

436. **Rendezvous with Life.** (A, P) The subject is kidney failure, the patient a man who is living a fairly normal life in the face of his chronic terminal illness by means of a home dialysis program. Information about kidney disease in general, dialysis, and related problems and treatment methods is clearly presented. Trainex Corporation, color film, 30 minutes.

437. **Retirement.** (HS, A) Current American habits and attitudes toward retirement, particularly the development of "retirement com-

munities" restricted to the elderly, come in for a measure of debate and criticism in this film. The manager of "Sun City" and Maggie Kuhn, founder of the Gray Panther Movement, are among the commentators. Cinema 5, color film, 50 minutes, 1978.

438. **Rick: An Adolescent Suicide.** (A) A 17-year-old high school senior committed suicide. The film tries to recreate events and to investigate Rick's mental and emotional state before the fact. Medical Media Network, black and white, 29 minutes, 1969.

439. **The Right to Die.** (HS, A) A general survey of issues related to euthanasia. Center for Cassette Studies, audiocassette, 45 minutes, 1977.

440. **The Right to Die (Career Aids).** (A) Now that our technology allows us to extend life (or at least the life processes) almost indefinitely, serious medical, legal, and moral questions arise about the initiation and the termination of such life support. The issues are discussed in this program with reference to several case histories. Career Aids, color filmstrip with audiocassette, discussion guide, 31 minutes.

441. **The Right to Die (CBS-TV).** (HS, A) Originally produced as part of the CBS News Closeup series, this film has the strengths and the faults of a typical network television documentary. A great variety of fascinating cases and people are introduced as the narrator takes up topics like extraordinary medical care in "hopeless" cases, truth-telling, mercy killings, and suicide in the face of an "undignified" terminal illness. Terminally ill patients, including children, report their feelings and their philosophies. Various experts—Dr. Kübler-Ross and other physicians, psychiatrists, clergymen—offer commentary on cases and various related issues. This is all good, fast-moving TV reporting, but no case history or issue is analyzed in any depth. As an introduction, however, the film is fine; available in two reels— one 30 minutes long, the other 26—and can be neatly integrated into at least a couple of discussion sessions. Macmillan Films, or University of Michigan, color, two reels, 56 minutes, 1973.

442. **The Right to Let Die.** (A) Four physicians discuss active and passive euthanasia, extraordinary care, the definition of death, and so on. Joseph P. Kennedy, Jr. Foundation, color film, 28 minutes.

443. **The Right to Live: Who Decides?** (HS, A) A stormy sea, an overcrowded lifeboat, and a captain who must decide who goes overboard are depicted in this segment from the Columbia Pictures feature film, "Abandon Ship" (starring, among others, Tyrone Power). The captain chooses the physically fit, but considering this and similar situations, audiences are forced to examine their own beliefs about who should live and who should die, whether in a lifeboat or in a hospital, on a stormy sea or in the daily life of our society. Learning Corporation of America, color film, 17 minutes, 1972.

444. **The Rights of Age.** (A) Based on the case history of a lonely elderly widow, this film introduces and explains a variety of

social and community services available to the aged. International Film Bureau, or University of Washington, black and white, 25 minutes, 1963.

445. **The Rite of Life and Death.** (HS, A) A young military officer and his wife dramatize the ancient Japanese ritual of hara-kiri. Washington State University, black and white film, 29 minutes.

446. **The Role of the Schools in Death Education.** (A) Schools at all levels should offer death education, argues Dr. Dan Leviton. He offers specific commentary on curricula as well as teacher and parent preparation in the subject matter, which should include crisis intervention. The Charles Press, audiocassette, 27 minutes.

447. **Ronnie's Tune.** (GS, HS) The film is a carefully detailed, realistic portrait of complex family reactions following the death of a teenaged son. Only with painful difficulty is it revealed to a visiting niece, Julie, that her cousin Ronnie's death was a suicide and that Ronnie's father has left his wife as a result. Ronnie's mother makes a great effort and is finally willing to talk freely about her response to the death and to share her grief. After tears, grieving, and much thought of her own, Julie decides to learn to play Ronnie's banjo. Wombat Productions, color, 18 minutes, 1978.

448. **The Rothe Tape.** (A) Dying of cancer despite several major operations to remove tumor growth, 22-year-old Marcus Rothe continues his college education. He makes this film record of his present life and attitudes toward his illness as a legacy for family, friends, and everyone sharing his last days. A minister conducts the interview. Shands Teaching Hospital, color videotape, 30 minutes.

449. **St. Christopher's Hospice: A Living Experience.** (A) Reporter Connie Goldman tours this world-famous London hospice, talking with staff, patients, and their family members as they describe the institution's philosophy and care procedures. The Charles Press, audiocassette, 38 minutes, 1975.

450. **Sallie: 1893–1974.** (A) Because some family members could not come to Oregon for Sallie McGinnis' funeral, the entire service was filmed. It is a "life-centered" service. Next to Sallie's casket are placed the big hats and golf clubs she enjoyed in life. There are eulogies, but joyful songs are sung and tea is served. The film reports thoroughly the positive reactions of family members to Sallie's life, death, and the funeral service. University of Oregon, color, 54 minutes, 1974.

451. **Sandcastle.** (GS, MS) This program for ages 10–12 presents a conversation between a father and his children on the unexpected death of their mother. Image Publications, color filmstrip and audiocassette or record, 1971.

452. **Science and Society: Biomedical Engineering.** (A) A variety of biomedical issues and their legal and ethical ramifications are introduced and explored in this program. Included are definitions of death especially vis-à-vis organ transplants, allocation of scarce medical resources, genetic experimentation, and extraordinary treatment.

Schloat Productions, two color filmstrips and audiocassettes or records.

453. **See No Evil: Portrait of a Late-Life Relationship.** (A) Two elderly people, both widowed and in failing health, try and fail to establish a relationship. This award-winning film can help sensitize medical professionals and counselors to the needs of the elderly and to the harsh realities of growing old in our society. Filmmakers Library, black and white, 15 minutes.

454. **Self-Destruction and Identity.** (A) Dr. Norman L. Farberow, a nationally recognized suicidologist, lectures. Psychology Today Cassettes, or Highly Specialized Promotions, audiocassette.

455. **A Service No One Else Provides.** (HS, A) The program is a neat, well-organized introduction to all the arrangements for the typical funeral provided by the funeral director. National Funeral Directors Association (or state F.D.A. or N.F.D.A. member), audio-cassette and filmstrip, 15 minutes.

456. **The Short Timer: A Cancer Patient with Relapse.** (A, P) The patient is carefully interviewed to try to discover the bases of his intellectual and emotional responses to his relapse. George Washington University, color videotape, 37 minutes, 1976.

457. **A Short Vision.** (HS, A) This fine animated film depicts the graceful, almost birdlike flight of an ICBM whose impact, of course, is catastrophic. The world burns totally, then flickers out like a snuffed candle, and nothing remains. Viewfinders, Inc., color, 7 minutes.

458. **Since the American Way of Death.** (A) The conclusion of this recent WTTW-TV (Chicago) documentary is that little has changed since Jessica Mitford's 1963 exposé of abuses in the funeral industry, *The American Way of Death.* Public Television Library, color videotape, 60 minutes.

459. **A Small Statistic.** (A) This film records the reactions of a young couple to the death of their first child. Association Instructional Materials, color, 27 minutes. (Recent correspondence with the distributor indicates that the film is now "withdrawn from circulation by sponsor.")

460. **Social Reconstruction after Death.** (A) It is hard enough for a survivor to reintegrate his or her life after a death, to make a fresh start, to assume new responsibilities, and to establish new relationships. But it is even more difficult, Dr. Jeannette Folta argues, because our society makes no provision for, and has little desire to assist, the survivor in those tasks. The Charles Press, audiocassette, 21 minutes, 1971.

461. **Sociology of Death.** (A) The Center for Death Education and Research at the University of Minnesota, under the direction of Professor Robert Fulton, created and presented for public television a series of 10 hour-long programs on death and dying in the fall of 1974. Examining the "social and historical developments that have

shaped current American attitudes toward death," the series was very well received. Each program comes with a discussion guide:

1. Death in American Society
2. Death and Denial
3. Death and Denying (The Dying Patient)
4. Grief
5. Death and Social Recuperation
6. Funerals
7. Death and the Child
8. Death and Contemporary Youth
9. Death and the Caregiving Professions
10. Death and Mortality

University of Minnesota, 10 videotapes, 60 minutes each, available as a set or individually, 1974.

462. **Some Day a Future.** (A) This is a film for and about widows. National Funeral Directors Association, color, 30 minutes.

463. **A Song Is a Gentle Thing.** (HS, A) See *Peacebird.*

464. **Soon There Will Be No More Me.** (HS, A) Lyn Helton is a 19-year-old wife and mother who is dying of bone cancer. She agrees to share her reactions to her death and her philosophy of life as a final gift for her daughter. Highly personal and very moving, the film would be most effective in triggering discussion. Churchill Films, or University of Washington, or University of California, Berkeley, or University of Illinois, color, 10 minutes, 1972.

465. **South Beach.** (HS, A) This film focuses on the large community of retirees living in South Miami Beach, old people typical of many in the country, fighting poverty, isolated from their families, often victimized by fear and despair, and now, many of them, angry and increasingly militant in the face of politicians who would tear down their homes to build hotels and condominiums. A fine film: finalist at the 1978 American Film Festival, and a winner at the 1978 San Francisco International Film Festival. Cinema 5, color, 30 minutes, 1978.

466. **Spare Parts for Human Bodies.** (A) A historical survey of transplants is followed by an introduction to current ethical and legal aspects of the issue. There are interviews with heart specialists Drs. Christiaan Barnard and Michael DeBakey, and brief filmed records of transplant surgery. University of Illinois, color film, 15 minutes.

467. **A Special Kind of Care.** (A) This film has two main purposes: to dramatize the effects on a family of a mother slowly dying of cancer, and the related problems of truth-telling; and to highlight the nature and functions of the National Cancer Foundation and its service arm, Cancer Care, Inc. (see Part III, this volume). With the counseling of Cancer Care, the father is finally able to meet the needs of his children and of himself in the crisis situation. Association Films, or American Journal of Nursing, color, 14 minutes, 1968.

468. **The Spirit Possession of Alejandro Mamani.** (A) A lonely 81-year-old widower, the last of his peer group, feels rejected by his children and everyone else. His mental decline is obvious, but he resists suicide—at first. This study of growing old, mental problems, and suicide in the Bolivian Andes provides valuable cross-cultural insights. Filmmakers Library, or University of California, Berkeley, color film, 27 minutes.

469. **Spiritual Needs of the Patient.** (A, P) Nurses are urged to be personally interested in patients, to relate well to patients' clergymen, and to understand how various religious faiths relate to sickness and health, dying and death. Trainex Corporation, color filmstrip and audiocassette or record, 20 minutes, discussion guide, 1969.

470. **Stages of Dying.** (A) Dr. Elisabeth Kübler-Ross presents a variety of insights from her pioneering research with the terminally ill: the "stages" of dying, verbal and nonverbal symbolic language, hope in dying, denial of patient and caregiver, and so on. Many case histories are used to illustrate her points. The Charles Press, audiocassette, 32 minutes, 1971.

471. **The Star Spangled Banner.** (HS, A) While the anthem is being played a soldier on patrol is shot. As he falls we see pictures of his family, friends, and a cross-section of Americans generally. This sensitive combination of song and imagery forces the audience to make connections they might otherwise ignore. Viewfinders, Inc., or Pyramid Films, color film, 5 minutes.

472. **The Stone Whistle.** (HS, A) This industry-sponsored film provides information on the customs and traditions of memorialization in America, and explains the process of making granite memorial stones. Allied Memorial Council, or Barre Granite Association, color, 30 minutes.

473. **Stop for a Moment . . . and Feel the Pain.** (HS, A) Here is an introduction to and survey of suicide and related issues, made for a general television audience. Canadian Broadcasting Corporation, color film, 60 minutes, 1972.

474. **Stopping Treatment with or without Consent.** (A, P) Dr. Joseph Fletcher, an ordained minister on a medical school faculty, makes a 30-minute presentation on the topic of euthanasia, drawing a series of fine distinctions in definition and application. Then follows a stimulating question-and-answer session between Dr. Fletcher and the physician members of the audience. Emory University, color videotape, 60 minutes, 1975.

475. **The Street.** (HS, A) Mordecai Richler's fine little book is turned into a delightfully moving animated film. A grandmother dies slowly in her son's home and the family, especially her grandchildren, reacts to her passing. The urban poor, ethnic Jewish atmosphere is faithfully reproduced. A 9-year-old grandson, loving but totally realistic and irrepressible, provides the main point of view. Living and dying in this family are real, ordinary, serious, and comic. These are individual people beautifully portrayed, experiencing death in

their own ways. National Film Board of Canada, color, 10 minutes.

476. **Sudden Death, Drugs, and Defibrillation.** (P) The program is for emergency personnel, and points out new techniques and procedures in the treatment of sudden death patients. Emory University, color videotape, 58 minutes, 1976.

477. **Sudden Infant Death Syndrome.** (A) A brief introduction to the topic. National Audiovisual Center, color film, 4 minutes, 1976.

478. **Sudden Infant Death Syndrome and the Pediatrician.** (P) Directed at physicians, this program presents guidelines for working with parents of SIDS-prone children, reports on recent research into the syndrome, and surveys parental responses to SIDS deaths. University of Arizona, color videotape, 43 minutes, 1974.

479. **The Suicidal Patient.** (A, P) A panel of four experts in suicidology address medical professionals and police officers. Basic suicide facts surveyed include methods, causes, warning signs, statistics, and a description of the work of suicide clinics. National Medical Audiovisual Center, or University of California, Los Angeles, Medical Center, black and white film, 60 minutes, 1968.

480. **Suicidal Patients.** (P) Varying causal factors in suicide are discussed by a group of doctors. Communications in Learning, audiocassette and seven accompanying slides, 31 minutes.

481. **The Suicidal Person—A Three-part Series.** (A, P) Here is general information about causal factors in suicide, and behavioral clues to watch for. The nurse's role in suicide prevention and intervention is also covered. Communications in Learning, audiocassette, 84 minutes, 10 accompanying slides, printed handouts.

482. **Suicide.** (A) Made originally for a general television audience, this program surveys causal factors, preventive measures, basic statistics, and other information on suicide for a general audience. Interviews with professionals, individuals who have attempted suicide, and relatives of "successful" suicides round out the presentation. Films, Incorporated, color film or videotape, 25 minutes, 1975.

483. **Suicide.** (A) Dr. Philip J. Allen, a sociologist, studies the causes of suicide and some typical circumstances and conditions. He tries to suggest a model of the typical suicidal individual. Jeffrey Norton Publishers, audiocassette, 53 minutes.

484. **Suicide.** (A, P) Causal factors are emphasized in this presentation, which also corrects mistaken notions about the suicidal individual. National Medical Audiovisual Center, or Videorecord Corporation of America, black and white videotape, 60 minutes.

485. **Suicide.** (A, P) Three color films or videotapes cover: prediction of suicide; treatment of suicide; and profiles of suicidal patients. Medi-Tel Communications.

486. **Suicide.** (A, P) This introductory survey is designed to instruct nurses working with suicidal individuals. Trainex Corporation, color filmstrip and audiocassette or record, teacher's guide.

487. **Suicide and Suicide Prevention.** (A, P) This thorough, well-written, and well-delivered series covers many aspects of suicide. Individual titles, available separately, are:

1. Suicide: An Overview
2. Assessment of Suicidal Risk
3. Suicide, Suicide Attempts, and Self-mutilation
4. Family Survivors of Suicide
5. Suicide and the Terminally Ill
6. Suicide in Prison
7. Management of the Suicidal Person
8. Examples and Discussion of Suicide Calls
9. Examples and Discussion of Suicide Calls, Continued
10. Suicide and Violence
11. How to Establish a Suicide Prevention Program
12. Current Issues and Problems in Suicide Prevention

Professionals in all helping fields will find these tapes valuable, as the focus is on the practical rather than the theoretical. The fifth audio-cassette is especially relevant. Behavioral Sciences Tape Library, 12 audiocassettes, 60 minutes each, 1972.

488. **Suicide: But Jack Was a Good Driver.** (HS, A) See *But Jack Was a Good Driver.*

489. **Suicide: Causes and Prevention.** (HS, A) This presentation for a high school audience includes issues and case studies carefully presented to foster discussion. Social Studies School Service, or Human Relations Media Center, two color filmstrips and audio-cassettes or records, teacher's guide, 1976.

490. **The Suicide Clinic: A Cry for Help.** (A) The work of a typical community suicide clinic serving a broad range of clients is described. The film shows how the clinic meets client needs, and some of the factors in the makeup of the suicidal individual which must be recognized and dealt with. Association Instructional Materials, or Indiana University, or University of California, Berkeley, black and white, 28 minutes, 1971.

491. **Suicide: Current Research and Prevention Efforts.** (A, P) Another series of audiocassette presentations like *Suicide and Suicide Prevention,* this more briefly surveys the field in moderate depth, providing a sound introduction for student caregivers. Titles of individual lectures are:

1. The Taxonomy of Suicide
2. Factors Which Predispose to Suicide
3. The Personality of the Suicidal Individual
4. Behavior Prior to Suicide
5. The Suicide Prevention Center
6. The Effectiveness of Suicide Prevention

Behavioral Sciences Tape Library, 3 audiocassettes, 60 minutes each, 1976.

492. **Suicide in the Classroom.** (HS, A) This videotape is available with a study guide by Professor Sandra Bertman. Highly Specialized Promotions, 1978.

493. **Suicide in the Elderly.** (A, P) This brief panel discussion on the subject focuses on behavioral clues and methods of intervention. McMaster University, color videotape, 30 minutes, 1974.

494. **Suicide Intervention.** (P) Here is brief introduction for nurses, using lecture and dramatized cases. American Journal of Nursing, color videotape, 30 minutes, 1975.

495. **Suicide: Practical Diagnostic Clues.** (P) This program is designed for the practicing physician. Network for Continuing Medical Education, black and white videotape, 13 minutes.

496. **Suicide Prevention.** (A, P) This is an introduction to the subject for nurses. Communications in Learning, audiocassette, 67 minutes.

497. **Suicide Prevention and Crisis Intervention.** (A, P) The author of this series, Dr. Allen J. Enelow, produced the film program of the same title. In these audiotapes designed primarily to train suicide clinic workers, several case studies are presented and analyzed. Michigan State University, or Charles Press, 6 audiocassettes, 1973.

498. **Suicide Prevention and Crisis Intervention: A Series of Case Histories.** (A, P) This film program is one of the most extensive audiovisual teaching resources available in the field. The heart of the program is six dramatized interviews with a variety of suicidal individuals. Paired with each case on separate reels are analyses of the content of the interview and of the interviewing and evaluation techniques used. Detailed suggestions for management of the patients, a test film, response sheets, and content checklist are also provided. With an emphasis on the practical, health care workers, social workers, policemen, clergy, teachers, and counselors will find this program, and even separate parts of it, valuable. The Charles Press, or Michigan State University, or Highly Specialized Promotions, 12 black and white films (plus test film), 20-35 minutes each, 1972.

499. **Suicide Prevention in the Hospital.** (A) Suicides do occur in hospitals, of course, and the purpose of Dr. Norman Farberow's presentation is to alert hospital staff—doctors, nurses, chaplains, volunteers, and others—to warning signs. "Successful" suicides should be studied carefully for further guidance. National Audiovisual Center—GSA, black and white film, 20 minutes, 1968.

500. **Suicide Prevention: The Physician's Role.** (A, P) Aimed primarily at physicians, these dramatized case studies illustrate warning signs of suicidal tendencies, and heighten awareness of both verbal and nonverbal communication. Background information on suicide in general is presented, and Dr. Karl Menninger concludes the film by urging doctors to become more aware of the suicide problem and its causes. Critics have suggested that less than professional acting detracts from this otherwise dramatically striking program.

Association—Sterling Films, or Network for Continuing Medical Education, black and white film or videotape, 20 minutes, 1967.

501. **Suicide: The Great Escape.** (P) Directed to health care professionals working with suicidal individuals, this lecture discusses causal factors of suicide in everyday life. Royal College of General Practitioners, reel-to-reel audiotape, 27 minutes, 1969.

502. **Suicide: The Unheard Cry.** (A, P) This film designed to train caregivers covers causes of suicide, behavioral clues, and modes of intervention. The context is military as the film was made by the Department of the Army. National Audiovisual Center—GSA, black and white, 45 minutes, 1969.

503. **Suicides: Causes and Prevention.** (A) Suicide among high school and college students is the focus of these two programs. Causal factors and varying scholarly theories about them are treated in the first program. In the second, the emphasis is on prevention and intervention. Human Relations Media Center, two color filmstrips with audiocassettes or records.

504. **Supportive Nurse-Patient Interactions in Cancer Nursing.** (A, P) American Cancer Society, audiocassette.

505. **Surviving Disaster: Psychological Effects.** (A) Robert Jay Lifton lectures on the subject. Highly Specialized Promotions, audiocassette.

506. **Sykes.** (A) The subject of this portrait is a gutsy, outspoken old fellow who works to supplement his pension as a piano player in a beer garden. He lives in a run-down Chicago Housing Authority apartment and gets little respect from a lot of people, but despite near blindness he is doing fine and expects to live a long time. Sykes can make audiences reexamine their stereotyped thinking about old age. Viewfinders, Inc., color film, 13 minutes, 1974.

507. **The Syndrome of Ordinary Grief.** (A, P) In an interview, a sophomore medical student describes his reactions to the accidental death of his only child, a 2-year-old boy, some weeks earlier. Included is a scholarly paper on this case history. University of Texas Medical Branch, color videotape, 32 minutes.

508. **Talking to Children about Death.** (A) Dr. George G. Williams argues that of course children should be taught about death. They almost automatically adopt parents' attitudes, so parents must straighten themselves out and then share openly with children. Otherwise children may have emotional problems in later life. Concrete suggestions for parents are offered. The Charles Press, audiocassette, 57 minutes, 1972.

509. **A Taste of Blackberries.** See *Understanding Death Series.*

510. **Teaching Death as a Process of Awareness and Coping.** (A, P) This series intends to teach basic lessons of caring for terminally ill patients, with particular emphasis on hospital nurses, and to teach future teachers of death and dying topics. The first program, "The Meanings and Orientations of Death," focuses on a variety of coping mechanisms and explains how to recognize them and how to use

them in patient care. "Terminal Illness as a Process of Awareness and Coping" analyzes Dr. Kübler-Ross's stages of dying by means of dramatized case studies. Finally, "Awareness, Assessment and Appropriateness of Coping Mechanisms" presents teaching methods that illustrate and foster understanding of coping mechanisms. Again, dramatized case studies help the lecturer make her points. Nebraska Television Council for Nursing Education, three black and white videotapes, 30 minutes each, with study manual and patient assessment and coping mechanism evaluation charts, 1973.

511. **Teddy Bear.** (A) The sudden choking death of a 30-year-old woman is graphically and silently portrayed. As she falls, flashbacks to her past are mixed with glimpses into her projected future life. The approach is imaginative and experimental, rather than realistic, and some critics have been left simply confused. The basic intent is to foster discussion by demonstrating the terrible, numbing shock of sudden death. There are not many audiovisual approaches to that subject. Imagesmith, color film, 10 minutes, 1973.

512. **Teen-age Suicide: A National Epidemic.** (A) Joseph Teicher lectures. Psychology Today Cassettes, audiocassette, 1977.

513. **Terminal.** (A) Members of the Open Theatre Ensemble of New York City perform in a frankly experimental production which combines acting, dancing, chanting, and pantomime. The theme is death and a wide variety of related issues, attitudes, and customs. Funeral ritual and hospital treatment of patients, for example, come in for a good measure of satire. Courses approaching death through literature and the other arts, or through philosophy or psychology will find this useful. Foundation of Thanatology, black and white videotape, 30 minutes, 1970.

514. **Terminal Cancer: The Hospice Approach to Pain Control (Part 1).** (A, P) Those familiar with the philosophy and practice of hospice care of the dying know that careful attention is paid to the alleviation of pain, physical as well as emotional and spiritual. This film recommends approaches to the administration of analgesics, and discusses a variety of medications in specific terms. The narrator is Dr. Sylvia Lack, Medical Director of Hospice, Incorporated, of New Haven. Network for Continuing Medical Education, color videotape, 19 minutes, 1977.

515. **Terminal Cancer: The Hospice Approach to the Family (Part 2).** (A, P) The hospice philosophy regards family members of a dying patient as essential members of the caregiving team. Whether the patient is dying at home or in the hospice facility, the staff works closely with the patient's relatives, who are charged with and trained for specific medical and nursing tasks, if they are willing and able. Furthermore, the hospice understands the patient as part of a family unit. Dying causes problems for the family, so the hospice wants to be involved. The patient is "treated" in medical as well as psychological, emotional, and social terms, as part of a family group. Dr. Sylvia Lack, Medical Director of Hospice, Incorporated, of New

Haven, narrates. Network for Continuing Medical Education, color videotape, 19 minutes, 1977.

516. **Terminal Illness: Reactions of a Patient, His Family, Friends and Physicians.** (A, P) This series is one of the most important audiovisual media in the field. It is a detailed, well-made tool for training health professionals, a study of the dying and death of one man, with careful analyses of the effects of these events on significant others. The first program is an "Introduction to the Patient," Dr. Gary Leinbach, a 39-year-old member of the faculty at the University of Washington Medical School. Diagnosed as having inoperable intestinal cancer, Dr. Leinbach and his wife share their emotional, familial, religious, and philosophical reactions to the disease and its prognosis. In "The Role of the Physician," Dr. Leinbach's doctors discuss their medical findings, treatments, and experiments in the case, and their emotional responses to the illness of a friend and colleague. "Pain Management" deals with pain as a continuing problem for the terminally ill. In "Religion and the Clergy" several of the ministers and others who discussed death and dying from various religious perspectives with Dr. Leinbach share their responses after his death, suggesting the values and the limitations of religious counsel for the dying. The last two videotapes called "The Grieving Process" present an in-depth study of the grief work of Dr. Leinbach's wife Arlene, both before the death and afterwards. The complexities of grief are demonstrated, and the responsibilities of caregivers to the surviving family members of their patients are emphasized. University of Washington Press, six color videotapes, 25–45 minutes each, 1972–74.

517. **Terminal Patients: Their Attitudes and Yours.** (P) Designed for health care professionals, this short film urges caregivers to examine their attitudes about working with the terminally ill. Filmed interviews with patients suggest that caregiver attitudes play an important role in the condition of the patient. Abbott Laboratories, color, 16 minutes.

518. **That Undiscovered Country.** (HS) The country "from whose bourn no traveler returns," as Hamlet tells us, is death. The audiocassette portion of this program presents readings of seven popular poetic interpretations of death, with musical background. An accompanying booklet contains these texts and other classic literary statements on death and dying. A detailed teacher's guide with many suggestions for use is included. Perfection Form Company, audiocassette, reader, teacher's guide.

519. **Themes in Literature: Death.** (HS, A) Professional readings from many authors—Chaucer, Shakespeare, Donne, Boswell, Gray, Wordsworth, Browning, Tolstoy, Dickinson, Synge, Millay, Gunther, Steinbeck, Agee, Stoppard—demonstrate a multiplicity of attitudes to human mortality. Guidance Associates, two color filmstrips and audiocassettes or records.

520. **Therapeutic Communication—A Series.** (P) This set of 8 filmstrip-audiocassette programs is designed to introduce nurses to the feelings and fears of dying patients so that more effective, more human professional-patient relationships can be established. J. B. Lippincott Company, 1976.

521. **They Need Not Die.** (A, P) This film illustrates emergency room treatment of critical cases, with emphasis on recent techniques in dealing with trauma. Creative Learning Center, color, 24 minutes.

522. **Things in Their Season.** (HS, A) Members of the Gerlach family, working a dairy farm in southern Wisconsin, were growing apart until the day that wife Peg was diagnosed as having leukemia. In the face of this tragedy the family forced itself back together, facing truth, finally speaking the unspoken, reevaluating their relationships, and eventually finding a measure of happiness. This is a fine film portrayal of the dynamics of death in the family situation. Learning Corporation of America, color, 79 minutes, 1975.

523. **Those Who Mourn.** (HS, A) Through carefully edited and juxtaposed flashbacks, the film presents a young woman, suddenly widowed, remembering her life with her husband, their baby, their courtship, the funeral, the coffin, and his saying long ago, in a lighthearted context, "You've got to lose sometime." Images of panic and despair are mingled with images of hope and renewed life in this effective stimulus for discussion. Teleketics, or Association-Sterling Films, color, 5 minutes, 1973.

524. **Though I Walk Through the Valley.** (HS, A) The title from Psalm 23 suggests the strong religious emphasis of this biography. Tony Brower, a 50-year-old college professor, has had stomach cancer for five years. The film begins at the end of Tony's last remission. As his condition worsens and he prepares for death, his strong faith sustains him and provides some comfort for his wife and daughters, who do not totally share his convictions. Though mainly about one man's dying, this is also a nice study in the family dynamics of death. Church Film Service, or Pyramid Films, or Gospel Films, or University of California, Berkeley, color, 28 minutes, 1972.

525. **The Threat of Suicide.** (P) Produced for an audience of nurses and doctors, this program discusses the warning signs of suicidal intent in patients, explains verbal and nonverbal clues, and suggests methods of intervention. Network for Continuing Medical Education, color videotape, 27 minutes.

526. **Threshold, H.S.** (A) This award-winning film suggests the possibilities of how much can happen in that split-second interval between life and death. As a young man is fatally shot, he relives his life and manages to project himself forward into a love relationship he never actually got to enjoy. University of Minnesota, color, 25 minutes, 1970.

527. **Through Death to Life.** (HS, A) Produced by Bauman Bible Telecasts, Inc., this series presents a detailed and comprehensive

treatment of the whole field of death and dying from the viewpoint of New Testament theology. Titles of separate programs are, for example, "The Denial of Death," "A Good Death," and "Life After Death." Accompanying the series is a 124-page study guide. One may also write for a free descriptive brochure. Bauman Bible Telecasts, Inc., 13 color films, 1977.

528. **Till Death Do Us Part.** (A, P) Five terminally ill cancer patients are interviewed by a psychotherapist to probe their emotional and psychological responses to their illness and treatment. Walter Reed Army Medical Center, videotape, 35 minutes, 1975.

529. **Till Death Do Us Part (Littman).** (A) A number of widows share their emotional reactions to the death of their husbands, and describe how they rebuilt their lives. Lynne Littman, color film, 30 minutes, 1977.

530. **A Time Out of War.** (HS, A) Calling a temporary truce, soldiers on opposite sides of a small stream that forms their battle line during the Civil War share conversation, tobacco, and the balmy, sunny day. Then a Union soldier who is fishing snags the body of a dead comrade. The Confederate soldier stands silently at attention during the burial, and both sides together fire the honorary volley of shots. The film is well made, the acting superb; and the story can trigger discussion on a variety of death and dying topics. Pyramid Films, black and white, 22 minutes.

531. **A Time to Mourn, A Time to Choose.** (A, P) See *Death and Dying: Closing the Circle.*

532. **To A Good Long Life.** (HS, A) Old age does not have to mean the weakening of intellectual or physical powers, or the withering of social contacts. One 67-year-old man still runs 17 miles a day and works as a hod carrier. An elderly lady who continues to teach painting points out one among many basic advantages to being old: one no longer needs to be driven by ambition. This film is effective in breaking down stereotyped thinking. Kent State University, color, 20 minutes.

533. **To Be Aware of Death.** (HS, A) This film surveys a number of young people on their feelings about death and their experiences with it. The commentary is made more attractive by means of accompanying color photography, still pictures, and folk music. University of Minnesota, or Billy Budd Films, color, 13 minutes, 1974.

534. **To Be Continued.** (HS, A) Here is a study of "little deaths," a topic not often treated in educational films. Life is filled with a constant series of losses, disappointments, and setbacks which may be helpful in teaching that we can begin anew, with fresh starts and second chances, even after a major loss. Indiana University, or University of Minnesota, color film, 14 minutes, 1976.

535. **To Be Growing Older.** (HS, A) In this thought-provoking film, the views of elderly people on the subject of their growing old, and their reports of experiences with the problems of aging, are nicely juxtaposed with opinions about growing and being old expressed by young people. Billy Budd Films, color, 13 minutes.

536. **To Die, to Live.** (A) The destruction of Hiroshima by the first atomic bomb detonated in wartime is the subject of this documentary film, produced by BBC-TV with Robert Jay Lifton as consultant. Emphasis is placed on those who survived the attack, and on the significance for humanity of its ability to destroy itself. Time-Life Films, color, 65 minutes, 1975.

537. **To Die Today.** (A) In the first section of this film Dr. Elisabeth Kübler-Ross lectures on her five-stage model of the dying process, and on difficulties with accepting dying and death that are widespread in our society. Occasionally while she speaks the camera records relevant scenes in busy hospital wards. Next, Dr. Kübler-Ross interviews a young man dying of Hodgkin's disease, and discusses his case—and his apparent acceptance of death—with a group of interns. This film, by now well known in the field, is essential Kübler-Ross. The patient interview and discussion section are available separately. Filmmakers Library, or University of California, or University of Michigan, or Ross Medical Associates, black and white film or videotape, 50 minutes, 1972.

538. **To Expect to Die: A Film about Living.** (A) Robert Hardgrove, a San Francisco journalist, is dying of cancer. Recorded here are his reactions to his disease, the prognosis, the treatments, temporary remissions and relapses. Of special interest are the efforts of friends and family members to cope with the prospect of Hardgrove's death. One conflict presented in some detail concerns one of Hardgrove's sons who, with his Christian fundamentalist religious beliefs, cannot accept his father's more liberal Unitarian views. Hardgrove's viewpoint is emphasized, however: his human life as he has lived it, and as he is dying out of it, is in itself important and valuable. Public Television Library, color videotape, 59 minutes, 1977.

539. **To Live until You Die: Two Aspects of Old Age.** (A) The life-style of an old Swedish lady, living alone in a one-room apartment, changes, but not necessarily for the better, when she moves into a government institution. As a contrast, a family in southern Italy demonstrates the traditional attitude towards the aged as elderly members of families retain their positions of respect in community and home. Kent State University, black and white film, 54 minutes, 1965.

540. **To Take a Hand.** (A, P) Nurse Carla cannot adjust to working comfortably with dying patients. Is it denial, fear, a faulty definition of professionalism or an unwillingness to care, to get involved? She comes to learn the necessity of allowing her emotions to happen, and then to use them meaningfully. There is good acting here, and a vivid climactic scene. American Cancer Society, color film, 22 minutes, 1971.

541. **To Think of Dying.** (A) See *Problem: To Think of Dying.*

542. **Today's Funeral Director: His Responsibilities and Challenges.** (A) The funeral service is an important element in the grief work of a family after the loss of a member. By providing an opportunity for family and community interaction, and through follow-up

contacts, the funeral director fosters survivor adjustment. Glenn Griffin, a funeral director, narrates. The Charles Press, audiocassette, 25 minutes, 1971.

543. **Tomorrow Again.** (A) This is a film to trigger discussion of old age and, in particular, the loneliness so often a major problem for the elderly. A resident of a retirement hotel, Grace looks forward every day to the attention she will receive when she enters the lobby wearing a favorite fur stole. The reality, of course, is that the old people there are lost in their own fantasies and loneliness, and they continue to stare into the television set or off into space while Grace has to turn away, still alone. Perhaps she'll come into the lobby again tomorrow. Viewfinders, Inc., or Pyramid Films, black and white, 16 minutes.

544. **Too Personal to Be Private.** (HS, A) Here are the reactions of a family to the death of a member, and an explanation of the importance of the funeral in helping meet their needs. National Funeral Directors Association, color film, 29 minutes.

545. **Tulip Garden.** (A) His wife always wanted to be buried in her tulip garden, so the elderly farmer arranges to do just that, in spite of his children and friends who insist on having the local funeral director and all the trappings. Canadian Broadcasting Corporation, audiocassette, 30 minutes.

546. **Two Daughters.** (A) In this evocative Swedish film, a mother mourns the death of her young daughter and remembers her own mother's death. This is a fine study of relationships and of generations, and an effective stimulus to discussion. University of California, Berkeley, color, 22 minutes, 1976.

547. **Two Worlds to Remember.** (A) This documentary film follows the progress of two elderly women as they close their apartment and move into a nursing home. Their reactions and problems in adjusting, as well as the help they receive and do not receive from professional staff, other residents of the home, and relatives, are recorded. Conditions of life in the home are graphically portrayed. Film Play/Data Bureau, color, 37 minutes, 1970.

548. **Uncle Monty's Gone.** (GS) Fat Albert and the Cosby Kids react to the death of someone close. Undine's Uncle Monty, a long-time entertainer, agrees to help the kids stage a fund-raising show. When he dies suddenly, Undine is crushed and angrily withdraws from her friends. Then her mother tells her more about Uncle Monty and his zest for life, and how he would have wanted them all to live with enthusiasm and joy. The show must go on, and with Undine and her friends back together, it does. University of Illinois, color film, 16 minutes, 1976.

549. **Understanding Changes in the Family: Playing Dead.** (GS, HS) This one of a series of filmstrip programs asks an audience of children to role-play. In the process, someone recalls the death of a grandfather and discussion takes up the idea. Guidance Associates, color filmstrip and audiocassette or record, 5 minutes.

550. **Understanding Death: A Basic Program in Death and Dying.** (MS, HS) Six filmstrips and three accompanying audiocassettes make up this introductory series on the subject for the schools. "Thinking About Death" gives general background and encourages students to examine their own experiences with and attitudes toward death. "Mourning," the second filmstrip, discusses grief as a normal human emotion, and one not exclusively associated with death. "Practical Guidelines," the next program, explains death certificates, wills, organ bequests, and so on. "Death's Moment and the Time that Follows" explains why "death" is so difficult to define in precise medical and legal terms, and that scientific advances constantly force changes in society's conception of death and of life. The fifth program, "Dying Occurs in Stages," builds on the theories of Dr. Kübler-Ross. Finally, "The Gift of Life" examines various types of "symbolic immortality" and argues that a well-spent life can rob death of some of its sting. Eye Gate Media, 6 color filmstrips (about 50 frames each) and 3 audiocassettes, available as a set or singly, 1976.

551. **Understanding Death Series.** (MS) Included in this series are four programs especially designed for middle school students, and an accompanying program for parents and teachers. In "Life-Death," death is presented as a natural part of the life cycle; natural, too, are feelings of grief. Causes of death and a number of other topics are covered. In both "Exploring the Cemetery" and "Facts About Funerals" a boy pays visits and gets background information from, respectively, a cemeterian and a funeral director. The fourth program, "A Taste of Blackberries," is adapted from a book by Doris Buchanan Smith. A boy loses his best friend, then works through his grief to an awareness of death as a natural part of the human experience. Finally, "Children and Death: A Guide for Parents and Teachers" offers advice on truth telling, death education, the changing stages and levels of children's understandings of death, and other matters. Educational Perspectives Associates, five color filmstrips and audiocassettes, also available separately.

552. **The Universal Flame.** (A) This introduction to the basic concepts of the religion called theosophy emphasizes its beliefs in reincarnation, karma, and the oneness of all human experience. Theosophical Society in America, color film, 29 minutes.

553. **University of California, Davis: A Series of Interviews With Mrs. Cieri.** (A, P) Mrs. Cieri is a middle-aged woman dying of cancer. In conversations videotaped over a period of time she shares her changing feelings about her disease and its prognosis, notes effective support she is receiving from her religious beliefs and friends, and reports on the effect her imminent death is having on her husband and other members of her family. She also comments on good and bad characteristics of the hospital care she is receiving. University of California, Davis, black and white videotape, 60 minutes, 1972.

554. **University of Southern California: A Series of Interviews with Terminal Patients.** (A, P) Each of the four interviews in the

series is named after the patient studied: "Bella" (50 minutes), "Mark" (25 minutes), "Mr. S." (60 minutes), and "Rocco" (60 minutes). Each patient reacts differently to his or her condition, and offers different insights into the process of dying. Bella, an essentially strong and courageous older woman dying of cancer, makes a number of important criticisms of her treatment as a patient and as an old person. Marc, an adolescent cancer victim, speaks articulately about his decidedly negative attitude toward hospitals in general and the treatment given him in particular. His anxieties offer important insights into the mind of the dying adolescent. Mr. S. aged 61, has been treated in various hospitals by several doctors, and none of them has built a decent personal relationship with him. His complaints should lead caregiving professionals to examine their consciences. Rocco is a young man who initially presents himself as cheerful and optimistic about his future, but in further discussion he reveals his fear about his bone cancer and its poor prognosis. University of Southern California School of Medicine, four black and white videotapes.

555. **Until I Die.** (A) Dr. Kübler-Ross opens this film by discussing her 5-stage model of the dying process and by offering general comments on the nature and effects of the tendency—among caregivers and lay people alike—to deny and avoid death. She then discusses problems encountered with dying children, and conducts interviews with two terminally ill patients. Like the film *To Die Today*, this is vintage Kübler-Ross, but here she makes the essential points in considerably less time. Ross Medical Associates, or American Cancer Society, or Association-Sterling Films, or University of Wisconsin, or University of Iowa Audiovisual Center, color film or videotape, 30 minutes, 1970. The sound track is also available on audiocassette from the American Journal of Nursing, Educational Services Division.

556. **The Upturned Face.** (HS, A) Stephen Crane's short story is transformed into a fine film. A young officer is killed in a war. His men have the painfully unpleasant task of going through his pockets, tugging him to a shallow grave, and filling it in. But the hardest task of all is shoveling the dirt onto the man's upturned face. Pyramid Films, or Viewfinders, Inc., color, 10 minutes, 1972.

557. **Very Good Friends.** (MS, HS, A) When her 11-year-old sister dies suddenly, a 13-year-old is tortured by grief, anger, and guilt. Her parents help her work through her feelings, accept the loss, and rest more comfortably with her memories. This fine study of a death in the family can stimulate discussion. Learning Corporation of America, color film, 20 minutes, 1977.

558. **Vestige or Value.** (HS, A) Two spokesmen for the funeral industry and two clergymen discuss death and dying, and the roles played by the two professions. Washington State Funeral Directors Association, or Allied Memorial Council, color film, 30 minutes.

559. **Viewpoint: The Dying Patient.** (A) See *Perspectives on Dying.*

560. **Viewpoint: The Nurse.** (A) See *Perspectives on Dying.*

561. **Walk in the World for Me.** (A, P) See *Death and Dying: Closing the Circle.*

562. **A Walk Up the Hill.** (A) At age 77 Dr. Allen Wakefield, about to retire from his medical practice to a small dairy farm, suffers two debilitating strokes leaving him totally paralyzed and unable to speak. After the first, less serious stroke Dr. Wakefield expressed his opposition to the use of extraordinary medical measures should his condition worsen. But when the time comes, the attending doctors and his wife and son all find it hard to act. The atmosphere of the dramatization, and of responses to the crucial questions, is obviously Christian. In the case of Dr. Wakefield the film does not offer a definitive answer, but it can spark further discussion. Gospel Films, or Church Films, or Family Films, color, 30 minutes, 1973.

563. **Warrendale.** (A) This documentary film is mainly the study of an institution for emotionally disturbed children, but its conclusion is of particular interest to death educators. One of the cooks at the institution, a favorite of the children, dies suddenly and unexpectedly. The children's grief reactions are astounding, from angry self-destructive activities to severe depression. Here are many aspects of grief which, in "normal" people, often do not surface, or which appear in more "acceptable" guises. Grove Press, or University of California, Berkeley, 105 minutes.

564. **Weekend.** (A) This short symbolic film was designed to discuss today's nuclear family faced with the problem of what to do with its aging members who are growing senile. Mass Media Associates, color, 10 minutes, 1973.

565. **What Can I Say?** (P) The question in the title is that posed by nurses when working with a seriously ill patient who asks about his or her condition. This film first dramatizes a nurse-patient encounter, then a training session at which that patient and others are discussed. Many aspects of truth telling and counseling are discussed, though specific answers to questions are not fully satisfying. Critics have noted also the comparatively weak acting, but the film would be valuable for heightening awareness and fostering discussion. American Journal of Nursing Company, or Association-Sterling Films, black and white, 31 minutes, 1968.

566. **What Is Death?** (A) Dr. John Theobald considers the fear of death, but reminds us that from a religious point of view death and life are both elements of a unified essence, God. Center for Cassette Studies, audiocassette, 30 minutes.

567. **What Man Shall Live and Not See Death?** (HS, A) Produced for a general television audience, this program has won prizes for documentary reporting but has also been described as a disjointed potpourri of death facts and issues. There are well over a dozen different topics and personalities presented, including Dr. Kübler-Ross, cryonics, St. Christopher's Hospice, a funeral director, grieving, and the ethics of extraordinary care. No single topic is explored in

any depth, but the film could still be valuable as an exciting introductory survey. NBC Educational Enterprises, or Films, Incorporated,
or University of California, Berkeley, or University of Illinois, color
film (two reels), 57 minutes, 1971.

568. **When Parents Grow Old.** (A) Here are selected scenes from
I Never Sang for My Father (q.v.). Learning Corporation of America,
color film, 15 minutes.

569. **When You See Arcturus.** (HS, A) An architect, bored with
his life, considers suicide. His son and daughter try to reason with
him, but to no avail. Only when the son is senselessly murdered does
the architect reconsider the value of his life and of life in general.
Paulist Productions, or Association Films, color film, 27 minutes,
1974.

570. **Where Is Dead?** (A) A 6-year-old girl, grieving at the accidental death of her brother, comes to understand death as part of the
cycle of life, and can then be happy with her memories of her
brother. The film is a fine study in the dynamics of grief, especially
in the child. While the reactions of the adult family members are not
emphasized, the adult-child relationships surrounding the death are
healthy. The acting and the whole production are first-rate. Encyclopaedia Britannica Educational Corporation, color, 19 minutes,
1975.

571. **Who Should Survive?** (A) The film opens with the birth of
a baby, a diagnosis of Down's syndrome, the parents' refusal to
permit life-saving abdominal surgery, and the subsequent starvation
of the infant in the hospital. A 19-minute panel discussion then
argues various legal, ethical, and scientific aspects of the case. A
teacher's guide and bibliography are available. Medal of Greatness,
or Joseph Kennedy Foundation Film Service, or University of California, Berkeley, color, 26 minutes, 1972.

572. **Who Speaks for the Baby?** (A) The case of a newborn
mongoloid infant who will die without corrective surgery is dramatized here. When the parents refuse their consent, the physician seeks
a court order to operate. In a panel discussion, professionals offer
their responses to the question of the title. See also *A Question of
Values* and *Who should Survive?* Network for Continuing Medical
Education, color videotape.

573. **Whose Life Is It Anyway?** (A) In an accident sculptor Ken
Harrison suffers a severed spinal cord. Concluding that his life is not
worth living, he demands to be released from the hospital and its
life-sustaining machinery. Has he the right to go home and die? May
his doctor and the hospital keep him imprisoned, as it were, for life?
Fine acting raises these and related issues in vivid fashion. Concern
for Dying, or Spectrum Motion Picture Laboratory, or University of
California, Berkeley, color film, 56 minutes, 1975.

574. **Widowhood.** (A) This panel discussion is led by author-
counselor Robert Buchanan, and includes a widow and a widower.

Reactions of those losing a spouse are shared, problems are recounted, and advice for outsiders trying to understand and help is suggested. Allied Memorial Council, color videotape, 30 minutes.

575. **The Widow-to-Widow Program.** (A) Dr. Phyllis Silverman founded this self-help organization for widows in the Boston area. In this presentation she provides background information on the history, philosophy, operation, and success of the group. The Charles Press, audiocassette, 35 minutes.

576. **Widows.** (A) Several widows discuss the effects on their lives of their husbands' deaths. They describe their emotional reactions and the often misguided responses of family, friends and professionals. Emphasis is also placed on what especially helped them, and information is provided about organizations for the widowed. Documentaries for Learning, or University of California, Berkeley, black and white film, 41 minutes, 1972.

577. **The Wild Goose.** (HS, A) The title character is an old gentleman who contrives an escape from a nursing home where he is badly treated. Not physically capable of being a "walkaway," he motorizes his wheel chair and rolls down the highway. The situation is funny enough, but the central problem—the cruel treatment afforded many old people in nursing homes—is made painfully obvious. Viewfinders, Inc., black and white film, 19 minutes.

578. **Wilf.** (HS, A) The hero is a solitary old farmer who is happy enough to be left alone on his land, living as he always has. Commercial interests, however, covet and finally get the land. The film ends with the problems Wilf has adjusting to an unfamiliar new life in the city. National Film Board of Canada, color, 21 minutes, 1970.

579. **Will Drafting.** (A) As he drafts two wills, providing for the desires of two very different clients, an attorney explains almost everything we have ever wanted to know about wills. University of California, Berkeley, black and white film, 40 minutes.

580. **The Will to Die (Parts I and II).** (A) In the first program, four nationally recognized authorities on suicide—Doctors Norman Farberow, Joseph Hirsh, Manuel Pardo, and Edwin Shneidman—present a general survey of suicide in America with special emphasis on "cries for help" and the proper attitudes and responses of caregivers. In the second program, a suicidal middle-aged woman describes her several suicide attempts and, in an interview with Dr. Hirsh, reveals her motives for her continuing desire to die. Dr. Hirsh then generalizes from this case study. Washington State University, or Association Instructional Materials, or Association—Sterling Films, two color films, 28 minutes each, 1972.

581. **With His Playclothes On.** (A, P) At 21 months Jerry dies suddenly of causes that, even after autopsy, are not completely understood. The immediate emotional responses of the parents and three older brothers are vividly presented. Two months after the death the family is still torn by unresolved shock, anger, and conflict, as the family members react on different levels and from incom-

pletely shared points of view. This study of grief in the family, one of the best available on the subject, includes extensive analytical commentary by Dr. Glen Davidson, Professor and Chief of Thanatology, Department of Psychiatry, Southern Illinois University School of Medicine. OGR Service Corporation, color filmstrip and audiocassette, 47 minutes, 1976.

582. **Writing a Will (Parts I and II).** (A) These two audiocassette programs offer a total of 52 minutes of expert instruction on the subject of wills: why, when, and how to draw up legally valid and acceptable wills. Center for Cassette Studies.

583. **You Are Not Alone.** (A) Sudden infant death syndrome is the topic of this program. Parents who have lost children to the disease, caregivers, and general audiences are reminded that causes of the syndrome are largely unknown, and that little can be done to prevent an attack. Specific advice is offered on dealing with emotional and other responses of parents, siblings, relatives, and friends. The cases of several couples are dramatized. Bureau of Community Health Services (HEW), or National Audiovisual Center—GSA, or National SIDS Foundation, or National Funeral Directors Association, color film, 25 minutes, 1976.

584. **You Have Six Months to Live.** (A) This audiocassette presentation studies the reactions of several individuals who have been told their lives are soon to end. It explores how, in the face of death, value orientations change or shift, how one's past life is summarized and evaluated, and how some people choose to spend the time that is left. Center for Cassette Studies, 26 minutes.

585. **You See—I've Had a Life.** (HS, A) At 13 Paul Hendricks is diagnosed as having leukemia. After some initial attempts at denial, the parents decide to tell Paul. The whole family shares the experience with him, working to enhance the quality of his life in the time remaining. The film records Paul's continuing school and athletic activities, treatments by medical staff, the caregiving activities, and the personal reactions of the parents and of Paul himself. This is a moving, well-made story of one family's togetherness in the face of death and of one child's courage. The words of the title, which accurately suggest the essence of his character and the quality of his response to death, are spoken by Paul to reassure a friend who came to offer sympathy. Viewfinders, Inc., or Eccentric Circle Cinema Workshop, or University of California, Berkeley, black and white, 32 minutes, 1973.

586. **The Young Man and Death.** (HS, A) Unique among audiovisual materials on death is this ballet danced to music of J. S. Bach by Rudolph Nureyev and Zizi Jeanmaire. The ballerina in the role of Death acts alternately as destroyer and as temptress. The Young Man, first fleeing then falling victim to her blandishments, gives himself up to her. Having won her victory, she scornfully turns away from him and offers him a noose. This film would be very effective

in classes studying death in the arts, or as a stimulus to discussion. Macmillan Films, color, 16 minutes, 1976.

587. **The Youth Killers.** (MS, HS) Leading causes of death in this age group are discussed in this program. A teacher's guide is included. Audiovisual Narrative Arts, two color filmstrips and audiocassettes or records, 1975.

588. **Yudie.** (HS, A) Yudie is a fascinating individual. Though she is well over 70 and though her life has been no bed of roses, she continues to be active in her community, on the job, and in her mind and spirit. This is a prize-winning film about a beautiful woman who is growing old in style. University of Michigan, black and white, 20 minutes.

Distributors

Abbott Laboratories
Professional Relations
Abbott Park
North Chicago, IL 60064

ABC News
7 W. 66th St.
New York, NY 10023

Academy of Health Sciences,
    U.S. Army
Attn: HSA-ZMD
Fort Sam Houston, TX 78234

ACI Films
(*see* Paramount Communications)

Alfred Shands Productions
334 E. Broadway, Suite 327
Louisville, KY 40202

Allied Memorial Council
P.O. Box 30112
Seattle, WA 98103

American Cancer Society
777 Third Ave.
New York, NY 10017

American College of Cardiology
9650 Rockville Pike
Bethesda, MD 20014

American Film Institute
John F. Kennedy Center for
    the Performing Arts
Washington, DC 20566

American Journal of Nursing
Educational Services Division
10 Columbus Circle
New York, NY 10019

American Journal of Nursing Company
267 W. 25th St.
New York, NY 10001

American Medical Association
535 N. Dearborn St.
Chicago, IL 60610

Association Films, Inc.
866 Third Avenue
New York, NY 10022

Association-Sterling Films
600 Gran.' Avenue
Ridgefield, NJ 07657

Association Instructional Materials
866 Third Avenue
New York, NY 10022

Audio Visual Medical Marketing, Inc.
850 Third Ave.
New York, NY 10022

Audiovisual Narrative Arts
Box 398
Pleasantville, NY 10570

Bailey Film Associates
(*see* BFA Educational Media)

Barr Films
P.O. Box 5667
3490 E. Foothill Blvd.
Pasadena, CA 91107

Barre Granite Association
51 Church St.
Barre, VT 05641

Bauman Bible Telecasts
3436 Lee Highway #200
Arlington, VA 22207

Behavioral Sciences Tape Library
485 Main St.
Fort Lee, NJ 07024

BFA Educational Media
Division of Columbia Broadcasting
   System, Inc.
2211 Michigan Ave.
Santa Monica, CA 90404

Billy Budd Films
235 E. 57th St.
New York, NY 10022

Brigham Young University
DMDP Media Business Services
W164 Stadium
Provo, UT 84602

Bureau of Community Health
   Services (HEW)
Program Services Branch
Parklawn Building
Room 7A-20
5600 Fishers Lane
Rockville, MD 20852

Canadian Broadcasting Corporation
Learning Systems
Box 500, Terminal A
Toronto, Ontario, Canada

Career Aids, Inc.
5024 Lankershim Boulevard
North Hollywood, CA 91601

Carlos Hagen
Box 342
Malibu, CA 90265

Carousel Films, Inc.
1501 Broadway
New York, NY 10036

Case Western Reserve University
Health Sciences Communications Ctr
2119 Abington Road
Cleveland, OH 44106

Center for Cassette Studies
8110 Webb Avenue
North Hollywood, CA 91605

The Center for the Humanities, Inc.
2 Holland Avenue
White Plains, NY 10603

Center for Mass Communications
Columbia University Press
440 W. 110 St.
New York, NY 10025

Centron Educational Films
P.O. Box 687
1621 W. Ninth St.
Lawrence, KA 66044

The Charles Press Publishers, Inc.
A Division of the Robert J. Brady Co.
Bowie, MD 20715

Children's Memorial Hospital
707 Fullerton Ave.
Chicago, IL 60614

Church Film Service
North 2923 Monroe St.
Spokane, WA 99205

Churchill Films
662 N. Robertson Blvd.
Los Angeles, CA 90069

Cinema 5
595 Madison Ave.
New York, NY 10022

Communication Research Machines
Del Mar, CA 90214

Communications in Learning, Inc.
2280 Main St.
Buffalo, NY 14214

The Compassionate Friends
1049 High Court
Carmel, IN 46032

Concept Media
1500 Adams Ave.
Costa Mesa, CA 92626

Concern for Dying
250 W. 57th St.
New York, NY 10019

Coronet Instructional Films
The Coronet Building
65 East South Water St.
Chicago, IL 60601

Creative Christian Communications
1855 South Shore Boulevard
Lake Oswego, OR 97304

Creative Learning Center
105 Edgevale Road
Baltimore, MD 21210

Creative Resources
Division of Word, Inc.
Box 1970
Waco, TX 76701

Current Affairs Films
24 Danbury Road
Wilton, CT 06897

Dana Productions
6249 Babcock Ave.
North Hollywood, CA 91606

Delores Ezers
P. O. Box 1048
La Jolla, CA 92038

Document Associates, Inc.
211 E. 43rd St.
New York, NY 10017

Documentaries for Learning
Harvard Mental Health Film Program
58 Fenwood Road
Boston, MA 02115

Documentary Photo Aids
P. O. Box 2237
Phoenix, AR 85002

Doubleday Multimedia
P. O. Box 11607
1371 Reynolds Ave.
Irvine, CA 92713

Eccentric Circle Cinema Workshop
P.O. Box 4085
Greenwich, CT 06830

Educational Enrichment Materials, Inc.
110 So. Bedford Road
Mt. Kisco, NY 10549

Educational Film Library Association
43 West 61st St.
New York, NY 10023

Educational Perspectives Associates
P. O. Box 213
Dekalb, IL 60115

Educational Record Sales
157 Chambers St.
New York, NY 10007

Edward Feil Productions
4614 Prospect Ave.
Cleveland, OH 44103

Emory University School of Medicine
A. W. Calhoun Medical Library
Woodruff Memorial Building
Emory University
Atlanta, GA 30322

Encyclopedia Britannica
    Educational Corporation
425 N. Michigan Ave.
Chicago, IL 60611

ETL Video Publishers, Inc.
1170 Commonwealth Ave.
Boston, MA 02134

Eye Gate Media
146–01 Archer Ave.
Jamaica, NY 11435

Family Films, Incorporated
5823 Santa Monica Blvd.
Hollywood, CA 90038

Film Communicators
11136 Weddington St.
North Hollywood, CA 91601

Film-Makers Cooperative
175 Lexington Ave.
New York, NY 10016

Filmmakers Library
290 West End Ave.
New York, NY 10023

Film Play/Data Bureau, Inc.
267 West 25th St.
New York, NY 10001

Films, Incorporated
1144 Wilmette Ave.
Wilmette, IL 60091

Foundation of Thanatology
630 W. 168th St.
New York, NY 10032

George Washington University
Medical Center
Audiovisual Services
2300 Eye St., N.W.
Washington, DC 20037

Georgia Regional Medical Television
Network
Emory University School of Medicine
69 Butler St., S.E.
Atlanta, GA 30303

Gospel Films, Incorporated
Box 455
Muskegon, MI 49443

Great Plains National Instructional
Television Library
Box 80669
Lincoln, NE 68501

Grove Press Film Division
53 E. 11th St.
New York, NY 10003

Guidance Associates
Communications Park
Box 300
White Plains, NY 10603

Hahnemann Medical College and
Hospital of Philadelphia
Department of Communications in
Medicine
230 N. Broad St.
Philadelphia, PA 19102

Harper and Row Media
2350 Virginia Ave.
Hagerstown, MD 21740

Highly Specialized Promotions
228 Clinton St.
Brooklyn, NY 11201

Human Relations Media Center
41 Washington Ave.
Pleasantville, NY 10570

The Humanist Alternative
7 Harwood Drive
Amherst, NY 14226

Illinois Funeral Directors Association
1046 Outer Park Drive, Suite 120
Springfield, IL 62704

Image Publications
Miles-Samuelson, Inc.
15 E. 26th St.
New York, NY 10010

Image Publishing Corporation
Box 14, North Station
White Plains, NY 10603

Imagesmith
123 Southeast Fourth St.
Minneapolis, MN 55514

Indiana University
Audio-Visual Center
Bloomington, IN 47401

Indiana University School of Medicine
Medical Education Resources Program
1100 W. Michigan St.
Indianapolis, IN 46202

Inland Empire Human Resource Center
2 W. Olive Ave.
Redlands, CA 92373

Interface
63 Chapel St.
Newton, MA 02158

International Film Bureau
332 South Michigan Ave.
Chicago, IL 60604

J.A.B. Press
Box 213-J
Fairlawn, NJ 07410

J. B. Lippincott Company
E. Washington Square
Philadelphia, PA 19105

Jeffrey Norton Publishers, Inc.
Audio Division
145 East 49th St.
New York, NY 10017

Joseph P. Kennedy, Jr. Foundation
1032 33rd St., N.W.
Washington, DC 20006

Joseph Kennedy Foundation
Film Service
999 Asylum Ave.
Hartford, CT 06105

Julian Morris Agency, Inc.
1350 Avenue of the Americas
New York, NY 10019

Kansas Department of Health
and Environment
Forbes Air Force Base, Building 740
Topeka, KA 66620

Kent State University
Audiovisual Services
330 Library Building
Kent, OH 44242

Learning Corporation of America
1350 Avenue of the Americas
New York, NY 10019

Library of Congress
Division for the Blind and Physically
Handicapped
1291 Taylor St., N.W.
Washington, DC 20542

Lynne Littman
6620 Cahuenga Terrace
Los Angeles, CA 90068

M. D. Anderson Hospital and
Tumor Institute
Medical Communications Department
University of Texas System
Cancer Center
Houston, TX 77025

Macmillan Films, Inc.–CCM Films
34 MacQuesten Parkway South
Mount Vernon, NY 10550

Marsh Film Enterprises
P. O. Box 8082
Shawnee Mission, KS 66208

Mass Media Associates
1720 Chouteau Ave.
St. Louis, MO 63103

Mass Media Ministries
2116 N. Charles St.
Baltimore, MD 21218

Maxi Cohen/Joel Gold
31 Greene Street
New York, NY 10013

McGraw-Hill Films
1221 Avenue of the Americas
New York, NY 10020

McMaster University Health Sciences
Co-ordinator, Learning Resources
Room 1G8
1200 Main Street West
Hamilton, Ontario, Canada L8S 4J9

Medal of Greatness
1032 33rd St., N.W.
Washington, DC 20007

The Media Guild
P. O. Box 881
Solana Beach, CA 92075

Medical College of South Carolina
Department of Medical Illustrations
Division of Continuing Education
80 Barre St.
Charleston, SC 29401

Medical Media Network
10995 LeConte Avenue, Room 514
Los Angeles, CA 90024

Medi-Tel Communications
565 Fifth Ave.
New York, NY 10017

Mental Health Training Film Program
Harvard University School of Medicine
58 Fenwood Road
Boston, MA 02115

Michigan State University
Department of Psychiatry
East Lansing, MI 48824

Michigan State University
Instructional Media Center
East Lansing, MI 48824

Milwaukee Regional Medical
    Instructional Television System, Inc.
5000 W. National Ave.
Milwaukee, WI 53193

Modern Talking Picture Service
5000 Park St. North
St. Petersburg, FL 33709

Montage Educational Films
P. O. Box 38128
Hollywood, CA 90038

National Audiovisual Center
General Services Administration
Washington, DC 20409

National Film Board of Canada
1251 Avenue of the Americas
16th Floor
New York, NY 10020

National Funeral Directors Association
135 W. Wells St.
Milwaukee, WI 53203

National Institute of Mental Health
Drug Abuse Film Collection
National Audiovisual Center, GSA
Washington, DC 20409

National Instructional Television
    Center
Agency for Instructional Television
Box A
Bloomington, IN 47401

National Medical Audio-Visual Center
Station K
Atlanta, GA 30324

National Naval Medical Center
Television Division,
    Naval Health Sciences
Education and Training Command
Bethesda, MD 20014

National Sudden Infant Death
    Syndrome Foundation
Room 1904
310 S. Michigan Ave.
Chicago, IL 60604

NBC Educational Enterprises
30 Rockefeller Plaza
New York, NY 10020

Nebraska Television Council
    for Nursing Education
P. O. Box 83111
Lincoln, NE 68501

Network for Continuing Medical
    Education
15 Columbus Circle
New York, NY 10023

New Dimensions Foundation
519 Montgomery St.
San Francisco, CA 94111

New Line Cinema
853 Broadway, 16th Floor
New York, NY 10003

Northern Illinois University
Media Distribution Department
Dekalb, IL 60115

O.G.R. Service Corporation
P. O. Box 3586
Springfield, IL 62708

Pacifica Tape Library
Pacifica Foundation
5316 Venice Blvd.
Los Angeles, CA 90019

Paramount Communications
5451 Marathon St.
Hollywood, CA 90038

Paramount Pictures, Inc.
1501 Broadway
New York, NY 10036

Parent's Magazine Films
Department F
52 Vanderbilt Ave.
New York, NY 10017

Paulist Productions
P. O. Box 1057
Pacific Palisades, CA 90272

Pennsylvania State University
Audiovisual Aids Library
17 Willard Building
University Park, PA 16802

Perfection Form Company
1000 N. Second Ave.
Logan, IA 51546

Perspective Films
65 E. South Water St.
Chicago, IL 60601

Phoenix Films
470 Park Avenue South
New York, NY 10016

Polymorph Films
331 Newbury St.
Boston, MA 02115

Prentice-Hall Media, Inc.
150 White Plains Rd.
Tarrytown, NY 10591

Professional Research, Inc.
American Video Network
660 South Bonnie Brae St.
Los Angeles, CA 90057

PSF Productions Corporation
1498 Sleepy Hollow Lane
New Braunfels, TX 78130

Psychology Today Cassettes
P. O. Box 278
Pratt Station
Brooklyn, NY 11205

Public Television Library
Video Programs Service
475 L'Enfant Plaza, S.W.
Washington, DC 20024

Pyramid Films
P. O. Box 1048
Santa Monica, CA 90406

Ross Medical Associates
1825 Sylvan Court
Flossmoor, IL 60422

Royal College of General Practitioners
Medical Recording Service Foundation
Kitts Croft, Writtle, Chelmsford
CMI 3 EH, England

San Diego Human Resource Center
P. O. Box 5322
San Diego, CA 92105

Serious Business Company
1588 Fell St.
San Francisco, CA 94117

Shands Teaching Hospital
Department of Pastoral Care
Box J-323
Gainesville, FL 32610

SL Film Productions
P. O. Box 41108
Los Angeles, CA 90041

Social Studies School Service
Human Relations Media
10,000 Culver Blvd., Dept. 20
P. O. Box 802
Culver City, CA 90230

Spectrum Educational Media
105 Beverly Ave.
Morton, IL 61550

Spectrum Motion Picture Laboratory
399 Gundersen Drive
Carol Stream, IL 60187

Stanford University School of Medicine
Division of Instructional Media
M 207
Stanford, CA 94305

Sterling Educational Films
241 E. 34th St.
New York, NY 10016

Sunburst Communications
39 Washington Ave.
Pleasantville, NY 10570

Teach 'Em, Inc.
625 N. Michigan Ave.
Chicago, IL 60611

Teleketics
1229 South Santee St.
Los Angeles, CA 90015

Thanatology Resource Center
of Massachusetts, Inc.
52 Ward St.
Worcester, MA 01610

Theosophical Society in America
Box 270
Wheaton, IL 60187

The Thomas More Association
180 N. Wabash Ave.
Chicago, IL 60601

Time-Life Films
Time-Life Building
1271 Avenue of the Americas
New York, NY 10020

Train-Aid Educational Systems
1015 Grandview
Glendale, CA 91201

Trainex Corporation
12601 Industry Ct.
Garden Grove, CA 92641

Trans Time, Inc.
Dept. KB
1122 Spruce St.
Berkeley, CA 94707

20/20 Media
P. O. Box 1062
Springfield, IL 62705

United Methodist Film Service
1525 McGavock St.
Nashville, TN 37203

University of Arizona
Health Sciences Center
Division of Biomedical
    Communications
Tucson, AZ 85724

University of California, Berkeley
Extension Media Center
2223 Fulton St.
Berkeley, CA 94720

University of California, Davis
School of Medicine
Medical Learning Resources
Davis, CA 95616

University of California, Irvine
Office of Medical Education
Irvine, CA 92664

University of California, Los Angeles
10962 Le Conte Ave.
Los Angeles, CA 90024

University of California, Los Angeles
Medical Center, Media Resources
Los Angeles, CA 90024

University of Illinois
Visual Aids Service
1325 S. Oak St.
Champaign, IL 61820

University of Iowa
Audiovisual Center
C-5 East Hall
Iowa City, IA 52242

Univeristy of Maryland
School of Medicine
Department of Psychiatry
Audio-Visual Section
Baltimore, MD 21201

University of Michigan
Audio-Visual Education Center
416 Fourth St.
Ann Arbor, MI 48103

University of Minnesota
AV Library Service
3300 University Ave., S.E.
Minneapolis, MN 55414

University of Nebraska/Lincoln
Instructional Media Center
Nebraska Hall 421
Lincoln, NE 68588

University of Oregon
Division of Continuing Education
    Film Library
P. O. Box 1491, 1633 S.W. Park Ave.
Portland, OR 97201

University of Pittsburgh
School of Medicine
1022 H. Scaife Hall
Pittsburgh, PA 15261

University of Pittsburgh
School of Nursing
Pittsburgh, PA 15213

University of South Florida
    Film Library
4202 Fowler Ave.
Tampa, FL 33620

University of Southern California
Division of Cinema, Films Distribution
    Section
University Park
Los Angeles, CA 90007

University of Southern California
School of Medicine
Instructional Media Services
2025 Zonal Ave.
Los Angeles, CA 90033

University of Texas
Health Sciences Center
7703 Floyd Curl Drive
San Antonio, TX 78229

University of Texas Medical Branch
Videotape Library of Clinical
  Psychiatric Syndromes
Galveston, TX 77550

University of Utah
Educational Media Center
207 Milton Bennion Hall
Salt Lake City, UT 84112

University of Virginia
School of Medicine
Charlottesville, VA 22904

University of Washington
Health Sciences Television Center
Seattle, WA 98195

University of Washington
Instructional Media Services
23 Kane Hall DG-10
Seattle, WA 98195

University of Wisconsin/Madison
Bureau of Audiovisual Instruction
1327 University Ave.
Madison, WI 53706

University of Wisconsin/Milwaukee
School of Nursing
Box 413
Milwaukee, WI 53201

Videorecord Corporation of America
180 East State St.
Westport, CT 06880

Viewfinders, Inc.
Box 1665
Evanston, IL 60204

Walt Disney Educational Media
  Company
500 South Buena Vista St.
Burbank, CA 91521

Walter J. Klein Co., Ltd.
Attn. Ms. Henny Brumberg
6301 Carmel Rd., Box 220766
Charlotte, NC 28222

Walter Reed Army Medical Center
Videotape Library
Room 1077, Building 54
Washington, DC 20305

Washington State Funeral Directors
  Association
4455 Aurora Avenue North
Seattle, WA 98103

Washington State University
Instructional Media Services
Pullman, WA 99164

WGBH/Distribution
125 Western Ave.
Boston, MA 02134

WKYC-TV
Public Affairs Department
1403 East Sixth St.
Cleveland, OH 44114

Wombat Productions, Inc.
Little Lake, Glendale Road
P. O. Box 70
Ossining, NY 10562

Zipporah Films
54 Lewis Wharf
Boston, MA 02110

PART III

Organizational Resources

Introduction

Teachers of death education at all levels should be familiar with the work of various national, regional, and local organizations. Most provide information to health professionals, teachers, and the general public through books or booklets, journals, newsletters, pamphlets, audiovisual materials, speakers, and the like. Some offer counseling and/or referral services for patients and their family members. Some are engaged in scientific and scholarly research; others are fund-raising organizations. Some represent the interests of professional and trade groups; others aim simply to provide a means for people with common interests, common needs, or common suffering to help one another. Many have local chapters or affiliates from which teachers can request further information. Indeed, a diligent survey in almost any community may very well discover local representatives of most of these or similar organizations who will be happy to bring the resources of their groups to bear for the benefit of the death educator and his or her students.

These organizations demonstrate that our communities—whether defined in local, regional or national terms—are indispensable sources of knowledge for students of death education. The variety of group interests and activities illustrates that death education is essentially an interdisciplinary study. Furthermore, the very existence and the ubiquity of such organizations offer hope that our death-denying society may come to regard dying and death, loss, grief and bereavement as enriching experiences in every individual's life, and as durable bonds uniting families, neighborhoods, and communities. Thus, to learn of death as the final stage of growth is to learn more of our humanity and of human societies.

The organizations are arranged in alphabetical order.

Listings

Alan Foss Leukemia Memorial Fund, *730 East 79th Street, Brooklyn, NY 11236*. This regional resource organization provides both economic and emotional support to leukemia patients and family members, and sponsors research. Write for further information.

ALSAC (Aiding Leukemia Stricken American Children), *St. Jude's Children's Research Hospital, 539 Lane Avenue, Memphis, TN 38105*. Originally known as American Lebanese-Syrian Associated Charities, this fund-raising group was founded by entertainer Danny Thomas. St. Jude's is a leading national center for the study and treatment of childhood cancers.

American Association of Homes for the Aging, *1050 17th St., N.W., Washington, DC 20036*. Extended care facilities in this group are voluntary, nonprofit, and government institutions. This nonprofit status in many cases makes a difference in the quality of care provided. Teachers of death education may want to become familiar with the work of this group and its affiliated institutions. The purpose of the association is "to provide unified means of identifying and solving problems of mutual concern so as to protect and advance the interests of the residents served." The group is also developing programs and curricula for administrator education, and it conducts workshops and institutes. Publications include the bimonthly *Concern*, and the *Directory of Nonprofit Homes for the Aged—Social Components of Care.*

American Association of Suicidology, *c/o Betsy S. Comstock, M.D., Department of Psychiatry, Baylor College of Medicine, 1200 Moursund, Houston, TX 77030.* The membership of this organization, the preeminent national group in the field, consists of nearly 600 professionals in various specialties devoted to the study of suicide and suicide prevention. The association supports basic research, educational programs and activities, and sponsors various publications: a quarterly journal, *Suicide and Life Threatening Behavior;* a triennial newsletter, *Newslink; Proceedings* of the annual meetings; a directory of suicide prevention centers; and a number of informative, low-cost booklets and pamphlets for general audiences. It is affiliated with the International Association for Suicide Prevention (see below).

American Cancer Society, Inc., *National Headquarters, 777 3rd Avenue, New York, NY 10017.* The very significant work of the society cannot be adequately described in brief space, nor can its importance to the teacher of death education be overemphasized. The society makes available a wealth of printed and audiovisual material for the general public as well as for health professionals and educators. The topics include various types of cancers and their treatments, rehabilitation programs, caring for the terminally ill, and bearing and sharing grief. There are very helpful and informed staff members on the local level as well as associated professionals and volunteers. Operating under the sponsorship of or in cooperation with the society are various other local and regional informational, self-help, and helping groups (listed below, International Association of Laryngectomees, Reach to Recovery, and United Ostomy Association) for patients with particular diseases or with particular physical and emotional needs. The society has divisional offices in every state and regional offices in many cities. For the death educator the A.C.S. is one of the most valuable resource organizations.

American Cemetery Association, *250 E. Broad St., Columbus, OH 43215.* Primarily a trade group of cemetery owners, administrators, and superintendents, the association collects data and sponsors a variety of publications for its members. Local cemeterian affiliates are happy to consult with death educators.

American Citizens Concerned for Life, *6127 Excelsior Boulevard, Minneapolis, MN 55416.* This anti-abortion, anti-euthanasia organization has a membership of over 4000 in a number of local and regional groups. Speakers, presentations, print and audiovisual materials of many kinds are readily available to educators. The group is involved in legislative action to limit abortion and to resist "death with dignity" proposals.

American College of Nursing Home Administrators, *4650 East-West Highway, Washington, DC 20014.* This group for professionals in the field certifies administrators, promulgates a code of ethics, and sponsors research in geriatrics. It maintains a speakers bureau and makes available a variety of publications and educational materials. Death educators covering nursing homes in their courses should contact this organization—it has a number of regional and state affiliates.

American Euthanasia Foundation, *95 North Birch Road, Suite 301, Ft. Lauderdale, FL 33304.* The "Mercy Will," a type of living will, is distributed by this organization, which is trying to get permission from the government to make the document available in V.A. hospitals. Also available is a booklet on euthanasia, "The Will to Die," which discusses both current issues and historical perspectives on the topic.

American Health Care Association, *1200 15th Street, N.W., Washington, DC 20005.* A national group with nearly 8000 members, the association is a federation of 50 state associations of nursing homes. It lobbies for the industry, offers continuing education programs for nursing home staff, and offers a wide range of publications: a bimonthly *Journal, Health Career Opportunities, Thinking About a Nursing Home,* weekly *Notes,* and a variety of bibliographies.

American Heart Association, *7320 Greenville Avenue, Dallas, TX 75231.* Here is the equivalent of the American Cancer Society for diseases and disabilities of the heart and circulatory system. Nationally well-known, the Association directs educational and public service efforts, sponsors and coordinates research, maintains a library, raises funds, and publishes educational materials including the monthly journal *Circulation.* There are major chapters in every state and many regional and local offices, which sponsor self-help and helping groups called Stroke, Heart, or Coronary Clubs. Inquire locally or write to the national office.

American Hospital Association, *840 North Lake Shore Drive, Chicago, IL 60611.* Working primarily on behalf of its members, over 6,500 institutions and 25,000 individuals in the field of hospital administration, the Association also publishes a large number of public service and patient service pamphlets, booklets, and other materials. Write for a copy of their materials catalogue, which lists both print and audiovisual resources available.

American Lung Association, *1740 Broadway, New York, NY 10019.* This nationally known Association fights diseases of the respiratory system: emphysema, tuberculosis, and other chronic, obstructive lung conditions. The organization conducts various educational programs for health professionals, sponsors research, helps provide for patient needs, and takes its messages into the schools and the community with publications, audiovisual programs, speakers, and resource personnel. The group also addresses the perils of smoking and pollution. See also Breath of Life Club.

American Medical Association, *535 North Dearborn Street, Chicago, IL 60610.* The major national association of physicians offers a uniform donor card and information on willing various organs to medical science. Write the Order Department, OP 371.

American Monument Association, *6902 North High, Worthington, OH 43085.* This trade association for quarriers, manufacturers, and wholesale distributors of cemetery monuments makes available for public distribution a variety of publications on the symbolism of various memorials and epitaphs. Death educators should also contact local cemeteries.

American Protestant Hospital Association, *840 North Lake Shore Drive, Chicago, IL 60611.* Write for copies of various forms on which a person may express his or her wishes about medical care provided in the case of terminal illness.

Association for the Scientific Study of Near-Death Phenomena, *P.O. Box 2309, East Peoria, IL 61611.* This recently formed organization promotes study and provides knowledge and understanding in this area. The Association plans to publish a quarterly newsletter and to sponsor small conferences for researchers and large symposia for the general public.

Barr-Harris Center for the Study of Separation and Loss During Childhood, *The Institute for Psychoanalysis, 180 N. Michigan Ave., Chicago, IL 60601.* The special concern of this organization is loss and grief as experienced by children under 10. It also sponsors research on the subject, consults with other community helping agencies, and works to educate the public through a speaker service.

Breath of Life Club (a service of the American Lung Association). Local chapters of A.L.A. sponsor this helping and self-help organization for patients with chronic lung problems and their families. The Club provides information, equipment, and encouragement.

Cancer Care, Inc., *One Park Avenue, New York, NY 10016.* This service arm of the National Cancer Foundation is a voluntary social welfare agency providing counseling and financial assistance to advanced cancer patients and their families within a 50-mile radius of New York City. It makes available a semiannual journal, *Lamp,* and various other publications.

Candlelighters Foundation, *123 C Street, S.E., Washington, DC 20003.* Formed in 1970, this is a loosely structured national federation of over 65 regional and local groups of parents with children suffering from or lost to cancer. While the member groups may have a variety of names and needs, the umbrella organization assumes larger tasks. It serves as a communications link among affiliated groups through newsletters, bibliographies, and other materials; helps in the formation of new local groups; sponsors regular gatherings of affiliates, many on the subject of new developments in research and treatment; conducts a parent-to-parent letter-writing program; and lobbies for increased federal funding for cancer research projects.

The teacher of death education should establish contact with Candlelighters and with a local parents' group. These people are most happy to share, and are invaluable sources of information and insight. As noted above, group names may vary locally; for example: LODAT (Living One Day at a Time), IMPACT (Interested, Motivated Parents Against Cancer Today), CURE (Children's United Research Effort–St. Louis), COPE (Cincinnati Oncology Parents' Endeavor), PALMS (Parents Against Leukemia and Malignancies Society–Kansas), Living With Cancer, Inc. (Grand Rapids, MI), Parents Who've Lost Children (Tucson), First Sunday (Detroit). For information inquire at a local hospital, doctor's office, chamber of commerce, or write Candlelighters.

Catholic Hospital Association, *1438 S. Grand Boulevard, St. Louis, MO 63104.* The monthly journal of the association, *Hospital Progress,* regularly covers death and dying topics with scholarly, theoretical, or practical articles. Reprints are available, as are a variety of other informational pamphlets and booklets. Through its Department of Health Services for the Aging, the association sponsors research, publishes findings, and conducts workshops and other educational programs on aging and caring for the elderly. It represents Catholic extended care facilities as well as Catholic hospitals.

Center for Death Education and Research, *1167 Social Science Building, University of Minnesota, Minneapolis, MN 55455.* The center sponsors research on all aspects of death and dying, grief and bereavement. It serves as a repository of relevant materials and as a focal point for the dissemination of information to professionals and to the public. The Center also provides speakers, conducts symposia and workshops, and develops and offers many publications and audio-visual materials for sale. Robert Fulton, an internationally known authority in the field of thanatology, is the founder and director.

Centre for Living with Dying, *1542 Los Padres Boulevard, Santa Clara, CA 95050.* The centre is a regional volunteer counseling service for patients and their families facing life-threatening illness, and for anyone deeply affected by the approaching or actual death of others. As an extension of training its own volunteers, the centre offers workshops on psychosocial issues for health professionals and provides a variety of presentations and seminars to community groups. In addition, it helps establish support or self-help groups for terminal patients and their families, widows and widowers, parents of dying and seriously ill children, and survivors of suicide. Most recently the centre has become involved in the work of an outpatient hospice. The centre has prepared an information package for anyone interested in the work of the Centre or in starting similar programs. Please send a $5.00 donation to cover printing and postage costs.

Concern for Dying, An Educational Council, *250 West 57th Street, New York, NY 10019 (800-223-7516).* Formerly known as the Euthanasia Educational Council, this nonprofit organization is dedicated to the creation of "an environment in which each individual can participate fully in decisions regarding his or her treatment during terminal illness." The group fosters humanistic application of medical treatment, argues against the use of heroic medical efforts in hopeless cases, and urges that painkilling drugs be given freely to terminally ill patients. The organization sponsors many conferences, symposia and workshops, and distributes a wide variety of printed and audiovisual materials for professionals, lay audiences and student groups at all levels. Concern for Dying publishes a quarterly newsletter for its membership, and distributes the Patient's Bill of Rights of the American Hospital Association as well as the Living Will, the concept of which it has popularized and for which it continues to lobby legislatively on a state-by-state basis. Note the toll-free telephone number.

Continental Association of Funeral and Memorial Societies, *1828 L Street, N.W., Suite 1100, Washington, DC 20036.* A memorial society is a kind of local cooperative whose purpose is to obtain dignity, simplicity, and economy in funeral arrangements through advance planning. It provides an alternative to traditional commercial funeral establishments and practices. There are over 150 local and regional groups in the United States and Canada, for which the continental association is the umbrella group for the U.S. In Canada write Memorial Society of Canada, Box 96, Weston, Ontario M9N 3M6. The national organizations offer a variety of printed literature, including information and help in establishing a local society, and a newsletter.

Council for Guilds for Infant Survival, *1800 M St., N.W., Washington, DC 20036.* This is one of several national groups working with Sudden Infant Death Syndrome. It offers help and counseling to parents, sponsors medical research, educates the public, and raises funds. There are well over 100 state, regional, and local affiliates, which operate autonomously. The Council offers a variety of publications including its newsletter, *Outcry.*

Cremation Association of North America, *15300 Ventura Boulevard, Suite 305, Sherman Oaks, CA 91403.* This is a national trade association for over 300 crematories. Write for information and the name and location of the crematory nearest you. The association promotes cremation through its publications, meetings, lectures, and other organizational means.

Cryonics Society of New York, Inc., *9 Holmes Court, Sayville, Long Island, NY 11782.* Write for information on this alternative method of body disposition and "symbolic immortality."

Cystic Fibrosis Foundation, *3379 Peachtree Road, N.E., Atlanta, GA 30326.* With over 100 regional chapters, the Foundation sponsors research, offers training programs for professionals and patients, operates care centers, informs the public about the disease, and raises funds. It publishes a quarterly magazine, *Profile,* and other educational materials.

Deafness Research Foundation, *366 Madison Avenue, New York, NY 10017.* In addition to its sponsorship of research and educational programs, the Foundation encourages individuals with hearing disorders to bequeath their inner ear structures to the National Temporal Bone Bank (see below) for research purposes. Write the Foundation for more information and necessary forms.

Equinox Institute, *159 Ward St., Newton, MA 02159.* A nonprofit, educational organization, the Institute plans and conducts seminars and workshops on various death and dying topics for teachers, counselors, and medical professionals.

Eye Bank Association of America, Inc., *3195 Maplewood Avenue, Winston-Salem, NC 27103.* Corneal transplant operations are now successful in about 90 percent of the cases, so there is good reason to expect that bequeathing one's eyes to an eye bank will result literally in the gift of sight. The association and its more than 60 cooperating regional eye banks can provide further information on eye donations as well as copies of the necessary form, the Uniform Donor Card. A New York City affiliate, Eye-Bank for Sight Restoration, 210 East 64th Street, New York, NY 10021, also publishes and distributes professional literature, conducts research and educational programs, and maintains a speakers bureau.

Forum for Death Education and Counseling, Inc., *P.O. Box 1226, Arlington, VA 22210.* This nonprofit organization of health professionals, educators, and counselors promotes death education and counseling, prepares and distributes educational materials, and sponsors periodic conferences and workshops for the dissemination of information and research. The forum has established a code of ethics and other standards, publishes a monthly newsletter, sponsors *Omega,* a major scholarly journal, and holds annual conferences for its members. There are currently 18 regional and local affiliates.

Foundation of Thanatology, *630 West 168th Street, New York, NY 10032.* The foundation is an educational and scientific organization with a largely medical, professional, and scholarly membership which studies the psychological aspects of dying, reactions to death, loss and grief, and recovery from bereavement. Through an ongoing series of symposia for professionals and an extensive publishing program, the foundation fosters its belief that death is a positive part of the living process and that patient care should be conceived of as a multidisciplinary task. Through its own model educational programs and leadership, the foundation is facilitates the establishment of death education courses at all levels. It conducts related educational and attitudinal research, provides speakers and consultants, and does medical referral work. In addition to the many books it has sponsored, the Foundation publishes the quarterlies, *The Archives of the Foundation of Thanatology* and *New Advances in Thanatology* and the bimonthly *Thanatology News.*

Gray Panthers, *3700 Chestnut Street, Philadelphia, PA 19104.* Organized by Maggie Kuhn, Gray Panthers is dedicated to consciousness-raising and activism in combating ageism in our society, and in making young and old alike aware of the importance of old people to our society. The group gives advice, referrals, and information, and assists in the establishment of local groups, of which there are now well over 50. It sponsors seminars and research on aging, and publishes a quarterly, *Network*, as well as other materials.

Grief Education Institute, *6198 South Westview, Littleton, CO 80120.* The institute was established over 2 years ago to offer grief counseling in support-group contexts to a whole range of clients, from survivors of suicide victims to parents who have lost children. Since then, additional activities have come to include a variety of educational programs, for both professional and public audiences, and scholarly research. Bibliographies and a newsletter are available at cost.

The Hastings Center: Institute of Society, Ethics and the Life Sciences, *360 Broadway, Hastings-on-Hudson, NY 10706.* Founded over 10 years ago to promote study of emerging bioethical issues, the center sponsors research, encourages establishment of ethical inquiry units in university and professional school curricula, and is involved in various public education programs. Death and dying is one of six major areas of emphasis, together with population control, genetic counseling and engineering, behavior control, health policy, and the foundations of ethics. The Center sponsors a variety of symposia and workshops for professionals, scholars, students, and the general public, and makes available a wealth of article reprints along with its bimonthly, *Hastings Center Report*, and annual annotated bibliographies.

Horizons in the Life Cycle, Inc., *c/o Riverside Church, 490 Riverside Drive, New York, NY 10027.* A ministry of the Riverside Church, Horizons provides referrals and a variety of counseling and educational services, including readings on death and dying.

Inland Empire Human Resources Center, *c/o Congregational Church, 2 West Olive Avenue, Redlands, CA 92373.* The center collects and distributes gifts and bequests of gold tooth fillings and pills from deceased persons. The gold is forwarded to dental schools serving the poor and the pills, needed by medical missionaries abroad, can be accepted if they are clean and properly labeled in original containers (such reuse is not legal in the United States and Canada).

International Association for Suicide Prevention, *University of California Medical Center, San Francisco, CA 94143.* With a worldwide membership of over 850 groups and individuals from a variety of disciplines and professions, the major function of the association is to provide an international forum for the exchange of research, information, and experience on suicide. It also sponsors and publishes research.

International Association of Laryngectomees, *Mr. Paul J. Scriffignano, Executive Secretary, American Cancer Society, 777 Third Avenue, New York, NY 10017.* In cooperation with the American Cancer Society, patients who have lost their natural voices due to the removal of the larynx are offered encouragement, therapy and related equipment and supplies, and training and rehabilitation, with the aid of speech therapists and people who have had the same surgery and have developed other speech skills. There are over 230 local clubs in 47 states, many with names like New Voice Club or Lost Cord Club. Available are a variety of educational and informational publications, and a bimonthly newsletter.

International Order of the Golden Rule, *c/o O.G.R. Service Corporation, P.O. Box 3586, Springfield, IL 62708.* This professional organization serving member funeral homes works to establish the funeral director as one of the primary resource people in his community regarding death, dying, grief, and funerals. Local member directors can provide a variety of printed and audiovisual materials, and are happy to consult with death educators.

International Work Group in Death, Dying, and Bereavement, *138 W. Walnut Lane, Philadelphia, PA 19144.* The Group's purpose is to "conduct meetings of workers who are active in the field of death, dying, and bereavement in which the level of competence is sufficiently high so that the atmosphere is one of shared collegiality and in which there is no 'audience.' It strives to "promote knowledge and test unproven theories and assumptions by empirical research." It is international in scope and plans to translate and disseminate its work to others. IWG holds annual meetings for the membership.

Jewish Funeral Directors of America, Inc., *1170 Rockville Pike, Rockville, MD 20852.* This organization aims to raise the standards for Jewish funerals as well as for funeral service practices in general. In conjunction with other organizations such as the Rabbinical Association, it sponsors conferences and seminars in death, dying, and bereavement for funeral directors, health professionals, students, and the general public.

Kara: Volunteer Emotional Support Services, *457 Kingsley Avenue, Palo Alto, CA 94301.* Using carefully trained volunteers, Kara offers counseling services on a nonprofit basis to terminally ill and near-death individuals, their families, and to the bereaved. Additional activities in the greater San Francisco area include involvement with groups of parents who have lost children, various community education projects, and referral services.

Leukemia Society of America, *211 East 43rd Street, New York, NY 10017.* With affiliated organizations in each state, the society provides help for needy leukemia patients, sponsors research, raises funds, and educates the public about the disease through a variety of publications and audiovisual materials. It is involved in professional education, sponsoring symposia and providing scholarships and awards. The Boston chapter (206 Park Square Building, St. James Street, Boston, Massachusetts 02116) sponsors a supportive program called OUTREACH for patients and family members that is typical of approaches used by other local affiliates.

O = Open doors of friendship
U = Unite patients and families
T = Trust one another
R = Reach out to understand others and oneself
E = Educate oneself to new ways of life
A = Approach life with new Awareness through sharing
C = Comfort one another at Crucial, Critical times in life
H = Hearing others talk about good days and bad days is how OUTREACH Helps families to cope

Life Extension Society, *2011 North Street, Washington, DC 20036.* Another group like the Cryonics Society of New York. Write for free information.

Living Bank, *P.O. Box 6725, Houston, TX 77005.* The bank is a nonprofit registry, coordinating and distributing agency, and information center for anatomical gifts. Write for further information and a Uniform Donor Card.

Make Today Count, *P.O. Box 303, Burlington, IA 52601.* Founded by Orville Kelly, a cancer patient desiring to combat his own feelings of isolation and rejection by others, this self-help organization promotes openness and honesty and works to improve the quality of life for persons with life-threatening illnesses and their family members. The group is also active in professional education, helping caregivers improve their work with seriously ill patients by better addressing their emotional needs. The national office provides an incorporation packet and other assistance in starting a local chapter (of which there are now well over 200), and publishes a newsletter and other materials.

Medic Alert Organ Donor Program, *Medic Alert Foundation International, 1000 North Palm Street, Turlock, CA 95380.* Like the Living Bank (see above), Medic Alert is a nonprofit registry for purposes of facilitating anatomical gifts. In addition, it provides its members with a wallet card and either a bracelet or a necklace on which is engraved one's basic medical information and a telephone number. Emergency personnel anywhere in the world can call that number collect to receive a full medical profile, as well as donor information if the situation warrants.

Mended Hearts, *721 Huntington Avenue, Boston, MA 02115.* In over 75 local groups the members of Mended Hearts are people who have had open-heart surgery. In addition to helping one another adjust, members also make contact with patients about to undergo the surgery and offer support and information. The organization publishes a newsletter and a periodical 6 times a year—*The Heartbeat.*

Monument Builders of North America, *1612 Central St., Evanston, IL 60201.* This trade association for memorialists publishes and distributes a variety of public relations materials and films. Write for information.

Mothers of Children with Down's Syndrome, *c/o Northern Virginia Association for Retarded Citizens, 105 East Annandale Road, Suite 203, Falls Church, VA 22046.* This regional parent-to-parent counseling and educational group is involved in sharing information on diagnostic testing, psychological, genetic and educational counseling, available clinics and therapies, and opportunities for schooling and recreation. The group works closely with medical professionals, and lobbies for federal funding of research. It has prepared and distributes, at cost, a parent information kit.

Muscular Dystrophy Association of America, Inc., *810 Seventh Avenue, New York, NY 10019.* Through its many local and regional offices the association provides medical examinations and treatments, orthopedic appliances, and recreational opportunities. It is involved extensively in sponsoring research, and publishes professional literature on the disease as well as public information materials.

NAIM, *U.S. Catholic Conference, Family Life Division, 1312 Massachusetts Avenue, N.W., Washington, DC 20005.* This national office organizes and coordinates the activities of local chapters, groups primarily Catholic in their sponsorship and activities which work to help the widowed. Local groups decide their own priorities and activities but the emphasis, at least in the greater Chicago area where NAIM originated in 1957, is on social, religious and informational activities. Chapters are not so much therapy as family.

National Abortion Rights Action League, *706 Seventh Street, S.E., Washington, DC 20003.* Claiming over 13,000 members in 51 state groups, NARAL is the most visible national proponent of the goal "to maintain the right of safe, legal abortion for all women." It is involved in political, social, and legal action, and publishes a newsletter and a periodical, *Abortion Law Reporter.*

National Alliance of Senior Citizens, *Box 40031, Washington, DC 20016.* Working on behalf of aged Americans, this group provides information to its members, alerts the public to the needs of the aged, and lobbies for legislation. It maintains a library and publishes a bimonthly journal, *Senior Independent,* and an annual for its members, *Senior Services Manual.* There are nearly 17,000 members in 150 regional affiliates.

National Association for Down's Syndrome, *Box 63, Oak Park, IL 60303.* With 1300 members, this is primarily a regional self-help group of parents of children with Down's syndrome. Publications include *Down's Syndrome, Family Management,* and *Mother to Mother.* The group is affiliated with the Illinois Association of the Mentally Retarded and, like Mothers of Children with Down's Syndrome (see above), may be typical of many other regional and local groups interested in the syndrome.

National Association for Mental Health, *1800 North Kent Street, Arlington, VA 22209.* With a million volunteers in over 900 state divisions and chapters, this is the only organization of its kind working on behalf of the mentally ill. The national office sponsors research and is involved in legislative and governmental agency activities in all related areas. It publishes informational materials and sponsors educational programs. While the association itself does not provide direct services, it works to ensure that quality mental health services are available to anyone who needs them. Locally, this goal means distribution of readings and films on such topics as aging, nursing homes, suicide, widowhood, and coping with deaths in the family. Local chapters also serve as referral centers and resource people to whom death educators may turn for information.

National Association of Cemeteries, *Suite 409, Rosslyn Building North, 1911 N. Fort Myer Dr., Arlington, VA 22209.* Members of this trade association—cemetery owners, administrators, and superintendents—are happy to consult with death educators and to make available a variety of printed informational materials.

National Association of Patients on Hemodialysis and Transplantation, *505 Northern Boulevard, Great Neck, NY 11021.* The association works to assist and to educate the patient, to make the public aware of kidney disease, and to encourage donations of kidneys. It publishes a quarterly journal, *News,* and other informational material.

National Cancer Foundation, Inc., *One Park Avenue, New York, NY 10016.* The foundation promotes and implements programs of improved professional and psychosocial services to advanced cancer patients and their families. It conducts social research, provides professional consultation, and sponsors educational programs for caregivers. The foundation "is dedicated to a more complete understanding of the psychological, emotional, economic and spiritual impact of catastrophic illness upon patients and families." See also Cancer Care, above.

National Catholic Cemetery Conference, *710 N. River Road, Des Plaines, IL 60016.* This trade association makes available a variety of public information material through member cemeteries.

National Council of Senior Citizens, *1511 K Street N.W., Washington, DC 20005.* A major organization of over 3,000,000 members distributed in some 3800 autonomous local groups, the council is both an educational and an action group. It supports, for example; continuation and improvement of Medicare; increased social security benefits; reduced drug costs for senior citizens; and improved housing, education, health and recreation programs for seniors. It lobbies for favorable legislation, sponsors rallies and workshops, maintains a speakers bureau, distributes films, and publishes a newsletter and other printed materials.

National Council on the Aging, *1828 L Street, N.W., Washington, DC 20036.* With a membership of representatives from business and industry, labor and the helping professions, and various governmental agencies and committees on aging, the Council works with a variety of other groups to develop awareness of the needs of older people— particularly the psychological, health and economic—and to improve methods and resources for meeting those needs. Much of the council's work is educational. It sponsors conferences and workshops, operates a national information and consultation center together with a national media resource center, and offers a wealth of printed and audiovisual material.

National Easter Seal Society for Crippled Children and Adults, *2023 W. Ogden Avenue, Chicago, IL 60612.* The society is the major national organization working on behalf of the physically handicapped. It cooperates with other agencies and with the government to provide services, and is involved in extensive activity to help patients, to educate the public, and to disseminate the results of research to professionals. Among its many publications are the periodicals *Rehabilitation Literature* and the *Easter Seal Communicator.*

National Foundation—March of Dimes, Box 2000, White Plains, NY 10602. The major purpose of this organization is to protect the unborn and the newborn through study and prevention of birth defects. It promotes research in perinatal and genetic medicine fields, and education on improving maternal and newborn health and the nature and treatment of such birth defects as Down's syndrome, spina bifida, cerebral palsy, and sickle cell anemia. It publishes a variety of pamphlets and other informational materials.

National Foundation of Funeral Service, *1600-1628 Central Street, Evanston, IL 60201.* Serving the funeral industry, the foundation operates a school of funeral service management, offers extension courses, maintains demonstration rooms, and conducts research programs. It has a large library devoted to funeral service, and offers some public education services. See National Selected Morticians, and National Research and Information Center.

National Funeral Directors Association, *135 West Wells Street, Milwaukee, WI 53203.* The major national trade association of funeral directors, this group is a strong spokesman and advocate for the industry and a vocal defender of traditional funeral customs and practices. Thus it and most local affiliated funeral directors are more than happy to cooperate in teaching death education units and courses, and to make available a wide variety of literature and audiovisual materials, most of which have been written and produced under association sponsorship. Write for a complete catalogue. The association sponsors research projects, preparation of books, and nationally known speakers for conferences on death and bereavement, with heavy emphasis on the merits of traditional funeral practices.

National Hospice Organization, *Tower Street 506, 301 Maple Avenue West, Vienna, VA 22180.* The organization was founded to serve the interests of the rapidly increasing number of hospices in the U.S. It acts as a communications link among hospices, works to educate both the public and health professionals about the hospice concept, recommends standards of care in program planning and operation, provides basic training materials and technical assistance to new hospice groups, and monitors relevant legislative activity on state and national levels. It plans to sponsor the *International Journal of Hospice Care*, a newsletter, and other publications.

National Information Center for the Handicapped, *1201 16th Street N.W., Washington, DC 20036*. Established to inform and assist parents of children with any type of physical or emotional handicap or defect, the Center offers information about services for the handicapped and provides referrals to appropriate local organizations. A variety of educational publications are available.

National Kidney Foundation, *116 East 27th Street, New York, NY 10016*. The foundation sponsors medical and scientific research, fosters improvement in patient services, and is involved in both public and professional education. It encourages the donation of kidneys and other body parts to medical science and coordinates its own kidney transplant program. Write for information on donating organs, for a Uniform Donor Card, and for other information about the work of the foundation.

National Multiple Sclerosis Society, *257 Park Avenue South, New York, NY 10010*. Organized to serve the patient through many regional and local chapters, the society supplies equipment, nursing services and therapy, arranges recreational and educational activities, and provides counseling and patient-to-patient and family-to-family contact. Publications include a newsletter and a variety of pamphlets. The society also sponsors research.

National Pituitary Agency, *Suite 503–7, 210 West Fayette Street, Baltimore, MD 21201*. This organization encourages and arranges for the collection of pituitary glands through donations and autopsies, and extracts from them a variety of hormones that are then distributed to researchers. The agency coordinates donations and research projects nationwide. Write for further information and a donor form.

National Research and Information Center, *National Foundation of Funeral Service, 1600 Central Street, Evanston, IL 60201*. This is a nonprofit organization that encourages and facilitates research into death-related issues in a variety of scholarly fields: sociology, economics, psychology, religion, psychiatry, and political science. Its services are free to those who write funded programs or dissertation proposals. Specific examples of assistance include help with bibliographic searches, access to one of the largest collections of literature on death in the world, information on funding sources for specific proposals, free access to major computer searches of the literature, and help in publishing and disseminating research findings. Joe A. Adams, Ph.D., is the director of the center. Telephone 312-328-6545.

National Right to Life Committee, *Suite 341, National Press Building, 529 14th Street, N.W., Washington, DC 20045*. The major goal of this anti-abortion, anti-euthanasia organization is to work for the passage of a human-life amendment to the constitution of the United States. Many local chapters will happily provide speakers and a variety of informational material, including the monthly *Right to Life News.*

National Selected Morticians, *1616 Central Street, Evanston, IL 60201.* This national association of over 900 individual funeral homes works to develop and maintain sound business and professional practices. Member funeral homes will provide a variety of pamphlet information on funeral planning, customs and costs, on practical concerns after a loss, and on grief and bereavement, and will be glad to consult with death educators.

National Sudden Infant Death Syndrome Foundation, *310 South Michigan Avenue, Chicago, IL 60604.* The major purposes of this group are to assist parents, to educate the public, and to promote research. It sponsors programs of professional counseling and, through its many local chapters, fosters parent-to-parent and self-help activities. It publishes a variety of educational and information literature as well as a quarterly newsletter, and makes speakers available. Consult your regional or local chapter.

National Temporal Bone Banks Program of the Deafness Research Foundation, *Johns Hopkins University, School of Medicine, Baltimore, MD 21205.* This nationwide organization encourages the donation of inner ear structures for teaching and surgical training purposes. Over 40 temporal bone banks across the country cooperate in the program. Write for information and necessary forms. See Deafness Research Foundation, above.

New Eyes for the Needy, Inc., *549 Millburn Avenue, Short Hills, NJ 07078.* This agency collects and distributes to the needy eyeglasses left by the dead.

Parents without Partners, *7910 Woodmont Avenue, Suite 1000, Washington, DC 20014.* This international nonprofit educational group works in the interest of single parents and their children. With a membership of over 160,000 in 1000 local affiliates, it is both a helping and self-helping organization studying the problems of single parents and sharing solutions, especially as regards upbringing of children and acceptance of the single-parent family by society. It publishes a variety of manuals and brochures, a periodical, *The Single Parent,* and maintains a speakers bureau.

Phoenix Society, *11 Rusthill Road, Levittown, PA 19056.* The society is a national self-help group for burn victims and their families. The executive director, Alan Jeffry Breslau, published a book called *The Time of My Death* (1977), about his extensive burn injuries in a plane crash, his treatment, and his rehabilitation.

Planned Parenthood Federation of America, *810 Seventh Avenue, New York, NY 10019.* The membership of this national group consists of nearly 200 affiliated organizations throughout the country. Its purposes are to make voluntary fertility control available to all, to conduct research into population control, to distribute information, to provide resource people, and to conduct educational activities. This is a group with a point of view radically different from that of, for example, National Right to Life Committee (see above).

Project Hear, *c/o Rodney Perkins, M.D., 1801 Page Mill Road, Palo Alto, CA 94304.* This eardrum and ossicle bank was established in 1969 by Dr. Perkins. It accepts gifts of inner ear structures for research purposes and possible transplantation.

Psychical Research Foundation, Inc., *Duke Station, Durham, NC 27706.* This nonprofit organization is concerned with the most profound mystery of our universe: Does consciousness continue beyond physical death? The foundation publishes the quarterly *Theta* in which research on near-death experiences, reincarnation memories, altered states of consciousness, and poltergeists and hauntings is reported.

Reach to Recovery. Through this program sponsored by the American Cancer Society, specially trained, physician-approved people who have had mastectomies offer new patients information and counseling. Reach to Recovery is also involved in professional education and in efforts to improve prostheses and make them more widely available. For further information contact a local office of A.C.S.

St. Francis Burial and Counseling Society, Inc., *1768 Church Street, N.W., Washington, DC 20036.* In its own words this nonprofit organization is "dedicated to all people who are concerned for spiritual rather than material values at the time of death." The options include simple wooden coffins and ash boxes, assembled or in kit form, and at reasonable prices. The society publishes a quarterly offering funeral planning advice, information on death and dying, book reviews, and provides counseling and public education programs.

Scientists for Life, *1908 Washington Avenue, Fredericksburg, VA 22401.* Like the National Right to Life Committee, Scientists for Life is an antiabortion, antieuthanasia group. It collects data and shares information with like-minded groups and with the public.

Shanti Nilaya, *26210 Lake Wohlford Rd., Valley Center, CA 92082.* Dr. Elisabeth Kübler-Ross has established this center for healing and the investigation of death. Workshops are offered.

SHANTI Project, *1137 Colusa Avenue, Berkeley, CA 94707.* The word means "inner peace" in Sanskrit, and summarizes the goals of the Project: "to offer direct community services consisting of counseling and companionship for patients and families and grief counseling for survivors of a death; to provide professional training and public education; and to conduct substantive research to evaluate the Project." Volunteer counselors have themselves experienced a loss and are specially trained. Write for further information and a copy of the Project newsletter *Eclipse.*

Society for the Right to Die, *250 West 57th Street, New York, NY 10019.* An arm of Concern for Dying (see above), the Society is engaged in legislative activity on behalf of "right to die" propositions. It also provides information on the current status of such legislation on a state-by-state basis, and publishes *Legislative Newsletter,* a monthly, and *Death with Dignity Legislative Manual.*

Society of the Compassionate Friends, *P.O. Box 1347, Oak Brook, IL 60521.* The Society was founded primarily to provide one-to-one communication, counseling, and self-help for parents whose children have died. There are nearly two dozen regional groups around the country.

Spina Bifida Association of America, *343 S. Dearborn Avenue, Suite 319, Chicago, IL 60604.* The cause of "open spine" is unknown, there is no complete cure, and the long-term prognosis is muscle weakness and paralysis. The association sponsors research, provides information, seeks to improve vocational training, and monitors legislation affecting the handicapped. It distributes a variety of publications including a bimonthly, *The Pipeline.*

Stroke Club of America, *805 12th Street, Galveston, TX 77550.* With over 5000 members, the club serves as a self-help organization for victims of strokes and their family members, providing patient-to-patient contact, and as a helping and educational resource, giving hope, encouragement, and practical information on rehabilitation. The club publishes a newsletter and a monthly, *The Stroke Memo.*

THEOS Foundation, *11609 Frankstown Road, Pittsburgh, PA 15235.* The group, founded as a nonsectarian Christian ministry to the widowed, derives its name from its motto: "They Help Each Other Spiritually." In over 40 church-affiliated chapters nationwide, members share experiences and feelings and help one another. Monthly meetings and occasional weekend conferences feature guest speakers and socializing. The foundation maintains a telephone hot line, publishes a newsletter, and has produced a book, *After the Flowers Have Gone.*

United Ostomy Association, *1111 Wilshire Boulevard, Los Angeles, CA 90017.* With over 500 affiliated groups nationwide, the purpose of the Association is to provide counseling, moral support, and information to people who have had, or are about to undergo, ostomy surgery (often as a result of cancer), with the goal of having the patient return to as normal a life as possible. Activities include a "visitor" program for new ostomates, speakers bureau, various educational services and materials, and support for enterostomal therapy educational curricula.

U.S. Coalition for Life, *Box 315, Export, PA 15632.* Members of the coalition are over 1200 anti-abortion organizations, agencies, and hospitals. This umbrella group conducts and sponsors research into various "population control" activities (family planning and genetic engineering as well as abortion and euthanasia) and keeps its membership informed by means of seminars, various publications, reprints, and monitoring of legislative activities. It helps local groups improve the quality and effectiveness of their work.

Widowed Persons Service, *c/o Leo Baldwin, Coordinator, National Retired Teachers Association, 1909 K Street, N.W., Washington, DC 20049.* Operating in 55 cities across the United States, this program depends upon the services of volunteer aides—specially trained widows and widowers of at least two years' duration—in reaching out to the newly widowed. Listening, sharing experiences, counseling, socializing, and providing information and referral are some of the tasks assumed by the aides. The organization is sponsored by the National Retired Teachers Association, the American Association of Retired Persons, and various other groups. Write for a copy of "Directory of Services for the Widowed in the United States and Canada," an annotated list of the names and addresses of regional and local organizations for the widowed.

PART IV

Community Resources

In the previous sections of this guide, we have presented a wide variety of resources that can be of assistance to death educators in their study of the wealth of knowledge that has accumulated in this field. These resources will also be helpful in the planning and development of a systematic course, unit, or module at various educational levels. They are equally relevant to educational programs dealing with death, dying, and bereavement as a whole, or to curricula restricted to specific subareas. To serve such diverse purposes, we have included a large range of printed materials and an even greater number of audiovisual items. We realize, of course, that both kinds of resources may be available to individual instructors to a limited extent. That is why we have made a special effort to identify organizational resources and periodicals for which the cost factor is unimportant, and have suggested ways to obtain audiovisual materials at the least cost. Where a well-stocked library is not available, a careful program of selected acquisitions can be planned on the basis of our annotations.

The community is a resource that can also be an inexpensive and invaluable aid to death education. We mentioned earlier that there are local chapters of many of the national organizations listed, but the community resources we have in mind go beyond these organizations. Continually engaged in daily tasks of coping with life and the implications of death, each community attracts, creates, or supports a whole spectrum of interesting resources: resident institutions and individuals, transient speakers or meetings, cultural events, persons with access to certain skills or materials, and so forth. These resources will be different in each community, but will always be present since they reflect common interests and needs growing out of a shared human condition.

Community resources are invaluable for a number of reasons. First, they are usually free. In many instances this is the decisive factor in determining whether or not a course or module on death and dying can be offered at all. Second, these resources are readily accessible, and often make themselves available to those engaged in death education. Third, these resources often possess unique competencies and perspectives. They help broaden our insights and deepen our appreciation of what death education really means. Fourth, the individuals, agencies, and institutions listed in this section are all engaged in interests and activities that concern them deeply. They are typically proud of the services they provide, and are happy to share them. Indeed, they may feel appreciated when invited to share their knowledge or experience with a student or a class. Fifth, such exchange between community and classroom may promote a sense of sharing. Finally, from a pedagogical perspective, active learning and interest is greatly enhanced when real life is brought into the classroom. Even with the best teacher, the classroom often bores students with its structure and monotony. Jerome Bruner, the scholar and author, has suggested that school curricula should include the community in a major way in every aspect of the educational process. We agree with Bruner and are convinced that a course on death and dying will be a richer, more interesting, and more realistic learning experience when teachers use community resources.

□   □   □

The following list of community resources is based on our own teaching about death, dying, and bereavement. It has grown out of our individual experiences which, in turn, depended on our particular institutions and communities. We discovered many of our best resources almost accidentally through suggestions from friends, colleagues, or students. Death education cuts across so many fields of interest and expertise that few can be aware of everything to which it is related. In fact, death educators themselves will benefit from a rich and varied education in the form of questions put to them, student projects, and the contacts that come their way in the course of this work. Our point is that opportunities abound for improving the quality of death education if we are only alert and imaginative enough to recognize them.

This list is not definitive. We offer it primarily as a point of departure from which each individual can launch his or her own survey of resources. What happened in our classes and workshops can not be precisely duplicated in other courses at other places, but similar resources are available in every community. With suitable modifications, most of the resources that we suggest could be applied to nearly any sort of course on death, dying, or bereavement. We intend this section, then, as a way of encouraging death educators to explore and use the local resources of their own communities. Consider the following as a sample of the resources available in most local communities and regional areas.

1. **Hospitals.** Because death and dying are so heavily institutionalized in our society, hospitals have become a rich source of information, expertise, and experience for death education. Hospital personnel can be recruited for guest lectures from a number of departments, including oncology, pediatrics, geriatrics, psychiatry, intensive care, cardiac care, emergency, burn center, family practice, and organ or body donation centers. In addition, we can use staff from a number of patient services, such as chaplains or pastoral care personnel, "floating" nurses, social services, psychological services, genetic counseling services, or outpatient clinics. Guided tours might be conducted through a typical ward or intensive care unit, the morgue or pathology laboratory, the emergency room, the radiology-oncology department, or the library.

2. **Hospices.** Hospices are new and rapidly growing developments in terminal care; where available, they supplement or provide an alternative to regular hospital care for dying persons and their families. Hospices specialize in the control of chronic pain or other discomforting symptoms that may accompany dying. Hospices range from free-standing institutions to volunteer programs coordinated from a telephone in a private home. We encourage readers to inquire about hospice programs in their own communities. Some programs are even located within hospitals as continuing care or palliative care units. Hospice staff and volunteers make good guest lecturers who are able to describe the needs of dying persons and their families, and to discuss the program of care which they require. Hospices also frequently have a special appreciation of the stresses that staff members encounter in working with death and dying.

3. **Nursing Homes.** Most nursing homes permit groups to make advance arrangements to tour their facilities. They might offer speakers from among their residents, nurses, administrators, social services directors, physical therapists and other rehabilitation personnel, and regular volunteers.

4. **Self-Help or Mutual-Help Groups.** These groups operate either alone or in cooperation with other organizations. They usually

function most effectively as a group of lay persons who have experienced trauma or loss themselves and who provide an opportunity for the sharing of experiences, thoughts, and feelings. For many persons, the concern and support of a group of people who have "been there before" can help them cope with their own problem. These groups also make available information concerning chronic or terminal illness and bereavement. For purposes of death education, it is striking to note the similarities in goals and means among these diverse groups. Many are local chapters of national or international organizations described in Part III. Among those whose concerns relate most directly to death, dying, and bereavement are such groups as "Make Today Count," "Candle Lighters," "Compassionate Friends," "Widowed Persons Service," "THEOS," and "Widow-to-Widow." Groups concerned with chronic illnesses, genetic deficiencies like Down's syndrome, or divorce ("Parents without Partners") can describe the larger range of trauma, limitation, and loss that occurs in human life and that constitutes a broadened context for discussions focusing on death, dying, and bereavement.

5. **Other Professional and Volunteer Services.** Usually, these are funded by federal, state, or local agencies. Among them are mental health clinics, suicide prevention centers, drug centers, cancer programs, education and counseling programs concerned with Sudden Infant Death Syndrome, "Youth Emergency Services" or "Call a Pal," and other hot line or crisis intervention services intended to help those in potentially life-threatening difficulties. Many of these services are directed to young people and are of particular interest to students.

6. **Various Professions.** Quite a large number of professional people work directly or frequently with persons involved in traumatic or life-threatening situations. These include psychiatrists, psychologists, social workers, counselors, lawyers, judges, policemen, firemen, penologists and wardens of correctional institutions, ambulance and rescue squad personnel, coroners, and clergy of all faiths. Obituary writers and others not likely to come to mind in an initial review of occupational categories also belong to this large and disparate group.

7. **Funeral Homes, Crematoria, and Cemeteries.** Many of those who work in the funeral industry are accustomed to speaking to groups about their activities and about funeral practices in the U.S. They include funeral directors, embalmers, cemetery and crematory operators, casket and monument makers, and others. Frequently, they will conduct tours through the funeral home, including its casket room, preparation room, parlors, and chapel, or through a crematory, cemetery, or mausoleum. These institutions often provide pamphlets and audiovisual materials that can be informative for students.

8. **Memorial Societies.** Many communities have local chapters of the Continental Association of Funeral and Memorial Societies. This organization, described more fully in Part III, was founded to

assist people in obtaining inexpensive and yet dignified funerals. Local chapters often encourage cremation or other forms of prompt disposal of the body, together with a subsequent memorial service. Their representatives can describe their goals and activities, and provide an alternative viewpoint to that of the typical funeral director.

9. **Dying or Bereaved Persons.** A person with a terminal illness or who has recently lost a loved one can be an invaluable resource for a course on death education. Their sharing of thoughts, feelings, and coping strategies can humanize and make concrete a subject that is sometimes impersonal and abstract. They can frequently convey important information and insights, and evoke deep emotion. At the same time, it must be remembered that not all such people have something they need or want to say, and not all are articulate or comfortable in speaking before a class. Nor should the success of a course on death education depend upon a kind of "thanatological voyeurism." However, a good deal of experience and the example of Elisabeth Kübler-Ross has taught us the twin values in having such people as our teachers and in providing them opportunities to perfrom this valuable service. The legitimate use of this sort of resource requires careful preparation and sensitivity on the part of the death educator.

10. **Other Faculty Members.** The professional expertise of other faculty members should be an obvious resource for death education. Typically, it will lead to team teaching or to guest lectures. We mention it here, however, especially to recall that other faculty members are likely to be an articulate source of avocational interests and personal experiences. The death educator needs to be alert to these possibilities, which will often be suggested initially in casual conversation or chance remarks.

11. **Students.** A parallel resource is our own students. It is not at all unusual for students enrolled in a death and dying course to have had significant death-related experiences in their work or personal lives that they are willing to share with a class. In our classes, students have reported on the following: part-time work as ambulance driver, member of a rescue team, firefighter, police officer, and nurse; intern at a correctional institution; volunteer in a crisis intervention service; assistant in a funeral home; aide or technician at a hospital or nursing home; personal involvement in serious accidents; loss of close family members; involvement in a case of Sudden Infant Death Syndrome or stillbirth; suicide in the family; and out-of-the-body experiences. Willingness to call upon one's own experiences is often contingent upon the establishment of a good atmosphere of sharing, and may need to be triggered by a particular topic or class discussion. But no death educator should neglect the resources embodied in his or her own students. Death education itself is a self-help and mutual-help experience.

Another set of materials that has recently become available for death education is a *Course by Newspaper* entitled, "Death and

Dying: Challenge and Change." This is an unusual resource, that is intended to be used with an explicit link to the community. Courses by Newspaper is a national program originated and administered by University Extension, University of California, San Diego, with primary funding from the National Endowment for the Humanities. This particular project was prepared by Robert Fulton and offered in newspapers throughout the country in winter 1979. The foundation of the course is a series of 15 articles of approximately 1200 words each designed to be published in local newspapers on a weekly basis. They constitute the "lectures" for the course; their authors are its visiting "faculty." The publication of these articles in newspapers serves the first aim of the project. Beyond that, the project seeks affiliation with local two- and four-year colleges and universities in order to achieve credit granting or noncredit arrangements. Alternatively, where no local institution participates or when classroom attendance would be impossible, extension credit can be accomplished through the University of California.

□   □   □

We conclude this section with a brief word of caution. Responsible death education is not an impersonal summation of syllabus, textbook, a few films, and some speakers or field trips. That is one reason why we have not included in this guide reproductions of course outlines or sample syllabi. We believe that individual instructors will want to shape their courses to their own strengths, the student population that is being served, the resources that are available, and the goals established for the particular course. In so doing, the instructor will want to test each resource for the advantages and disadvantages that its use will offer. Ordination to the ministry does not make every member of the clergy capable of effectively resolving the profound mysteries of death, just as a medical or nursing degree does not guarantee its holder to be a caring person, and not every dying patient or bereaved survivor will have something profound or even articulate to say. Some potential speakers are willing to appear as part of their own coping (which may only be a passing need); others have a financial, personal, or ideological stake in their presentation. Thus, teaching an effective course on death, dying, and bereavement is not like being ringmaster at a circus composed of an unrelated series of speakers, trips, and events. The instructor must choose from among many possible resources. He or she must be willing to modify those choices in light of their tested effectiveness and in the interests of long-term growth and development. And the death educator must make a special effort to integrate all of the elements that are selected into a meaningful organic whole. This hard work of preparation and follow-up is necessary if the goals of the educational process are to be properly respected. Our object here is to suggest resources, but it is important to take care in the use of these potential riches for the task of education about death.

Appendix: Additional Entries

The following entries were received as the book was going to press.

PRINTED RESOURCES

Adams, D. W. *The psychosocial care of the child and his family in childhood cancer: An annotated bibiography.* Hamilton, Ontario: McMaster University Medical Centre, 1979.

Anabiosis. A regular digest of news for the membership of the Association for the Scientific Study of Near-Death Phenomena. P.O. Box 2309, East Peoria, IL 61611.

Barton D., Crowder, M. K., & Flexner, J. M. Teaching about dying and death in the multidisciplinary student group. *Omega*, 1979-1980, *10*, 265-270.

Beinecke, J. A. *Death and the secondary school student.* Washington, DC: University Press of America, 1979.

Berg, C. D. Life and death drawings in adolesence. *Illinois School Arts*, 1979, *79*, 42-44.

Birx, C. R. *Concepts of death presented in contemporary realistic children's literature: A content analysis.* Unpublished doctoral dissertation, Northern Arizona University, 1979.

Bryant, E. H. Teacher in crisis: A classmate is dying. *Elementary School Journal*, 1978, *78*, 232-241.

Cappiello, L. A., & Troyer, R. E. Study of the role of health educators in teaching about death and dying. *Journal of School Health*, 1979, *49*, 397-399.

Cook, M. J. B. *Effect of bibliotherapy on college students as revealed in their emotional acceptance of death and dying.* Unpublished doctoral dissertation, 1979, University of Akron.

Crase, D. Exemplary resources for students and teachers of death education. Ten pages, privately circulated by the author from the College of Education, Memphis State University, Memphis, TN 38152.

Dorr, R. F. *Death education in McGuffey's readers, 1836-1896.* Unpublished doctoral dissertation, University of Minnesota, 1979.

Duncan, C. C. *Teaching children about death: A rationale and curriculum guide to grades K-12.* Unpublished doctoral dissertation, Boston College, 1979.

Frederick, D. L., & Frederick, D. *Death education and counseling: A training manual.* New York: Pilgrimage, 1978.

Freeman, J. T. *Aging: Its history and literature.* New York: Human Sciences Press, 1979.

Hargrove, E. L. *An exploratory study of children's ideas about death, with a view toward developing an explanatory model.* Unpublished doctoral dissertation, North Texas State University, 1979.

Kane, B. Children's concepts of death. *Journal of Genetic Psychology*, 1979, *134*, 141-153.

Langley, S. *An exploratory study of the effects of age, ethnicity, religion, education, sex, and health on the formation of death-related behaviors.* Unpublished doctoral dissertation, New York University, 1979.

Mayans, A. A workshop: Coping with death and dying for educators and school counselors. *The School Counselor*, 1978, *26*, 62-63.

McClam, P. A. *The effects of death education on fear of death and death anxiety among health-care and helping professionals.* Unpublished doctoral dissertation, University of South Carolina, 1978.

Myers, J. E., Wass, H., & Murphey, M., Jr. Ethnic differences in death anxiety among elderly persons. *Death Education*, in press.

Pope, A. J. Children's attitudes toward death. *Health Education*, 1979, *10*, 27-29.

Rosenthal, N. R., & Terkelson, C. Death education and counseling: A survey of counselors and counselor educators. *Counselor Education and Supervision*, 1978, *18*, 109-114.

Schachter, S. C. Death and dying education in a medical school curriculum. *Journal of Medical Education*, 1979, *54*, 661-663.

Steinhausen, G. W. *Indentification of variables which predict college student acceptance of described teaching approaches for death education.* Unpublished doctoral dissertation, Southern Illinois University at Carbondale, 1979.

Taylor, S. *Personalization of the death, dying, and grieving processes in a selected group of student nurses.* Unpublished doctoral dissertation, East Texas State University, 1979.

Wass, H. Aging and death education for elderly persons. *Educational Gerontology*, 1980, *5*, 79–90.

Wass, H., & Towry, B. J. Children's death concepts and ethnicity. *Death Education*, in press.

Wass, H., Richards, R. S., Angenendt, S., Fitch, M., Drake, D., & Stergios, J. Effectiveness of short-term death education programs for adults. *Essence*, submitted for publication.

Watkins, B. T. Bias charged in a course on death and dying: Courses by newspaper. *Chronicle of Higher Education*, 1979, *18*, p. 9.

Wittmaier, B. C. Some unexpected attitudinal consequences of a short course on death. *Omega*, 1979–1980, *10*, 271–275.

AUDIOVISUAL RESOURCES

And We Were Sad, Remember? (HS, A) In a 20-minute dramatized episode, a small family group (mother, father, and 2 young children) reacts to grandmother's death. Then there is a 10-minute discussion involving various children and adults about what it is like to lose a parent. The major point made is that it is not easy, but that children must always know the truth. This program is one of a series called "Footsteps," sponsored by the U.S. Office of Education, on approaches to parenting. A viewer's guide to the whole series may be obtained from Consumer Information Center, Pueblo, CO, 81009. The film is available from the National Audiovisual Center, Reference Department, National Archives and Records Service, Washington, DC 20409, color film, 30 minutes.

Attitudes toward Death. (HS, A) Dr. David C. Thomasma, director of the University of Tennessee Program on Human Values and Ethics, is the author of this set of six hour-long television programs: "Funeral Practices, Rituals and Grief"; "Death as a Foreign Policy Tool"; "The Death Penalty"; "Sickness, Aging and Dying"; "Euthanasia"; and "American Attitudes about Death". Write Jerry Franklin, Production Manager, WKNO-TV, Box 80,000, Memphis, TN 38152.

Basic Principles of Terminal Care. (P) This is a general introductory survey for medical professionals. Communications in Learning, audiocassette, 28 minutes.

Begin with Goodbye. (A,P) This is a six-film series of dramatizations, starring noted actors, of various life crises, including dying and death. Write for descriptive brochure. Mass Media Ministries.

Children and Death. (A) The topic is introduced and explored with an audience of parents, teachers, counselors, medical personnel, and clergy in mind. Wolfelt Productions, 814 W. Charles St., Muncie, IN 47305, color filmstrip (or slides) and audiocassette, discussion manual, 15 minutes, 1979.

The Connecticut Hospice Training Film. (P) To provide a detailed analysis of the interdisciplinary nature of the hospice caregiving team, this program focuses on the treatment given one patient, from admission to point of death. The Hospice Institute for Education, Training and Research, 765 Prospect St., New Haven, CT 06511, 1980.

Death and Dying as Related to Staff Interaction. (P) In this lecture, caregiving staff are urged to view terminally ill patients as whole persons, and are offered insights into the nature and effects of various types of pain (physical, social, spiritual). Communications in Learning, audiocassette with handout, 30 minutes.

Death and Dying: Emotional Components. (P) Nursing assistants are the intended audience of this lecture surveying the nature of grief, the "stages" of dying, caregiving for dying patient and the family, truthtelling, and other basic topics. Communications in Learning, audiocassette with six slides and printed handout, 21 minutes.

Death and Dying: Euthanasia: The Right to Live and the Right to Die. (A, P) Dr. C. Charles Bachmann clarifies various definitions of the term *euthanasia*, differentiates between "active" and "passive" euthanasia, and then discusses the "living will" and the patient's right to refuse medical treatment. Communications in Learning, audiocassette, 52 minutes.

Death and Dying: From the Perspective of One Intimately Involved—The So-Called Terminal Phase. (A, P) Dr. C. Charles Bachmann interviews a terminally ill patient who seems to have reached a level of acceptance, in part through strong religious faith. Communications in Learning, audiocassette, 58 minutes.

Death and Dying: Physical Components. (P) Nursing assistants are the intended audience of this lecture surveying the physiological and psychological signs of imminent death and outlining the nursing assistant's duties in preparing the body after death. Communications in Learning, audiocassette with six slides and printed handout, 16 minutes.

Death and Dying: The Funeral: Its Function and Place in Society—Life's Fitting Tribute. (A) As its title suggests, this lecture by Dr. C. Charles Bachmann presents the funeral as a necessary and valuable part of the mourning process. Communications in Learning, audiocassette, 59 minutes.

Death and Dying: When a Child Dies. (A, P) Dr. C. Charles Bachmann interviews a mother who has lost several of her children to a genetic disease. Communications in Learning, audiocassette, 43 minutes.

The Denial of Death: No Time for Heroes. (A, P) This lecture presentation addressing professional caregivers is a detailed analysis of death denial, both in society generally and in terminally ill patients. Communications in Learning, audiocassette, 43 minutes.

A Documentary News Series on Hospice Care. (A) KWGN-TV in Denver produced this news report on the Boulder County Hospice. The focus is on one patient and his family as they receive treatment. Write to Mr. Eric Schmidt, KWGN Television, 550 Lincoln, Denver, CO 50203.

Dust to Dust. (HS, A) Armageddon has happened. The earth is barren, ash-strewn, scoured of civilization and life—except for a latter-day Adam and Eve who state bleakly about them and, in evocatively poetic language, wonder how it all came about. Mass Media Associates, color film, 15 minutes, 1972.

The Dying Patient. (P) Hospital housekeeping staff are the intended audience of this lecture, which surveys the "stages" of dying and other general background information about dying patients. Housekeepers are helped to know when to call for medical help, and are given a series of do's and don't's when working in a dying patient's room. Communications in Learning, audiocassette and 13 slides, 17 minutes.

Ethical Issues and Dilemmas. (A) The producers advertise this audiocassette program as a "minicourse" in a variety of ethical issues of concern today—for example, abortion, euthanasia, and extraordinary care. The focus is on the practical: ethical decisions cannot always be divorced from political or economic concerns. Lansford Publishing Company, P.O. Box 8711, 1088 Lincoln Ave., San Jose, CA 95155. Six audiocassettes, printed outlines for students, teacher's manual.

Euthanasia: Pro or Con. (P) Nurses are the intended audience of this lecture, which surveys various definitions and applications of the term *euthanasia*, discusses the nature and extent of individual choice, and outlines the responsibilities of nurses in these matters. Communications in Learning, audiocassette, 33 minutes.

Family Reactions to Stillbirth. (P) This lecture presentation urges medical professionals to deal more sympathetically with such situations, and offers useful background information and suggestions. Communications in Learning, audiocassette, 16 minutes.

Four Women: Breast Cancer. (A) Four women who underwent mastectomies are interviewed before and after their surgery. General audiences, individuals in similar situations, and caregiving professionals can learn useful lessons from this film, "a remarkable testimony to the ability of people to find strength and comfort in crises." Filmmakers Library, color film, 55 minutes.

Good Grief. (A) This comparative study of contemporary U.S. funeral practices focuses initially on the needs of survivors immediately after a loss. Mourners must be allowed, first, to fully express their grief; second, to make major decisions about funeral, burial, and memorial arrangements; and third, to actively participate in the funeral ceremonies. The thesis of this program is that neither traditional U.S. funerals nor memorial society arrangements meet these needs as well as the approach of what is called "the liberating funeral director," typified by Mr. Roy Nichols of Chagrin Falls, Ohio. Nichols, other funeral directors and representatives of memorial societies, and survivors who have experienced the three funeral modes in question participate in discussion of these issues. Write WBGU-TV, Bowling Green State University, Bowling Green, OH 43403, color videotape, 60 minutes.

The Grief Phenomenon: A Therapy for Bereavement. (A, P) This lecture surveys grief and mourning as both natural and necessary processes in coping with loss. Communications in Learning, audio-cassette, 47 minutes.

Handle with Care. (HS, A) A total of 42 elderly people, some weak, bedridden, and institutionalized, others still vigorously active in home and community, are asked three questions and are filmed as they reply: (1) What is the hardest thing you must face when dying? (2) When it comes time for you to die, what would make the experience easier for you? (3) In your opinion, what happens to you after you die? The simple format of this program belies the tremendous impact it has on all audiences, young or old, layperson or professional caregiver. Extension Media Service, c/o Administrative Office, Berkeley Public Library, 2090 Kittredge St., Berkeley, CA 94704, color film or videotape.

Hospice: An Alternative Way to Care for the Dying. (A) Focusing on the work of the Riverside Hospice in Boonton, New Jersey, this documentary program introduces general audiences to the hospice concept. Billy Budd Films, color film, 26 minutes.

Hospice Care: An Alternative. (A, P) The Boulder County Hospice Home Care Program is introduced in this slide-audiocassette presentation. Problems in grief and bereavement are covered, as are components of staff training. Patients and their families are interviewed. General audiences unfamiliar with hospices, as well as community and professional groups planning their own hospice programs, will find this introduction to the concept informative. Boulder County Hospice, Inc., 2118 14th St., Boulder, CO 80302, 25 minutes.

Hospice Training Film. (A, P) This new film introduces the hospice concept and describes a particular home care program in California. Write Hospital/Home Health Care, 23228 Hawthorne Blvd., Torrance, CA 90505, 12 minutes.

An Introduction to the Hospice Concept. (P) This lecture traces the growth of hospice, describes its characteristics and its advantages, defines various models of hospice care, and points to areas needing further study. Communications in Learning, color filmstrip and audiocassette, 22 minutes.

Just Hold My Hand. (A, P) Two middle-aged women, both dying of cancer, are filmed during the last 6 months of their lives. One is a widow, a mother of seven, whose "most horrifying thought is having to leave my family." Pressures, problems, and conflicts in the family group and in the individual children are revealed. The other woman, a professional research biologist, is especially troubled by her inability to work and the concomitant (for her) loss of human dignity; thus she decides to stop her chemotherapy treatments. Both women discuss euthanasia at some length. The mother of seven would never consider interfering with the plan of God, but the scientist disagrees: "I say I'll never do it, but I know it's in my medicine cabinet. Maybe I will. . . ." The overall theme of this impressive and very moving filmed documentary is how two people overcome great odds to live their last months meaningfully. Doctors Ned Cassem and Melvin Krant, involved in the care of these patients, comment. Write Mr. Howard Finkelstein, Boston Broadcasters, Inc., 5 TV Place, Needham Br., Boston, MA 02190, color videotape, 60 minutes.

Life, Death and the American Woman. (A) The thesis of this documentary is that "most women give little attention to their bodies until they begin to register pain." The cases of 10 women suddenly facing a variety of crises—cancer, complications in pregnancy, career hazards, and menopause—are presented. Best Films, P.O. Box 725, Del Mar, CA 92104, color film with discussion guide, 51 minutes.

Live for Life. (A) Thinking his life has lost its meaning, a man attempts suicide, only to discover new insights into handling the real problems in his life. This short animated film would be useful in triggering discussion. Filmmakers Library, color film, 12 minutes, 1979.

Minnie Remembers. (A, P) Now that she is old, institutionalized and alone, Minnie remembers painfully the caring and sharing of her youth and her marriage. Her grown children, infrequent and uncomfortable visitors, call her "Mother" or "Grandma"; no one knows her name anymore. This very striking program, excellent for triggering discussion, is based on a poem by Donna Swanson. Mass Media Ministries, color film, 5 minutes, 1976.

Minnie: This Is the Life. (A, P) The subtitle is ironic. Minnie's life, especially in her old age and in her dying, was impoverished, painful, and lonely. Most people ignored her; those who came to help came too late. There are important insights here for caregivers. Mid-America Resource and Training Center on Aging, 5218 Oak St., Kansas City, MO 64112, color film, 30 minutes.

Murder One. (A) Six convicted murders are asked why they killed. These portraits of personalities and motives offer valuable insights into a particular kind of death not fully explored in audiovisuals. Best Films, P.O. Box 725, Del Mar, CA 92140, color film with teacher's guide, 46 minutes.

An Overview and Perspective: The Pornography of Death. (A, P) This is an introductory lecture survey of basic issues in death and dying in the United States. Communications in Learning, audiocassette, 45 minutes.

Patient's Attitude to Death. (A, P) Despite a mastectomy for breast carcinoma, Alison is dying of the disease. Her feelings about her prognosis, her fears for herself and her family, and the role of her religious faith in her experience are reported in this interview. Communications in Learning, audiocassette, 31 minutes.

The Question of Euthanasia. (A, P) Dr. C. Charles Bachmann and the founders of Hospice, Buffalo, discuss "euthanasia," meaning "good death," in a hospice context. Communications in Learning, audiocassette, 59 minutes.

The Question of Suicide. (A, P) A panel of professionals discusses the causes and prevention of suicide, and surveys society's atttudes toward it. Communications in Learning, audiocassette, 66 minutes.

Religion Update: A Panel Discussion. (P) Nurses are the intended audience of this program which surveys the attitudes of the three major faiths toward various life crises. By knowing something of the religious orientations of their seriously ill and dying patients, nurses can better meet their needs. Communications in Learning, audiocassette, 36 minutes.

Richie. (HS, A) The theme of this story is teen-age drug addiction and its impact on a family. Richie's parents cannot comprehend his increasing dependency on drugs and his resulting behavior changes. Disintegrating communication results in incresingly hostile confrontations in the home, climaxing in the father's shooting of Richie. This program is an edited selection from the feature film, "The Death of Richie," based on a book by Thomas Thompson. Learning Corporation of America, color film, 31 minutes, 1978.

Significant Loss: The Grief Phenomenon in Losses other than Death. (A, P) Our own dying and the death of someone close are perhaps the most painful losses we may experience in this life, but they are not the only ones. For example, a divorce, loss of a job, an amputation, or a house fire give rise to various levels of grief. These experiences, too, must be mourned, must be accepted, and life must begin again. General audiences and professional caregivers are offered a broad and useful concept of grief in this presentation. Communications in Learning, audiocassette, 46 minutes.

Smiles. (A) This is a film on aging developed by Dan Leviton and George Callaghan. Adults' Health and Developmental Program, University of Maryland, College Park, MD 20740, color film, 29 minutes.

Some Days It's Harder to Say Yes: Suicide in the Classroom. (HS) Offered here are interviews with two high school students who are suicidal, together with related information and insight into teens and suicide. Highly Specialized Promotions, color videotape, 30 minutes, 1979.

Why Me? (MS, HS, A) The "stages" of dying described by Dr. Kübler-Ross are dramatized in this prize-winning cartoon story of a man informed that his death is imminent. The surprise ending has been called "uplifting," offering a positive message for "living our remaining moments to their fullest." Pyramid Films, color film or videotape, 10 minutes.

Note. Item numbers 57, 67, and 356 in the Audiovisual Resources section now have a U.S. distributor: Communications in Learning. Item number 356 has a new title: *Nature and Management of Pain in Terminal Malignant Disease* (3rd Ed.).

AUDIOCASSETTES

Big Sur recordings, the official tape recording service for the Esalen Institute, the Association for Humanistic Psychology, the C. G. Jung Institute of San Francisco, and other groups, has available nearly 40 audiocassettes in many areas of death and dying, recordings of presentations made at meetings of the sponsoring organizations. A list of titles, speakers, and dates follows:

Are Fears of Dying Fears of Living in Disguise? Hank Kavanaugh, 1974.

The Art of Dying: An Overview. Hank Basayne, Patty Driver Scott, Joseph Chilton Pearce, Robert Kavanaugh, 1974.

Attitudes toward Death. Edgar Jackson, 1974.

Beyond Death and Dying. Rev. James Diamond, Raymond Moody and Panel, 1976.

Blacks, Chicanos, Oriental-Americans and Death. Mokusen Meyuki, Ronald Lunceford, Richard Kalish, 1974.

Choosing Your Death: An Experiential Exercise. Hank Basayne, 1974.

Clinical Evidences of Reincarnation. Ernest Pecci, 1976.

Cultural Aspects of Death and Dying. Jonathan Garfield, 1975.

Death Personalization Exercises. Charles Garfield, 1976.

Experiences of Dying: A Matter of Style. E. Mansell Pattison, 1974.

Fear of Death and Terminal Illness Counseling. Keith Kerr and Peggy Kerr, 1975.

Free Fall and Death. Joseph Chilton Pearce, 1974.

The Function of the Death Guide. Charles Garfield, 1975.

Human Values and the Death Rite. Jay Calhoun, 1974.

An Invitation to Explore the Art of Dying. Hank Basayne and Edgar Jackson, 1974.

The Last Hours of Life. Elizabeth Kübler-Ross, Rev. James Diamond, Viola Reibe, Samuel Weinstein, 1976.

Letting Go. Edith Stauffer, 1974.

A Life Span View of Death. Richard Kalish, 1974.

Models of After-Life in Esoteric Traditions. Pascal Kaplan, 1976.

The One Real Death. Murshida Ivy Duce, 1976.

Optional Ways of Dying. Stanislav Grof and Joan Halifax Grof, 1975.

Overcoming the Fear of Death: The Life Counseling Approach. David Cole Gordon, 1975.

The Parabola: A Jungian Viewpoint. Reverend Bishop Edward Crowther, 1974.

Parents and the Dying Child. Eugenia Waechter, 1974.

Perspectives on Death, Dying and Beyond. Pascal Kaplan; Dying as an Altered State of Consciousness. Charles Garfield, 1976.

Presentation and Discussion of "Art of Dying." Edgar Jackson, 1974.

Professional/Personal Involvement with the Dying Patient. Lillian Pearson, 1974.

Professionals are Mortal, Too. Lillian and Leonard Pearson, 1974.

A Psychic Looks beyond Death. Mro and Allan Cohen, 1976.

The Psychology of Karma. Gina Cerminara, 1976.

The Sage Project: Growth Experiences for the Elderly. Ken Dychtwald, 1975.

Ten Years Teaching on Death and Dying. Leonard Pearson, 1974.

Terminal Illness Counseling Experience. Keith Kerr, 1975.

The Transpersonal Experience of Death. Viola Davis, 1974.

Understanding Hallucinations of the Dying. Allan Cohen, 1976.

A Zen Approach to Dying. David Cole Gordon, 1974.

Zen View of Dying. Rev. Jiyu Kennett, Roshi, 1975.

Each audiocassette runs between 1 and $1\frac{1}{2}$ hours, and sells for $8.95. Write Big Sur Recordings, P.O. Box 91, Big Sur, CA 93920 for detailed descriptions of the content of these tapes, and for further information about the work of its sponsoring organizations.

DISTRIBUTORS

American Friends Service Committee, 407 South Dearborn St., Chicago, IL 60605.

ORGANIZATIONAL RESOURCES

Association for the Care of Children in Hospitals, *3615 Wisconsin Avenue, N.W., Washington, DC 20016.* Founded in 1965 the association "seeks to foster and promote the health and well-being of children and families in health care settings by education, interdisciplinary inter-action and planning, and research." Members are chiefly medical and administrative professionals, but interested parents are joining in increasing numbers. The association's publications (a quarterly journal, a newsletter, various bibliographies, and other books) as well as its yearly conventions and study sections address themselves to a whole range of child-care issues, including, for example, the seriously ill child, the dying child, the child with cancer, and children in hospice settings.

Grief Center, Inc, write *Chaplain John Paolini, 4848 Summer St., Lincoln, NE 68506.* This regional community service organization, devoted to grief education and counseling, is run by the clinical pastoral education program staff of the Bryan Memorial Hospital in Lincoln, Nebraska.

Institute for the Seriously Ill and Dying, *Henry Avenue and Abbottsford Road, Philadelphia, PA 19129.* This nonprofit educational and research organization provides training and clinical experience on emotional aspects of terminal disease. Institute programs are designed especially for workers in various medical and psychological disciplines—physicians, psychiatrists, psychologists, psychiatric social workers, nurses, and counselors.

Shell of Hope Institute, *2584 National Drive, Brooklyn, NY 11234.* This organization offers death education and counseling services for a whole range of audiences, from preschool through professional, under the auspices of hospitals, community organization centers, schools, and colleges. The institute also provides personal counseling for dying patients and their families, and for the grief-stricken.

The Tissue Bank, *Naval Medical Research Institute, NNMC, Bethesda, MD 20014.* This facility accepts donations of needed bodily organs and tissues.

Topical Index:
Audiovisual
Resources

Numbers refer to entry numbers.

Aging and old age:
  the aged and their families, 9, 256,
    346, 390, 539, 564, 572
  caring for the aged, 8, 10, 85, 132,
    161, 251, 262, 281, 329, 360,
    390, 392, 397, 444, 539
  general, 10, 11, 232, 244, 251, 252,
    281, 342, 346, 353, 362, 370,
    375, 380, 384, 392, 437, 453,
    465, 468, 532, 535, 543
  institutions for the aged, 42, 197,
    209, 244, 286, 371, 390, 392,
    437, 539, 543, 546, 564, 577
  personal experiences and attitudes
    of the aged, 9, 10, 26, 27, 28,
    161, 209, 224, 256, 284, 286,

Aging and old age, personal experiences
    and attitudes of the aged (*Cont.*):
    312, 329, 342, 360, 361, 372,
    373, 404, 453, 465, 468, 506,
    532, 535, 539, 543, 547, 554,
    577, 578, 588
Attitudes toward life and death in our
    society, general discussions and
    surveys of a variety of topics, 17,
    83, 91, 116, 124, 126, 131, 136,
    147, 149, 151, 157, 162, 163,
    165, 173, 183, 191, 220, 226,
    261, 290, 297, 299, 302, 311,
    331, 332, 363, 380, 394, 395,
    427, 461, 513, 531, 533, 536
Autopsy, 31, 32, 358

Bioethical topics and issues:
  birth defects, 343, 349, 410, 424,
    571, 572
  death with dignity, 30, 149, 151,
    161, 169, 190, 441
  definition of death, 196, 221, 334,
    394, 428, 442, 452
  euthanasia, 38, 135, 190, 221, 335,
    338, 339, 388, 394, 423, 439,
    441, 442, 474
  extraordinary care, 30, 189, 388,
    423, 440, 441, 442, 452, 562
  general, 30, 75, 132, 158, 165, 189,
    190, 196, 221, 271, 344, 388,
    394, 400, 403, 410, 423, 427,
    428, 439, 441, 442, 452, 474,
    562, 571, 572, 573
  patient's refusal of treatment, 82,
    190, 403, 562, 573
  transplants and related issues, 74,
    158, 221, 233, 334, 428, 452,
    466

Cancer:
  caring and caregiving, 19, 20, 21,
    50, 51, 52, 53, 54, 55, 60, 77,
    78, 80, 91, 182, 184, 205,
    253, 325, 330, 366, 416, 417,
    456, 504, 551
  family reactions, 90, 205, 242, 283,
    287, 330, 359, 402, 585
  in children, 20, 65, 90, 287, 359,
    366, 554, 585
  personal reactions to one's diagnosis
    and treatment, 44, 89, 90,
    115, 182, 242, 273, 283, 298,
    304, 327, 359, 377, 402, 413,
    448, 456, 528, 541, 553, 554,
    585
Caring and caregiving (this heading
  identifies those many audiovisual
  materials developed to teach
  understanding of the nature of
  the dying experience, thoughtful
  sympathy for the dying patient,
  and the ability to relate with and
  effectively meet the needs of the
  patient and family members—
  whether those needs are medical,
  emotional, psychological, social,
  spiritual, or practical. Each item
  is labeled for potential audience
  appeal, but the reader will have

Caring and caregiving (*Cont.*):
  to assess his or her own needs
  and experience in making
  choices. Some items obviously
  appeal to sophisticated medical
  professionals with specialized interests, but most of these audiovisuals, even those ostensibly
  addressed to caregivers, have
  value for any audience of mature
  adults who want to relate better
  with the dying. By the same
  token, many AV items addressed
  to general adult audiences have
  much to offer medical professionals who have not had occasion to acquire the relevant skills
  or experience:
  fo: the bereaved: family members
    and/or survivors, before and
    after the death, 56, 57, 59,
    61, 69, 87, 95, 124, 146, 152,
    164, 171, 193, 200, 204, 206,
    235, 263, 385, 416, 419, 421,
    433, 461
  (*See also* Caring and caregiving
    for the dying; Grief and
    bereavement)
  for the dying, 56, 57, 58, 59, 60,
    61, 76, 79, 80, 86, 91, 92,
    97, 112, 115, 119, 121, 122,
    123, 124, 129, 130, 147,
    161, 163, 165, 171, 175,
    176, 177, 178, 183, 184,
    193, 199, 200, 201, 203,
    212, 218, 223, 237, 246,
    253, 263, 278, 282, 285,
    296, 301, 310, 323, 333,
    340, 341, 356, 367, 376,
    377, 386, 395, 398, 399,
    400, 409, 415, 417, 418,
    419, 420, 422, 430, 433,
    461, 463, 470, 510, 516,
    517, 520, 537, 540, 553,
    554, 555, 559, 560, 565
  (*See also* Cancer; Hospice)
  for the dying child, 65, 69, 70, 81,
    91, 130, 174, 178, 183, 287,
    314, 400, 554, 555
Cemeteries and burial customs, 63,
  124, 179, 198, 240, 311, 369,
  382, 551
  (*See also* Funerals; Memorialization)

Children's attitudes and responses to
     death (general), 66, 67, 68, 72,
     73, 81, 91, 107, 127, 180, 257,
     264, 303, 314, 350, 425, 426,
     461, 475, 533, 554, 570
Children's attitudes and responses to
     death of someone close—parent,
     grandparent, sibling, other
     relative, friend, 14, 24, 25, 69,
     103, 141, 144, 147, 150, 264,
     294, 314, 348, 425, 451, 475,
     509, 548, 551, 557, 563, 570,
     581
     (*See also* Bereavement; Grief)
Clergymen as caregivers of the dying
     and the bereaved, 14, 77, 97,
     122, 178, 385, 387, 558
Cross-Cultural Aspects of Death:
     general, 98, 118, 139, 165, 214,
          216, 231, 248, 305, 370, 393,
          429
     in particular countries or areas:
          Africa (Bantu tribes), 231
          Africa (Botswana), 139
          Africa (Ghana), 227
          American Indian (Navajo), 25
          American Indian (Nez Perce),
               284
          Australia (Aborigines), 347, 411
          Bolivia, 313, 468
          Canada (Eskimo), 255
          India, 139
          Japan, 445
          Mexico, 106
          Montenegro, 383
          Moro, 319
          New Guinea, 108, 139
          New Hebrides, 319
          Solomon Islands, 319
          Trobriand Islands, 231
          Venezuela, 315
Cryonics, 102, 211, 260
Cystic Fibrosis, 96

Death and dying, general introductory
     surveys of a variety of basic con-
     cepts and issues, 84, 142, 163,
     165, 289, 291, 302, 303, 355,
     395, 414, 441, 461, 550, 551,
     555, 567
Death themes in art, 156, 165, 393

Death themes in literature:
     general, 128, 143, 154, 165, 393,
          513, 518, 519
     poetry on audiocassette or film,
          236, 247, 312, 374, 392,
          404, 405, 518
     short stories and novels on film, 14,
          23, 25, 35, 64, 107, 207,
          220, 248, 308, 309, 311,
          314, 328, 368, 379, 475,
          509, 551, 556
Death themes in music, 155, 165, 389,
     393, 463, 513, 586
Donating the body or body parts after
     death, 233, 270, 279, 302
Drug abuse and death, 104, 137, 219,
     354, 587
Dying and death in the family (the
     dynamics of terminal illness and
     death, modes of grieving, con-
     flicts, exploration of the "life
     cycle" or "the generations"), 12,
     14, 23, 24, 25, 40, 90, 103, 115,
     144, 147, 150, 172, 186, 203,
     206, 223, 253, 256, 264, 272,
     287, 299, 314, 352, 359, 390,
     402, 407, 433, 447, 467, 475,
     516, 522, 524, 538, 545, 546,
     548, 551, 557, 562, 568, 569,
     581, 585
Dying and death of a spouse, personal
     responses, 23, 87, 88, 192, 242,
     294, 308, 310, 401, 522, 523,
     541, 545
Dying and death of one's child,
     parental reactions, 12, 90, 110,
     113, 124, 134, 148, 150, 152,
     207, 208, 230, 235, 287, 294,
     326, 432, 459, 507, 546, 561,
     581, 585
     (*See also* Dying and death in the
          family; Grief and
          bereavement)

Funerals:
     alternative, contemporary, or
          humanist, 254, 292, 302,
          450, 545
     objections to traditional funeral
          customs and funeral directors,
          225, 311, 458

Funerals (*Cont.*):
  traditional, (many of these materials
    are sponsored and distributed
    by the funeral industry), 18,
    22, 40, 118, 124, 125, 133,
    136, 163, 165, 167, 187,
    202, 213, 214, 215, 216,
    217, 225, 229, 240, 267,
    276, 280, 295, 311, 313,
    336, 369, 382, 391, 393,
    455, 458, 461, 542, 544,
    551, 558

Grief and bereavement (The emphasis
  is on the emotional dynamics):
  experienced by children, 14, 24,
    25, 69, 103, 147, 150, 318,
    352, 570, 581
  experienced by family members
    (*see* Caring and caregiving for
    the bereaved; Dying and
    death in the family)
  experienced by parents, 110, 148,
    150, 152, 207, 208, 230,
    326, 432, 459, 507, 581
    (*See also* Dying and death of
    one's child)
  experienced by a spouse, 23, 39,
    87, 88, 238, 308, 310, 352,
    421, 516, 522, 523
    (*See also* Dying and death of a
    spouse; Widow and
    widower)
  general, 40, 95, 125, 136, 140,
    144, 165, 172, 228, 229,
    238, 294, 306, 307, 318,
    320, 322, 460, 461, 516,
    520, 534, 541, 563, 570,
    581

Hospice care, background information,
  philosophy, treatment policies,
  and practices, 164, 170, 245,
  275, 356, 449, 514, 515
Hospitals, 115, 246, 263, 385
  (*See also* Caring and caregiving)

Kidney disease, 175, 333
Kübler-Ross, Dr. Elisabeth, presenting
  her own views, 80, 84, 91, 112,
  122, 123, 174, 278, 285, 323,
  376, 470, 537, 555

Kübler-Ross (*Cont.*):
  (*See also* Caring and caregiving for
  the dying)

"Life and life" experiences and
  phenomena, 123, 265, 368, 526

Memorialization (gravestones and
  markers), 124, 214, 225, 240,
  311, 337, 472
  (*See also* Cemeteries; Funerals)
Music therapy for the dying, 389,
  463

Organizations:
  Make Today Count, 317
  National Cancer Foundation (Cancer
    Care, Inc.), 467
  SHANTI Project, 200
  Suicide Clinics, 490
    (*See also* Suicide, intervention
    and prevention)
  Widow-to-Widow Program, 575

Pain, 50, 321, 340, 356, 395, 429,
  514, 516
Personal experiences, Suicide attempts
  (first-person accounts) (*see*
  Suicide)
Personal experiences with diagnoses of
  terminal illness and related
  attitudinal changes (First-person
  responses to one's imminent
  death), 44, 74, 89, 90, 115, 145,
  166, 172, 186, 191, 242, 247,
  255, 259, 272, 273, 278, 283,
  296, 298, 301, 304, 317, 327,
  377, 402, 413, 448, 464, 516,
  522, 524, 528, 538, 541, 553,
  554, 562, 584
Personal experiences with near-death
  and related attitudinal changes
  (first-person accounts), 2, 3,
  293, 505

Religion and death (religious responses
  to death; religion as providing
  comfort or consolation to the
  dying and/or to the bereaved),
  14, 82, 114, 123, 165, 166,
  226, 261, 297, 300, 314, 341,

Religion and death *(Cont.)*:
  344, 351, 369, 381, 394, 431,
  433, 434, 469, 516, 524, 527,
  538, 552, 553, 562, 566

Sudden and/or accidental death,
  attitudes, responses, treatment
  modalities, 43, 76, 91, 100,
  357, 476, 505, 511, 521, 523,
  536, 581
Sudden Infant Death Syndrome
  (SIDS), 7, 49, 93, 94, 378, 477,
  478, 583
Suicide:
  in the aged, 4, 322, 468, 493
  causal factors, 15, 33, 47, 62, 101,
    153, 159, 168, 480, 481,
    483, 484, 487, 489, 491,
    501, 502, 503, 569
  for a cause, 149, 151, 445
  effects on survivors, 6, 62, 153,
    192, 406, 447, 482, 487, 569
  general, 15, 16, 29, 47, 101, 153,
    168, 169, 222, 239, 258,
    268, 322, 324, 354, 406,
    408, 412, 454, 473, 479,
    482, 485, 486, 487, 490,
    491, 492, 494, 496, 497,
    498, 499, 580
  intervention and prevention, 6, 16,
    48, 239, 268, 481, 487, 491,
    494, 496, 502, 503, 525
  personal experiences, suicide and
    attempts, 159, 168, 482, 580
  warning signs, 15, 16, 48, 101, 239,
    258, 406, 408, 438, 481,
    483, 487, 488, 491, 495,
    499, 500, 502, 525, 580
  in the young (adolescents,
    teenagers), 5, 6, 16, 48, 159,
    222, 239, 438, 447, 461,
    488, 492, 503, 512, 587

Teaching children about death, audiovisuals for preschool, grade
  school, and middle school levels
  (high school teachers may be
  guided by the HS audience labels
  given with many AV items, or
  use their own judgment concerning items marked A, for adult
  audiences), 25, 107, 117, 141,
  180, 181, 196, 248, 264, 348,

Teaching children about death, audiovisuals for preschool, grade
  school, and middle school levels
  (Cont.):
  350, 364, 451, 548, 549, 550,
  551, 557, 587
Teaching children about death,
  discussion and techniques, 67,
  68, 69, 127, 138, 195, 249, 364,
  446, 508
Trigger films (These are on a variety of
  topics, to foster discussion or
  "break the ice," and are effective
  for most audiences at the
  beginning of units of instruction
  on death and dying, especially
  where members of the audience
  are not familiar with one another
  or with the teacher. Many of
  these audiovisual materials are
  less than 20 minutes long and do
  not claim to be thorough surveys
  of their topics. Headings offered
  here are suggestive only: the
  concept of what could be a
  "trigger" will vary with
  individual teachers, their classroom goals, and the perceived
  needs of students.):
  aging gracefully, 375, 588
  aging ungracefully, 543
  attitudes toward life and death,
      185, 188, 210, 220, 266,
      309, 435, 513, 530, 553, 586
  autopsy, 32
  concentration camps, 257, 363
  dead body, 109, 556
  death of a father, 210
  death of a mother, 435
  death of a son, 12
  dying for a cause, 274
  life cycle, the generations, 41, 99,
      180, 181, 210, 277, 288,
      365, 546
  living on death row, 293
  mass death, 328, 363
  nuclear holocaust, 13, 241, 243,
      457
  overcrowded lifeboat, 1, 443
  responsibility for the lives and
      deaths of others, 188, 236,
      250, 274
  sudden death, or close calls, 2, 3,
      43, 76, 379, 511, 523

Trigger films (*Cont.*):
  suicide, 4, 33, 149, 586
  vulgarization of death in society,
    266
  war, violence, and related issues,
    34, 36, 45, 46, 99, 105, 157,
    160, 243, 250, 316, 379,
    471, 530, 553
  what is important in life and what
    is not, 33, 149, 460

War and death, attitudes to war, to
  killing, to violence, 13, 34, 36,
  37, 46, 64, 108, 160, 241, 243,
  269, 274, 316, 368, 379, 457,
  471, 530, 536, 556

War and death, attitudes to war, to
  killing, to violence (*Cont.*):
  (*See also* Attitudes toward life and
    death)
Widow and widower, 39, 87, 88, 192,
  238, 252, 294, 310, 352, 401,
  413, 462, 468, 516, 523, 529,
  541, 574, 575
  (*See also* Dying and death of a
    spouse; Grief and bereave-
    ment; Grieving and adjusting;
    Living as a widow or widower)
Wills, insurance, estates, and other
  practical matters, 133, 165, 276,
  579, 582
  (*See also* Cemeteries; Funerals;
    Memorialization)

Topical Index:
Organizational
Resources

Numbers refer to page numbers.

Abortion (educational and/or pressure
    organizations with various points
    of view on abortion, family
    planning, population control and
    related topics: definition of life,
    quality of life, definition of
    personhood, and so on), 252,
    261, 264, 265, 266, 267
    (*See also* Euthanasia)

Body disposition (organizations
    concerned with the body or
    parts of it after death; groups
    under Funerals may also be
    involved in helping survivors of a
    death):

Body disposition (*Cont.*):
    cemeteries, 252
    cremation, 256
    cryonics, 256, 260
    donation to medical science (Most
        medical schools throughout
        the country need cadavers for
        scientific research and to
        train physicians, and are
        happy to receive bequests.
        The degree of need may vary,
        however, and each school
        may impose its own
        restrictions.):
    bodily organs: eyes, 257
        general, 254, 260

Body disposition, donation to medical
    science, bodily organs (*Cont.*):
        inner ear structures, 256,
            265, 266
        kidneys, 262, 264
        pituitary glands, 264
        other donations: eyeglasses, 265
        gold fillings, 258
        pills, 258
    funerals, alternative, 256, 266
    funerals, traditional, commercial,
        259, 263, 265
    monuments (memorialization), 254

Educational, research, scholarly
    organizations (All of the
    organizations discussed in this
    book are educational in the
    broad sense of the term. Many
    conduct or sponsor research in
    addition to their other activities.
    Those organizations noted here,
    however, exist exclusively to
    engage in specialized educational
    programs: conducting and
    publishing scholarly and
    scientific research, developing
    and implementing professional
    training programs, and creating
    curricula and learning materials
    for various audiences. Death
    educators at all levels should be
    familiar with the work of these
    groups, which include American
    Association of Suicidology;
    Center for Death Education and
    Research; Concern for Dying,
    An Educational Council;
    Equinox Institute; Forum for
    Death Education and Counseling,
    Inc.; Foundation of Thanatology;
    The Hastings Center: Institute of
    Society, Ethics and the Life
    Sciences; International
    Association for Suicide
    Prevention; National Hospice
    Organization; National Research
    and Information Center; and
    Widowed Persons Service), 252,
    255, 256, 257, 258, 263, 264,
    268

Euthanasia (educational and/or
    pressure groups with various
    points of view on euthanasia and
    related topics: death with
    dignity, the living will, allocation
    of scarce medical resources,
    definition and application of
    extraordinary treatment,
    definition of life, definition of
    death, quality of life, definition
    of personhood; some are also
    active in abortion issues), 252,
    253, 255, 264, 266, 267

Helping organizations (depending on
    the individual group, helping can
    take various forms: medical and
    other professional treatment,
    guidance, counseling, education,
    rehabilitation, training, funding,
    sponsorship of research, and/or
    assisting in the problems of
    survivors):
    the aged, 251, 257, 261, 262
    the dying, the seriously ill and the
        disabled from various causes,
        and/or their families: Birth
        defects, 266
    cancer, 251, 252, 254, 258, 259,
        260, 262, 263, 266, 267
    cystic fibrosis, 256
    Down's syndrome, 261, 263
    emotionally handicapped, 261,
        264
    general, 255, 260, 262, 266
        (*See also* Body disposition)
    heart-circulatory system disease,
        253, 260, 267
    kidney disease, 262
    laryngectomees, 258
    leukemia, 251, 259
    mastectomees, 266
    mental illness, 261, 263
    multiple sclerosis, 264
    muscular dystrophy, 261
    ostomates, 267
    physically handicapped, 263,
        264, 267
    respiratory diseases, 253, 254
    sickle cell anemia, 263
    spina bifida, 263, 267

Helping organizations, the dying, the
   seriously ill and the disabled
   from various causes, and/or their
   families (*Cont.*):
      stroke, 267
      sudden infant death syndrome,
         259, 265
   parents who have lost children (As
      noted in these listings, there
      are many national
      organizations and their local
      affiliates devoted to helping
      parents whose children fall
      victim to particular diseases.
      For example, groups of
      parents of children with
      cancer have the Candle-
      lighters as their national
      umbrella organization. Many
      other groups, are formed and
      operate regionally and locally,
      often in conjunction with
      social service or pastoral care
      departments of hospitals and
      clinics. Death educators
      should inquire locally for
      parent-to-parent organiza-
      tions serving their area.), 252,
      254, 255, 259, 262, 265,
      266, 267
   widows, widowers, 255, 261, 265,
      267, 268
   (*See also* Self-help)

Institutions (The national organizations
   listed here may be of limited
   help to the death educator. Ask
   at local facilities for tours and/
   or presentations by professional
   personnel.):
   hospices, 263
   hospitals, 253, 255
   nursing homes, 251, 253

Self-Help (patient-to-patient, person-
   to-person) (These organizations
   are listed elsewhere in this index,
   most of them under Helping.
   They are presented separately
   here to underline the potential
   importance and value of these
   groups and their members as
   resouces in death education
   courses. Since members of these
   groups have had the experience
   (whether a serious disease,
   surgery, or loss of a loved one)
   upon which the group focuses,
   their work, counseling, and
   presentations to students of
   death education are more
   immediate, less abstract and
   academic. Those who have been
   closest to death can probably
   teach more effectively about
   it, especially in courses of
   limited duration. For further
   information about self-help
   groups write The National
   Self-Help Clearinghouse, 184
   Fifth Avenue, New York, NY
   10010. For a scholarly analysis
   of the nature and function of
   self-help groups, together with
   an extensive bibliography, see
   Alan Gartner and Frank
   Riessman, Self-Help in the
   Human Services, Jossey-Bass,
   1977), 253, 254, 255, 258, 259,
   260, 261, 265, 266, 267, 268
Suicide, suicide prevention (Note that
   in most cities suicide prevention
   bureaus, crisis hot lines and/or
   other counseling services are
   available. The death educator
   should inquire locally.), 252,
   258, 261

Index

Numbers refer to page numbers.

Abortion, 57, 105, 106, 107, 117,
    121, 252, 261, 264, 267
Aging/the aged, 24, 40, 42, 45, 113,
    124, 127, 128, 160, 162, 188,
    189, 190, 194, 199, 200, 201,
    203, 204, 206, 207, 213, 214,
    216, 217, 218, 222, 226, 228,
    231, 232, 235, 251, 257, 261,
    262
    (*See also* Dying; Nursing homes)

Bereavement, 37, 47, 48, 49, 80, 84,
    86, 103, 106, 108, 110, 111,
    117, 118, 126, 142, 163, 168,
    175, 180, 196, 217, 222, 225,
    232

Bereavement (*Cont.*):
    adolescent, 18
    caregivers, 29, 39, 84, 198
    child, 7, 9, 11, 14, 15, 20, 47, 108,
        160, 177
    counseling, 46, 49, 187, 258
    elderly, 30, 44
    family members, 160, 177, 183,
        185, 224, 228
    follow-up, 216
    impact of, 42, 178
    spouse, 47, 160, 163, 188, 197, 202
    (*See also* Widowhood)
Bibliographies about death-related
    topics, 95–121
Bioethics, 53, 57, 101, 105, 114, 121,
    125, 128, 183, 186, 206, 209,

Bioethics (*Cont.*):
    211, 212, 213, 214, 215, 231,
    232, 258
Body disposal, 43, 109, 110, 256
Books about death:
    for adults, 16, 104, 109, 114, 116
    for the bereaved, 42, 49
    for children and adolescents, 9, 13,
        15, 16, 17, 19, 41, 103, 104,
        107, 109, 111, 113, 116, 117
    for parents, 41, 104

Capital punishment, 57, 103, 195
Caring for the dying (*see* Learning;
    Terminal care)
Children's literature and death, 8, 9,
    10, 17, 18, 19, 104, 105, 111,
    121
Community resources, 109, 184, 214,
    273–276
Coping (*see* Helping people to cope
    with death)
Counseling, 105, 126, 127, 130, 180,
    231, 266
    bereaved, 46, 47, 49
    children, 17
    the dying, 195
    the elderly, 45
    families, 39, 180, 185
Cross-cultural studies, 14, 19, 139,
    172, 173, 176, 179, 187, 189,
    190, 194, 196, 197, 198, 201,
    206, 207, 211, 213, 215, 218,
    227
Cryonics, 171, 185, 191, 256

Death anxiety [*see* Death fears
    (anxiety)]
Death and the arts (music, poetry,
    drama), 13, 15, 24, 92, 113,
    120, 152-254, 176, 178, 179,
    199, 204, 205, 206, 207, 210,
    223, 224, 234
Death attitude(s), 5, 6, 42, 53, 87, 89,
    103, 116, 135, 137, 139, 140,
    143, 161, 162, 175, 179, 181,
    197, 201, 208, 213, 216
    adolescents, 7, 16, 31, 119, 134,
        141
    children, 7, 9, 11, 16, 46, 119, 134,
        167, 172

Death attitude(s) (*Cont.*):
    college students, 21, 22, 23
    counselors, 46
    the elderly, 12, 45, 135, 138, 139,
        143, 144, 175
    medical students, 34, 37, 138
    nurses, 27, 33, 34, 43
    nursing students, 27, 31, 33, 34,
        37, 40
    paramedical staff, 31, 34
    parents, 12
    pediatricians, 34
    physicians, 28, 30, 34, 37, 136,
        175, 209
    social workers, 28, 30
    teachers, 8, 16, 41
Death attitude changes, 53
    through counseling (*see* Counseling)
    through death education, 5, 6, 20,
        21, 22, 23, 29, 32, 35, 37,
        135
    through development, 9, 12, 13,
        14, 17, 18
    through personal experiences, 13,
        15, 31, 159, 163, 169, 183,
        189, 191, 192, 215, 217, 234
Death concepts, 187
    of children, 9, 10, 11, 12, 13, 14,
        15, 17, 19, 134
Death denial, 18, 91, 107, 199, 208,
    230
Death fears (anxiety), 134, 138, 139,
    140, 142, 144
    adolescents, 15, 23, 31
    adults, 46, 135, 136, 142
    children, 7, 17, 19, 23, 38, 39, 47
    college students, 21, 22, 23, 24, 25,
        135, 136, 137, 138, 142, 144
    the elderly, 41, 45, 135
    medical students, 34
    nurses, 33, 35
    physicians, 32, 34
    terminal patients, 34, 41, 137, 193
Death of a pet, 9, 13, 16, 42, 201, 212
Death-related journals and newsletters,
    111, 124-132
Definition of death, 57, 87, 90, 208,
    231
Dying:
    adolescent, 29, 107, 234
    child, 13, 20, 25, 27, 28, 29, 31,
        34, 37, 38, 107, 167, 169,
        173, 175, 181, 204

Dying (*Cont.*):
  and old age, 12, 24, 40, 42, 43, 45,
    57, 187, 191, 193
  patient, 29, 76, 111, 181, 194, 204,
    208, 224, 225

Educational organizations, 111, 237–
  245
Emotional support 20, 182
  for the bereaved, 26, 32, 39, 47,
    48, 49, 170, 184, 185, 188,
    234, 259
  for caregivers, 27, 166, 169, 194,
    204, 227
  for the dying, 26, 29, 31, 170, 182,
    186, 259
Euthanasia, 57, 59, 87, 90, 105, 107,
  109, 110, 116, 120, 126, 163,
  186, 200, 208, 214, 218, 252,
  253, 267

Family:
  and child's death concerns, 9, 10,
    12, 13, 19, 28, 30, 42, 43,
    44, 45, 109, 167, 187, 201
  and dying patient, 26, 27, 28, 29,
    30, 32, 37, 39, 177, 191,
    192, 197, 198, 203, 210,
    218, 223, 225, 228, 230, 234
  and health care personnel, 28, 30,
    184, 211
  and physician, 28, 29, 30, 37, 184,
    209
Funeral (cemetery) industry, 40, 43,
  102, 109, 110, 125, 161, 166,
  174, 179, 182, 183, 185, 186,
  187, 188, 192, 194, 195, 197,
  200, 204, 206, 207, 216, 227,
  230, 256, 259, 262, 263, 265,
  274

Helping institutions, 111
  (*See also* Hospice)
Helping organizations, 47, 48, 49, 111,
  126, 128, 130, 184, 217, 233,
  251–268
Helping people to cope with death, 7,
  9, 13, 28, 30, 36, 38, 39, 42, 45,
  47, 60, 104, 170, 171, 176, 177,
  179, 184, 222

Hospice, 27, 32, 62, 90, 106, 119,
  129, 179, 180, 189, 193, 215,
  223, 263, 273
Hospitals, 26, 39, 118, 179, 189, 204,
  273

Laws and death, 40, 46, 117, 128,
  192, 193, 200, 233, 234
Learning:
  about death (*see* Teaching—where;
    Teaching—who)
  to care for the dying, 25, 27, 35,
    36, 39, 47, 54, 82, 107, 165,
    166, 212
  to care for family of dying, 26, 27,
    54, 84, 165, 166
  to cope with death and grief, 7, 9,
    27, 30
  (*See also* Bereavement)
  to face death, 28, 30, 31, 45, 169,
    184, 208, 212, 227, 234
  to live with death, 49, 128, 176,
    189, 191, 194, 196, 206
Life-threatening disease, 25, 28, 36,
  87, 116, 126, 128, 161, 165,
  171, 181, 182, 189, 190, 194,
  199, 200, 204, 205, 209, 212,
  213, 229, 251, 252, 254, 255,
  256, 259, 261, 262, 264, 267

Media exchange, 102, 106
Mediagraphies, 101, 102, 103, 115,
  154–157
Media guides, 17, 102, 103, 106, 117
Medical ethics, 6, 113, 114, 121, 168,
  179, 183, 186
  (*See also* Bioethics)
Memorial societies/Memorialization,
  43, 109, 125, 200, 218, 254,
  256, 260, 274

Nursing homes, 31, 40, 43, 184, 185,
  204, 228, 233, 253, 273

Organ donation, 188, 192, 193, 257,
  260, 264, 265
Organ transplantation, 109, 178, 186,
  192, 213, 215, 217

Personal death awareness, 22, 24, 31, 78, 169, 190, 226
Philosophy, 19, 21, 60, 195, 201, 209
Preparation:
  for dying, 28
  (*See also* Laws and death)
  for living, 6, 40, 73, 108, 186, 227
Psychology of death, 7, 23, 24, 35, 65, 66, 67, 76, 86, 90, 113, 115, 117, 177, 179, 208

Religion and death, 16, 23, 41, 77, 113, 114, 137, 141, 145, 160, 169, 179, 180, 204, 205, 213, 218, 225, 229, 230

Study of death, 202
  assessment instruments, 134-145
  methodology, 134, 137-145
Sudden death, 49, 120, 159, 168, 176, 177, 202, 215, 219, 223, 230, 231, 232, 233
Sudden infant death, 26, 120, 160, 164, 170, 205, 219, 234, 256, 265
Suicide, 23, 57, 104, 107, 115, 130, 136, 159, 160, 161, 162, 164, 166, 171, 176, 178, 179, 180, 186, 188, 191, 192, 198, 210, 211, 214, 215, 216, 218, 219-222, 225, 233, 252, 258

Talking about death:
  with children, 12, 13, 28, 41, 42, 44, 109, 113, 121, 183, 187, 189, 201, 203, 222
  in the classroom, 7, 8, 9, 13, 189, 215, 229
Teaching curricula, 6, 7, 8, 18, 35, 37, 47, 74
  course(s), 11, 12, 21, 22, 23, 27, 44, 69, 176
  course outlines, 8, 11, 14, 19, 21, 24, 41, 44
  curriculum (course) content, 9, 17, 34
  curriculum materials, 11, 12, 18, 33, 92, 103, 119, 159-235
  discussion topics, 7, 12, 19, 20, 28, 41

Teaching curricula (*Cont.*):
  format, 27
  interdisciplinary approaches, 10, 11, 24, 37, 92
  laboratory approach, 32, 35
  seminars, 39, 44
  units (teaching, instructional, study), 8, 10, 11, 12, 14, 15, 20, 40
  workshops, 29, 32, 33, 35, 40, 41
Teaching effectiveness, 6, 8, 15, 21, 37
Teaching goals and objectives, 5, 6, 7, 13, 23
Teaching methods and techniques, 6, 8, 14, 23, 26
Teaching personnel, 6, 7, 11, 21
Teaching rationale (need for), 7, 16, 20, 37
Teaching—where?, 7
  college, 6, 21, 22, 23
  community, 6, 42
  continuing education centers, 29, 44
  home, 43, 45, 121
  medical schools, 25, 27, 28, 33, 37
  nursing schools, 27, 28, 30, 38, 82
Teaching—who?
  adults, 40, 41, 43
  clergy, 43, 168, 171
  college students, 21, 22, 23
  counselors, 44, 46, 47, 48
  educators, 7, 8, 9, 10, 11, 44, 48, 117
  the elderly, 44, 45
  elementary school children, 8, 9, 10, 11, 13, 14, 15, 16, 17, 20, 48, 175, 229, 235
  health professionals, 25, 26, 27, 34, 35, 36, 37, 39, 40, 48, 59, 63, 82, 117, 162, 174, 204, 207, 210, 225
  high school students, 8, 10, 11, 12, 14, 16, 17, 18, 19, 20, 173, 207, 235
  physicians, 27, 56, 71, 205, 207, 209, 210
  the public, 42, 44, 111, 112, 231
  social workers, 28, 31, 34, 81
Terminal care, 25, 26, 27, 32, 33, 34, 36, 38, 59, 63, 71, 82, 115, 118, 165, 166, 168, 173, 174, 185, 191, 192, 198, 200, 202, 204, 206, 208, 211, 212, 213, 222, 223, 224

Truth telling in terminal illness, 25, 35, 36, 39, 231

Violence, 143, 160, 163, 164, 176, 178, 186, 188, 203, 216

War, 160, 163, 164, 166, 179, 188, 189, 190, 192, 193, 198, 218, 226, 227, 230
Widowhood, 21, 47, 49, 87, 103, 111, 112, 119, 132, 163, 169, 172, 209, 217, 226, 232, 233, 267, 268